A Caregiver's
Bible to Excellence!

A Caregiver's
Bible to Excellence!

VOLUME I

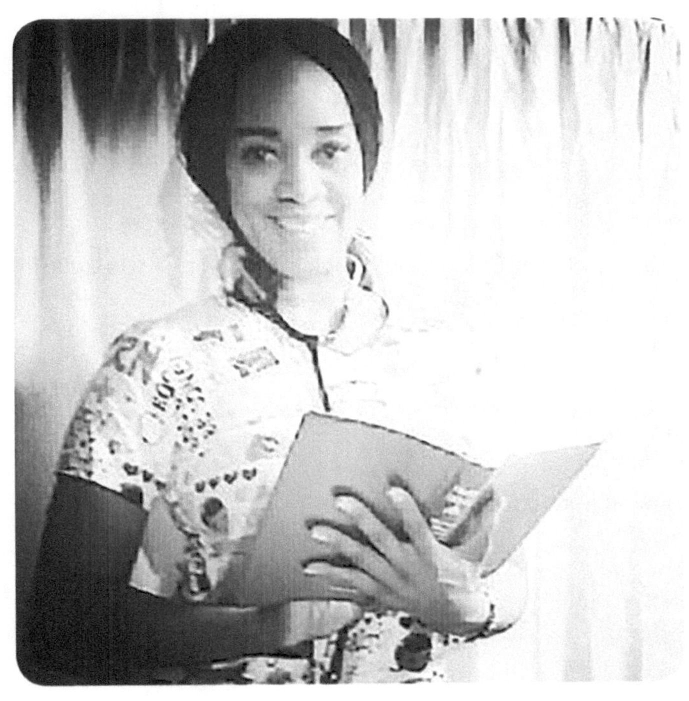

Miss Asondra StarN'air

Library of Congress Control Number: 2021923835

PAPERBACK: 978-1-956803-61-7
EBOOK: 978-1-956803-62-4

Ordering Information:

For orders and inquiries, please contact:
1-888-404-1388
www.goldtouchpress.com
book.orders@goldtouchpress.com

Printed in the United States of America

CONTENTS

Then I heard the voice of the Lord saying, "Whom shall I send? And who will go for us?" And I said, "Here am I. Send Me!"

—Isaiah 6:8

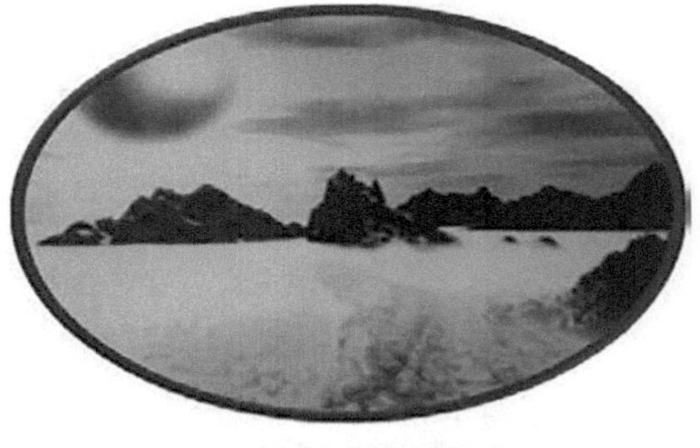

The Purpose

To help win souls for Christ, the excellent way!

Take my yoke upon you and learn from me, for I am gentle and humble in heart, and you will find rest for your souls.

—Matthew 9:22

The Mission

It's Simple As Pie, "We Want Our Share Of It", Don't Deny!

Code of Ethics
Straight out of "The Book"

As God's messenger, I give each of you this warning. Be honest in your estimate of yourself, measuring your value by how much faith God has given you. Just as our bodies have many parts and each part has a special function, so it is with Christ's body. We are all parts of his own body, and each of us has different work to do. And since we are all one body of Christ, we belong to each other, and each of us need all the others.

—Romans 12:3–5

Here She Comes, World.

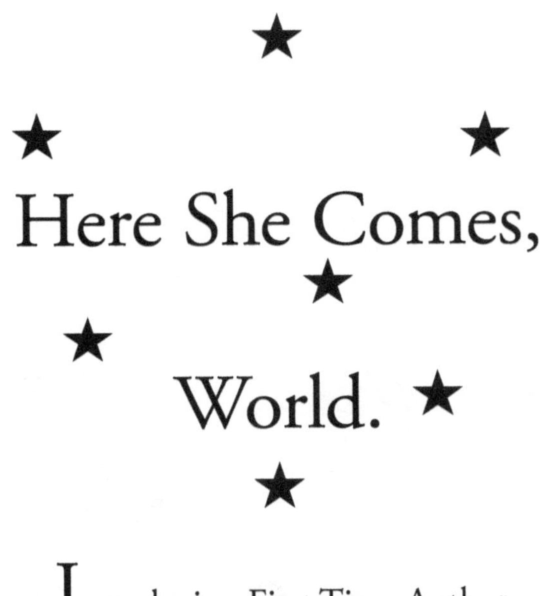

Introducing First-Time Author

Miss Asondra StarN'air

A CAREGIVER'S BIBLE TO EXCELLENCE!

Miss Asondra StarN'air

All are Called, Few are Chosen.

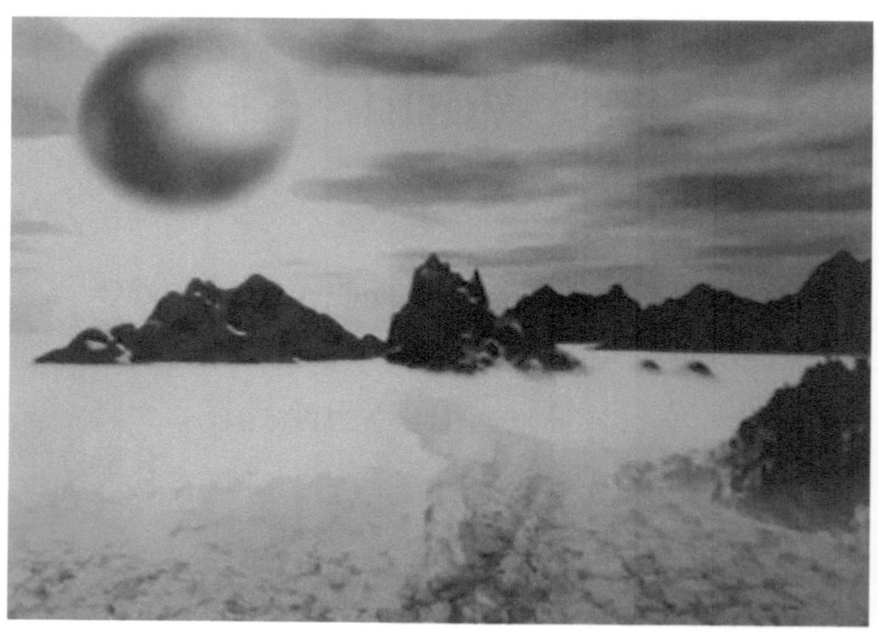

Hello and Welcome to the World of Caregiving!

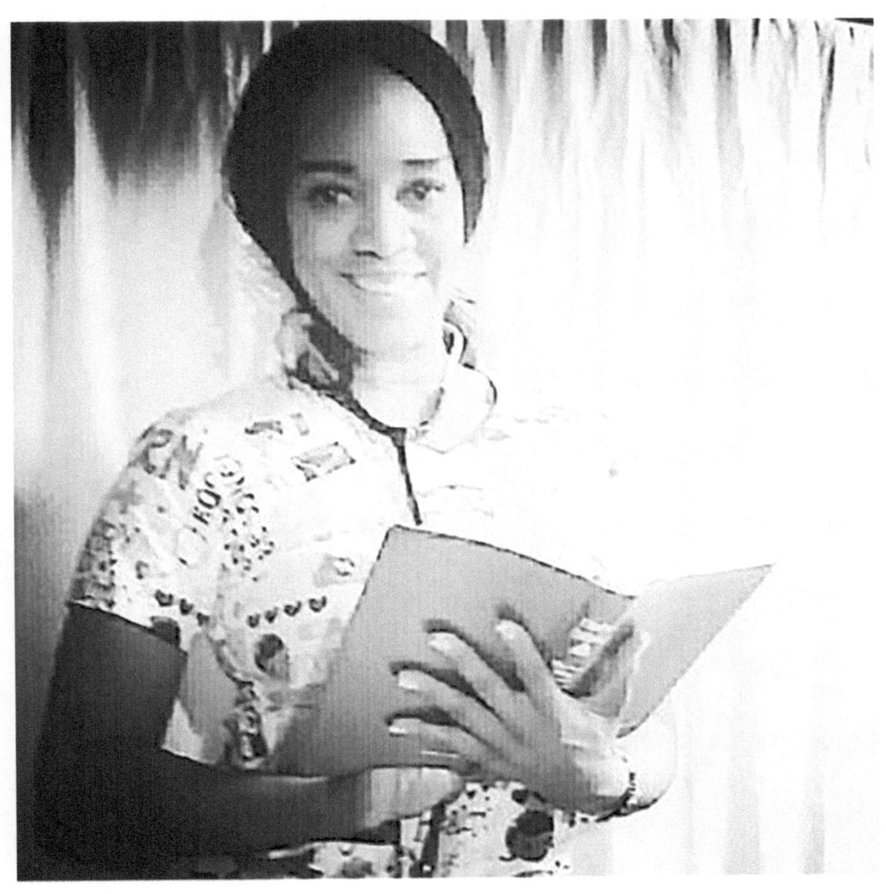

INTRODUCTION

FOR MORE THAN twenty years now, I have worked and observed the world of caregiving. I have traveled from place to place throughout the state of Ohio, providing care in just about every area of healthcare I am a State Tested Nurse Assistant (STNA). I've worked in Hospitals, Nursing homes, Home-care, and Hospice. I've also worked with the Department of Developmental Disabilities (DODD) prior to all that I ran a type A daycare center. I worked with children 0 to 5 years old. I did this for 14 years and guess what? I'm a pet parent too, I know what to do, so you see, I have a lot of experience and know how when it comes to providing care.

And before all that, I spent my younger years in hospitality, I worked in the restaurant industry for many, many years. So how did I get here? How did I become a "Caregiver"? Sadly and unfortunately my dad got sick, he was diagnosed with lung cancer and given only 3 to 6 months to live and I was devastated, shocked and unprepared. Suddenly I became his caretaker because he wanted no one else but me, he wanted me to handle all of his affairs too.

"Caregiver", what's that? I Knew how to take care of children, and pets but, adults? And someone whose dying and not just someone, my dad, oh help me Jesus, I thought, because I had no clue of what to do or how to care for my dad, until Jesus showed me. Yes, all he said was "pretend like you are taking care of me." From that moment on, I wasn't taking care of my dad, I was taking care of Jesus! World, that's how Miss Asondra StarN'air me, Became a "Caregiver". And not just any caregiver either, I became a caregiver in Jesus name. Excellence care, no excuses, no one to blame. But little did I know, that God would use me to write a book. He took all the love I had inside my heart for him and my earthly dad and placed a brand new calling on my life. Next thing I knew I was hooked, I wanted to start caring for seniors like my dad. I wanted to make sure that the elderly was well cared for under my watch. So I entered the world of Caregiving and never looked back.

But it wasn't easy you see, shortly after my dad died, a part of me died too; and it took a great while for me to get over it and heal but, when I finally did, I starting taking health care classes. I became a home health aide. (I hate that word 'aide', it leaves a dark feeling each time I hear it.) while still doing my daycare business, I started taking care of seniors on the weekends, I thought that was going to be it, daycare during the week and senior care on the weekends but the new calling that God was placing on my life kept saying bye -bye daycare, hello senior care. So eventually, I gave it all up, the daycare business, money and all. I was making a lot of money too almost fourteen thousand dollars a month when I decided to go with God's new call on my life, I must admit, the money mattered, but God's call on my life mattered the most. I am here on this planet to do his will, not mine. I trust God, He said to me, "Don't Worry"! Be at peace and rest assure I will always take care of you with money or without money. (God and I are best friends, we talk everyday, "a lot" and about everything) He said he will make sure that I have enough to I eat, have shelter and he'll keep shoes on my feet. And like Abraham in the bible, I believed God! Like I said, I made a lot of money, I went from a little under fourteen thousand dollars and thousands a month to a little over minimum wage; I know that's crazy but that's the choice I made, "I don't sweat it" God is with me, He's leading the way. Too, I'm no longer a prisoner of this world, I'm not in a cage.

As I see it, I'm with Christ, I'm changing lives in so many ways and if you want to, so can you!

Listen up, listen, if you are a caregiver, or thinking about becoming a caregiver my advise to all of you out there is this: Let Christ lead not you, let Him do for you what He did for me, He showed me the "Excellent Way"! So if you have lots of love inside of you to give and a caring heart, like me, become a caregiver for Christ. Reach out, help serve and care for others, be a team player too, if you do, god will surely bless you. Nevertheless, **"ALL"** are called, but few are chosen. This book "A Caregivers Bible To Excellence" is my contributions to the world, a once shy and timid girl. Now I'm in a different world! Today I'm a caregiver for Christ. And let me tell you this, all the hard work and time spent on this book,in my heart, it was truly worth the sacrifice. It is finished! It's yours now and I hope that this book will change the way you think about care-giving forever. I tell you the truth, nobody does it better than the man above. And I must say this, I believe that in order to care for someone completely you must not do it for the money, you must do it with a full heart of love.

Dear love, it's my hope that you will get so much out of this book and agree that it is truly a ***Caregiver's Bible to Excellence!*** *Let's go.....*

Jesus, "The Almighty Caregiver"

There has never been or will ever be a "Caregiver" like our Lord Jesus Christ. He healed the sick, let the blind see, made the cripple walk—miracles after miracles!

When I began my careers as a caregiver out in the world, I had no real role model. Although I received hundreds of hours in training and eventually became a certified nurse assistant. Still I saw no one whom I could look up to or mimic. On the contrary, I saw more disturbing things I do not care to mention.

With no real role model, I began listening to that still small voice inside, guiding me, telling me what to do. The voice inside me said each patient was Jesus: love and care for each one like you are caring for Jesus. "Remember, you are not working for man; you're working for me."

Check this out, when something would come up and I was not sure of what to do because it was unusual or out of the norm, like pulling a rabbit out of a hat, Jesus got that! He would give me creative ways to handle anything that came my way. My job was to listen to the master and do what he say—everything turned out better than Okay.

Soon, people started noticing that I was no ordinary caregiver, certainly not their typical aide, there was something different and special about my work, and the people I took care of said so. All through my care giving career, and still holds true today, customers would call back to the office and demanded I be the one assigned to them. I was in great demand, so much so, that I couldn't get a day off, I was booked up seven days a week. Little did they know, Jesus was running the show!

He became my role model in every way, I took him on each assignment and so should you. Truth be told, I take him everywhere I go, whether I'm working or not, he's my everyday role model for life!

I cannot say this enough, and this goes out to the entire health-care team—doctors included. There is only one role model for "Caregiving," and that is Jesus Christ. As caregivers, we must start to look to him to help us help others and ourselves; only then will we truly be saving lives and providing excellent care.

One Body With Many Parts

1 Corinthians 12:12–27

The human body has many parts, but the many parts make up one whole body. So it is with the body of Christ. Some of us are Jews, some are Gentiles, some are slaves, and some are free. But we have all been baptized into one body by one Spirit, and we all share the same Spirit.

Yes, the body has many different parts, not just one part. If the foot says, "I am not a part of the body because I am not a hand," that does not make it any less a part of the body. And if the ear says, "I am not part of the body because I am not an eye," would that make it any less a part of the body? If the whole body were an eye, how would you hear? Or if your whole body were an ear, how would you smell anything?

But our bodies have many parts, and God has put each part just where he wants it. How strange a body would be if it had only one part! Yes, there are many parts, but only one body. The eye can never say to the hand, "I don't need you." The head can't say to the feet, "I don't need you."

In fact, some parts of the body that seem weakest and least important are actually the most necessary. And the parts we regard as less honorable are those we clothe with the greatest care. So we carefully protect those parts that should not be seen, while the more honorable parts do not require this special care. So God has put the body together such that extra honor and care are given to those parts that have less dignity. This makes for harmony among the members, so that all the members care for each other. If one part suffers, all the parts suffer with it; and if one part is honored, all the parts are glad. All of you together are Christ's body, and each of you is a part of it.

My message to field workers (me included) is this: As "Caregivers" of the Body of Christ, let there be no strife among us. Our first job is to take care of each other. Yes, love and work well with each other as a team. We are—again—one body. Without love, peace, and harmony between us, *"The Body"* how can we really serve and take care of others? Therefore, we need each other!

Hello, my name is Miss Asondra StarN'air, I'm a caregiver too! Everybody can call me Star; it is a pleasure meeting all of you too. This book was written by a caregiver, **"ME"** I wrote it with caregivers in mind. I tried to put in everything I could think of to help aid you into becoming an excellent caregiver, but it still won't happen if Jesus is not the role model. Jesus is **"The Greatest Caregiver of All"** and the one who inspired me to write this book for you. We have a lot of ground to cover, so let's get started.

Again, Welcome to ***A Caregiver's Bible to Excellence!***

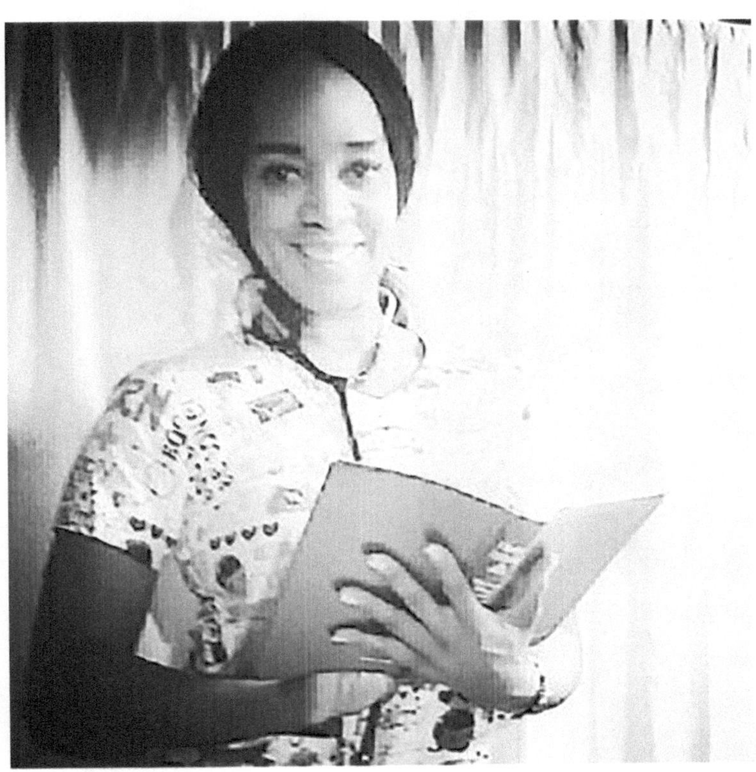

Welcome To The World Of Caregiving!

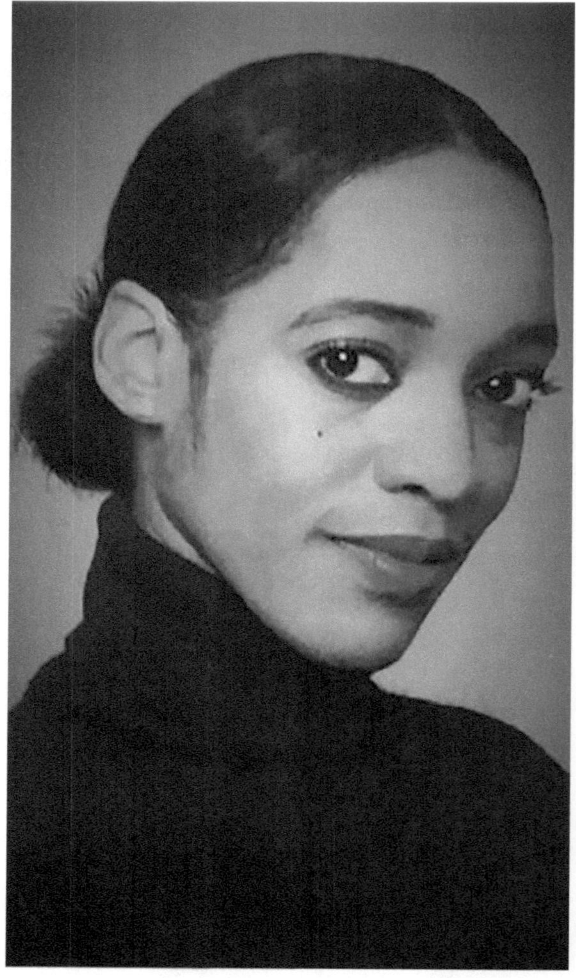

No longer a shy and timid girl
I'm a light, I want to help change the world!

Here We Go....

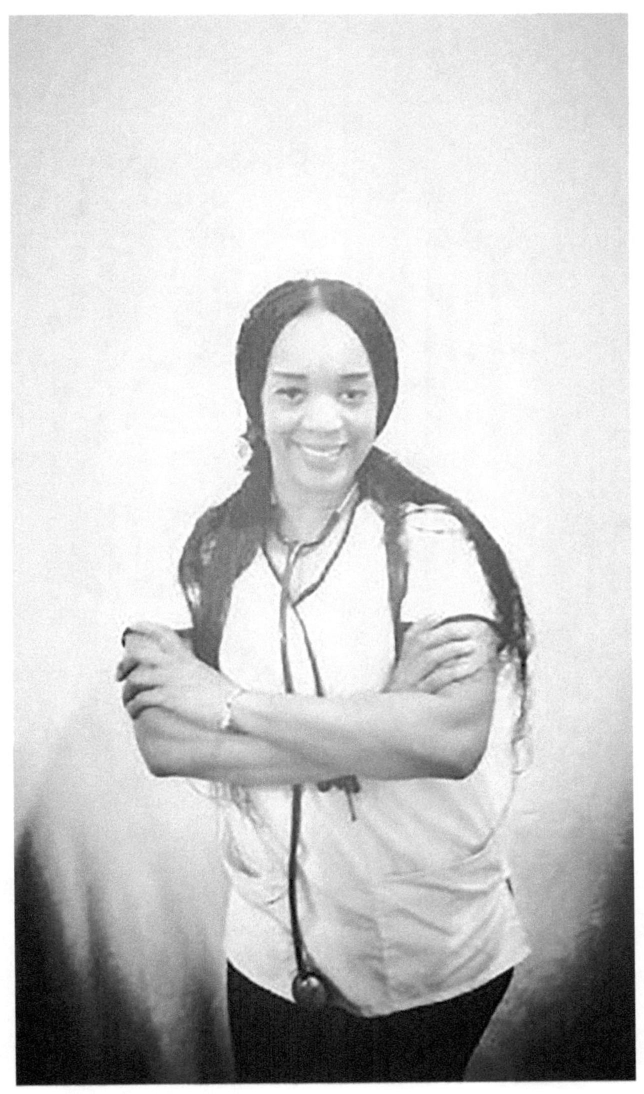

Meet

The HealthCare Team

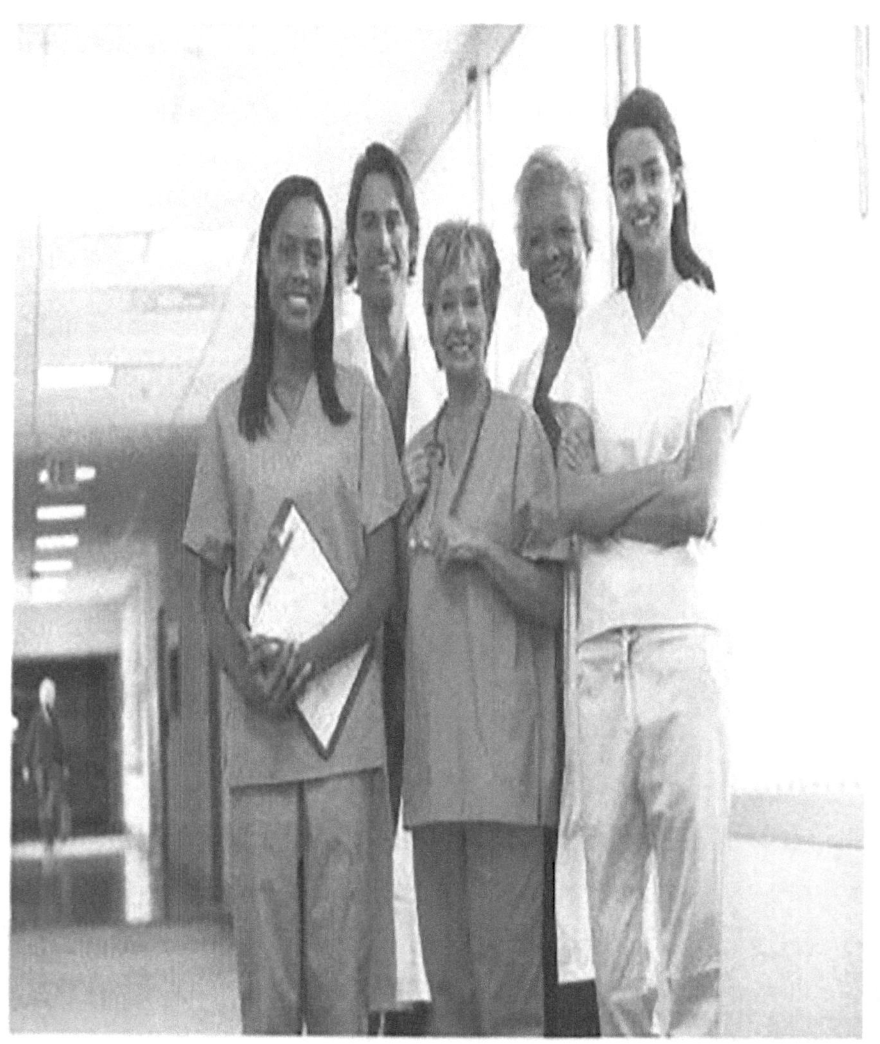

Health Care Is A Team Effort

Each health-care provider is like a member of the team with a special role. Some team members are doctors or technicians who help diagnose diseases. Others are experts who treat disease or care for the patients' physical and emotional needs.

Doctor (Dr.)—Qualified practitioner of medicine, a physician.

Physician Assistant (PA)—Practice medicine on a team with physicians and surgeons and other health-care workers.

Registered Nurse (RN)—Is tasked with the protection, promotion, and optimization of health and abilities, prevention of illness and injury, facilitation of healing, alleviation of suffering through diagnosis and treatment of human response and advocacy in the care of individuals, family, groups, communities, and populations.

Nurse Practitioner (LPN)—A nurse who cares for people who are sick, injured, convalescent, or disabled. LPNs work under the direction of registered nurses or physicians.

State-Tested Nurse Assistant (STNA)—Individuals who have taken and successfully passed their state's examination; put on their state's registry. In Ohio, they're called STNAs. In other states like Michigan and Georgia, STNAs are called CNAs (certified nurse assistants). Nurse assistants are the eyes and ears of the RN and LPN. They play a vital role in making sure patients receive the hands-on care they need.

Home Health Aides (HHA)—Supported care provided in the home. May or may not be certified; depends on company's policy.

Pharmacist—A person who is professionally qualified to prepare and dispense medical drugs.

Dentist—A person qualified to treat the diseases and conditions that affect the teeth and gums, especially the repair and extraction of teeth and insertion of artificial ones.

Technologists —Encompasses several occupations, diagnostics, imaging, laboratory testing, or surgical assisting while job duties vary by specialization, these individuals typically assist physicians.

Therapist and Rehabilitation Specialist

*****Physical Therapist (PT)**—Helps patients reduce pain and improve or restore mobility in many cases without the expense of surgery and often reducing the need for long-term use of prescription medications and their side effects.

*****Occupational Therapist (OT)**—Is a health and rehabilitation professional. They work with people of all ages who need specialized assistance to lead independent, productive, and satisfying lives due to physical, developmental, social, or emotional problems.

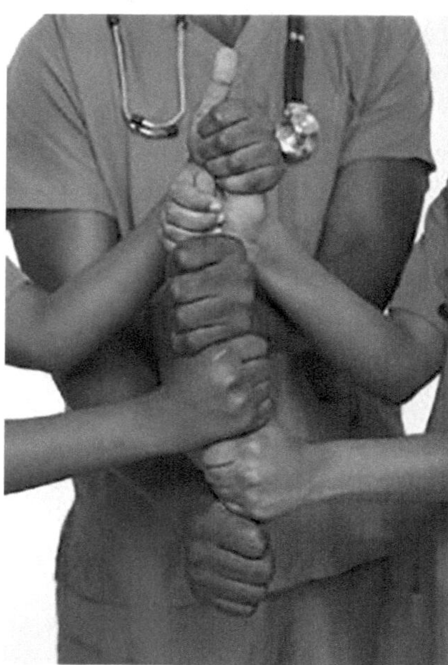

Remember, **"Teamwork Makes The Dream Work"**!

SECTION I

Home Care

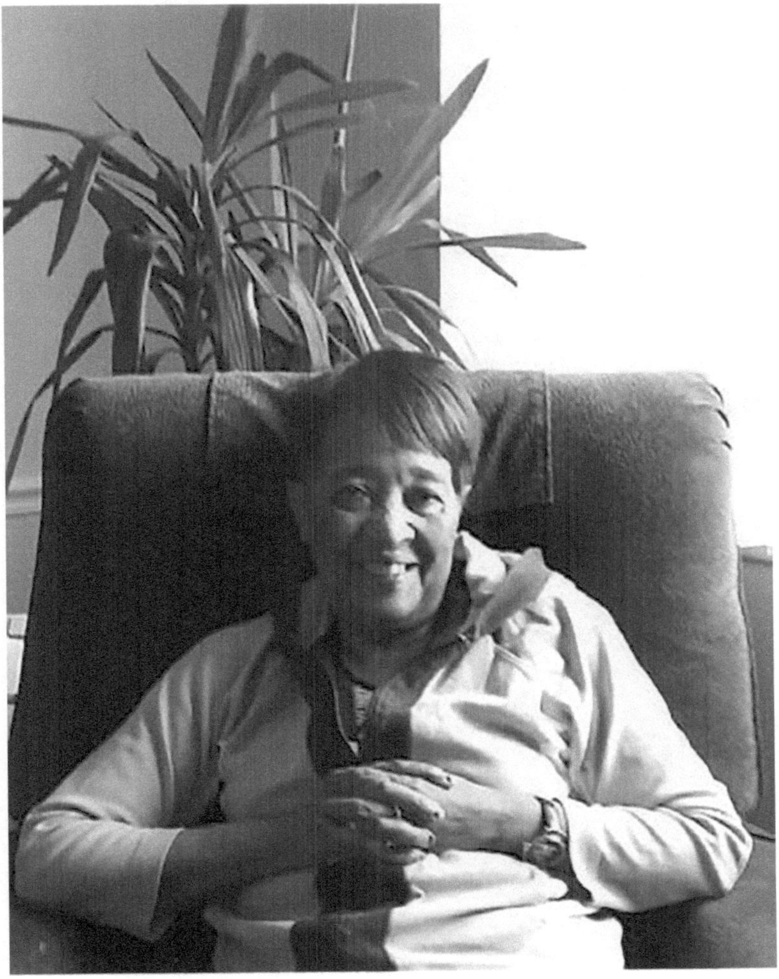

Caregiving at it's Fineness!

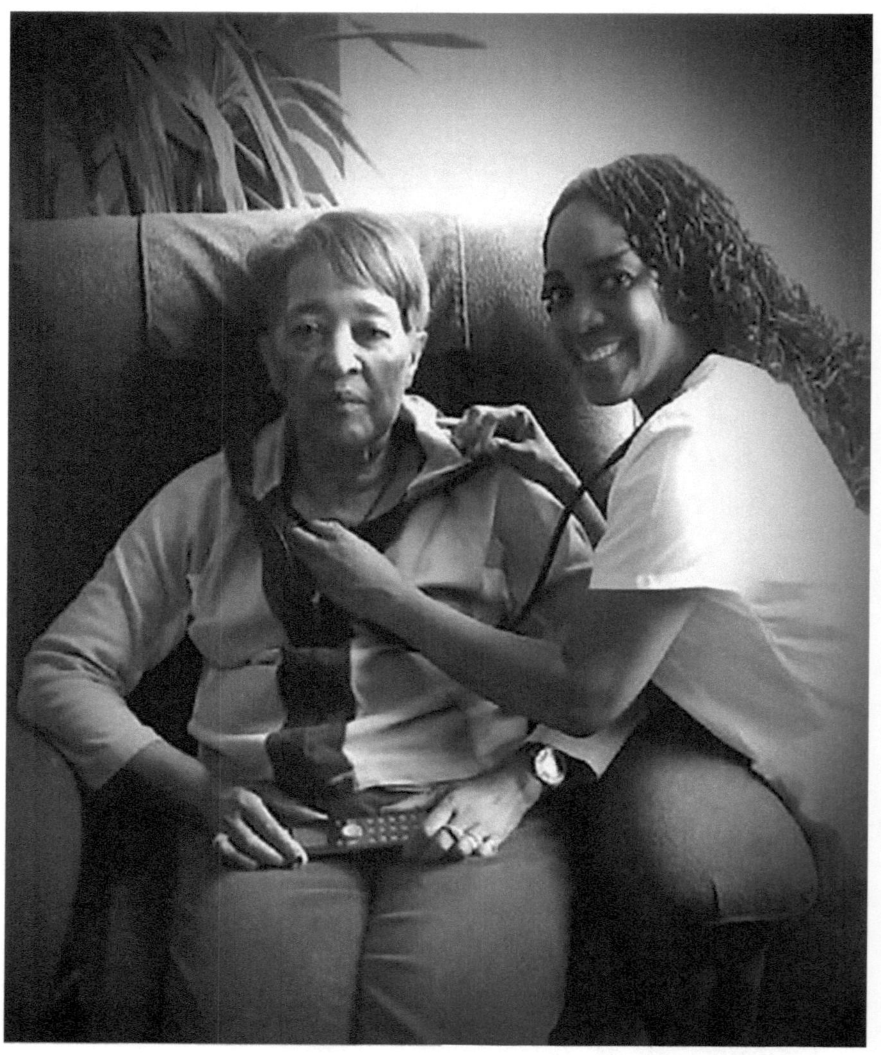

 Miss Asondra StarN'air

ADLs
Activities of Daily Living

As caregivers, we need a solid understanding of activities of daily living, what it means, how it was proposed and our role as caregivers.

Activities of Daily Living is a term used in health care to refer to people's daily self-care activities.

The concept of **ADLs** was originally proposed in 1950 by Dr. Sidney Katz and his team at Benjamin Rose Hospital in Cleveland, Ohio, and has been added to and refined by a variety of researchers since that time.

Health-care professionals often use a person's abilities or inabilities to perform **ADLs** as a measurement of the individual's functional status, particularly in regard to people with disabilities and the elderly.

And of course, younger children often require help from adults to perform **ADLs** as well; they have not yet developed the skills necessary to perform them independently.

There are two components to activities of daily living. One is called the basic, which consists of the following ADLs:

- Bathing and showering
- Dressing
- Self-feeding
- Personal hygiene and grooming
- Toilet hygiene (getting to the toilet, cleaning oneself, and getting back up)

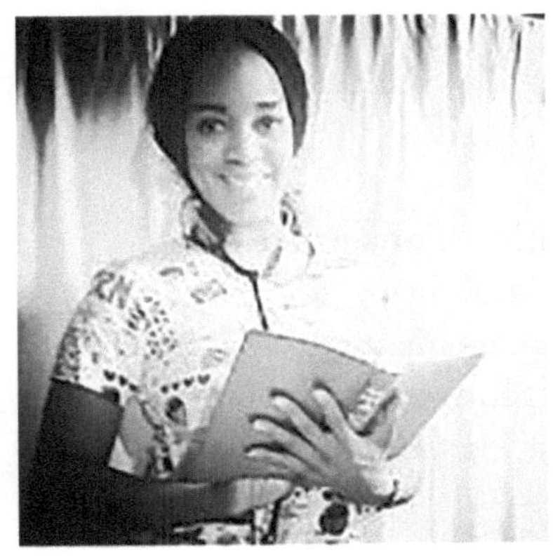

The other component is what we call Instrumental Activities of Daily Living IADLs and that consist of the following:

- Housework
- Preparing meals
- Taking medications as prescribed/medication reminders
- Managing money (family only)
- Shopping for groceries, clothing, etc.
- Use of telephone or other form of communication
- Transportation

Here is a useful mnemonic caregivers can use: **SHAFT**.

- **S**hopping
- **H**ousekeeping
- **A**ccounting
- **F**ood preparation
- **T**ransportation/telephones/devices

And be advise, only assigned family members should handle money management affairs, not employed caregivers.

Now, when it comes to deciding what is needed for an individual receiving care, it is often the occupational therapist or registered nurse (**RN**) that evaluates **IADLs** when completing patient assessments.

The American Occupational Therapy Association identifies twelve types of **IADLs** that may be performed as co-occupation with others.

- Care of others (including selecting and supervising caregivers)
- Care of pets
- Child rearing
- Communication management
- Community mobility
- Financial management and maintenance
- Home establishment and maintenance
- Meal preparation and cleanup

  Miss Asondra StarN'air

- Religious observances
- Safety procedures and emergency responses
- Shopping

Anyone caring for a loved one or employed by another company still can be assessed by an occupational therapist at their discretion. Occupational therapists have been given the freedom to decide what should be done in a particular situation. **"WE"** as caregivers, must adhere to advice given by other professionals at that time.

Our role as caregivers is to ensure we do an excellent job at meeting the needs of individuals who are in our care. Continuing education will be the key to our success.

Daily Routine
Morning Care Vector Set

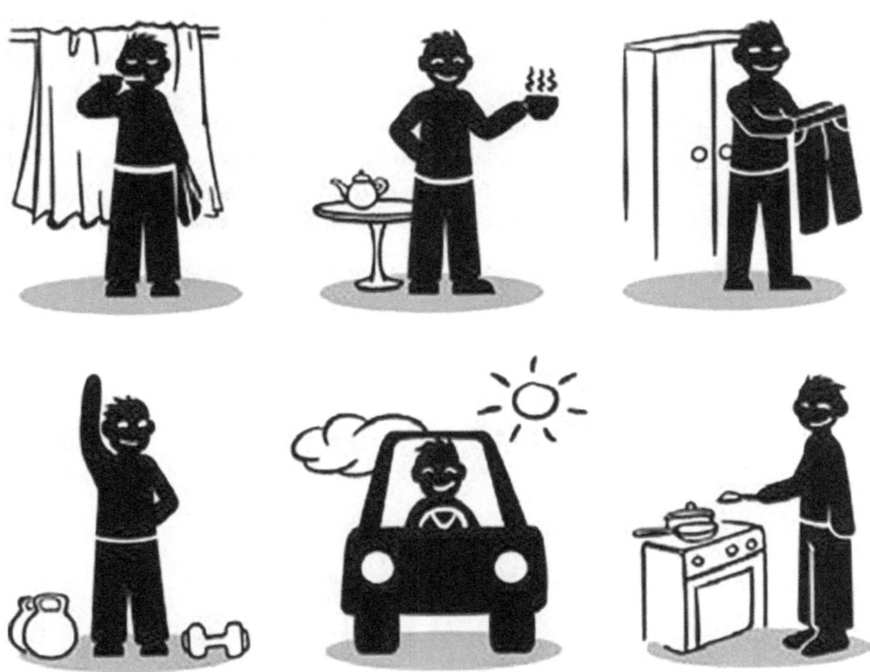

PHASES OF AGING

In the United States all people over the age 18 are considered adults but there is a very large difference between say an 21 year old and a 50 year old wouldn't you agree, most people would. So we separate them. **"Young Adults"** and **"Middle Adults"**.

But what some of you caregivers may not know is the elderly population has been divided into what's known as **'Life Stage Subgroups.'**

- **The Young Old.**   65-74
- **The Middle Old.** 75-84
- **The Old Old.**   **85 and Older**

Reason for this is because today's seniors are not the seniors of their generation these seniors are living a lot longer and thriving too especially **'The Young Old'**. Many in this subgroup need very little help or none at all. They still drive and live relatively normal and independent lives. Some of these movers and shakers however, live in assistant living communities, downsizing and preparing for the time they will need help, but until then this age group is still having a good time living life to the fullest. The next subgroup **'Middle Old'** is starting to need some assistance, However, may not be ready for long term care (LTC) facilities. But still, very important that caregivers keep close eyes on changes that may be taking place. This group is more prone to falls and may show some early signs of memory care impairments, such as Dementia and Alzheimer's Disease but not all, just keep close watch on this group.

Now we have the last sub group **'The Old, Old'** I think that says it all!

This Group is old, old, and very frail and venerable.

It is our responsibility as Caregivers to help love and take care of the sick, elderly, poor, widowed and anyone else that is in need of care. Whether Formal or Informal we must step in and lend a helping hand. *Leviticus 19:32 you shall stand up before the gray head and honor the face of the old man. and you shall fear god: I Am the Lord.*

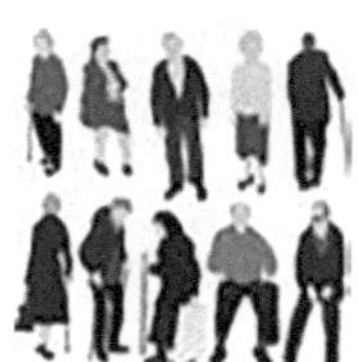

Help The Seniors, The Poor and The Very Old, 'Jump On Board!'

Dementia

Dementia is a general term for loss of memory and other abilities severe enough to interfere with Activities of Daily Living (**ADL's**) it is caused by physical changes in the brain.

Alzheimer's disease is the most common type of dementia, accounts for 60-80 percent of cases.

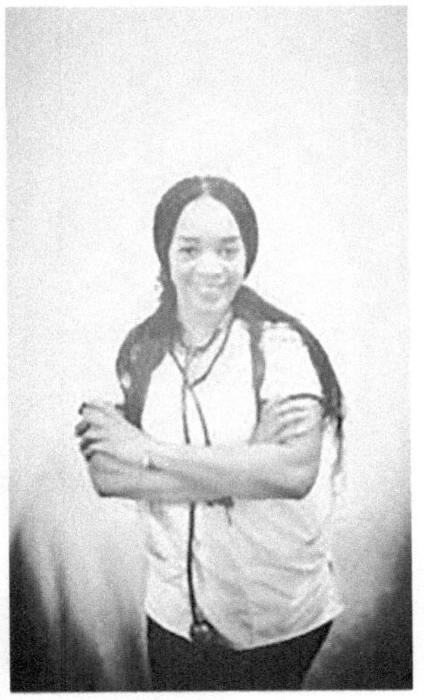

- There are more than 3 million cases per year and growing.
- Dementia can't be cured but treatment may help.
- Dementia is chronic can last for years or be lifelong.
- Also, Dementia requires a medical diagnosis, lab test or imaging often required.

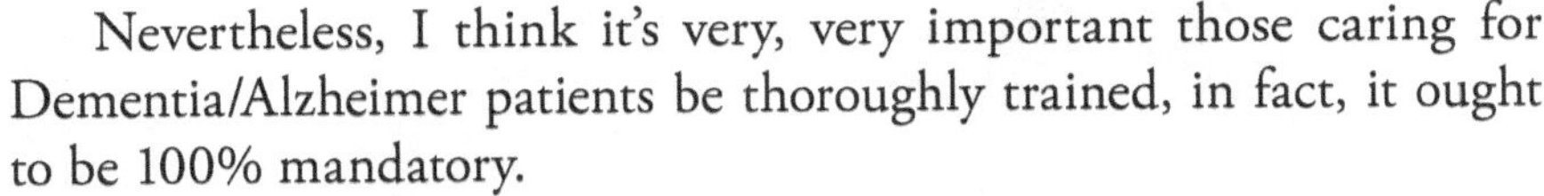

Nevertheless, I think it's very, very important those caring for Dementia/Alzheimer patients be thoroughly trained, in fact, it ought to be 100% mandatory.

Dementia caregiving is a world of its own, normal rules don't apply.

Therefore we need all the training and support we can get. Caregivers **WE** will be the ones to motivate and help keep them safe. Family Caregivers and Professional Caregivers alike, must master working with memory care individuals if you are going to be effective.

We must stay informed, competent, and professional at all times.

Welcome to the world of Caregiving, we are not the caregiver's of our parents' generation. Today we are truly "Healthcare Professionals" stay educated!

Care

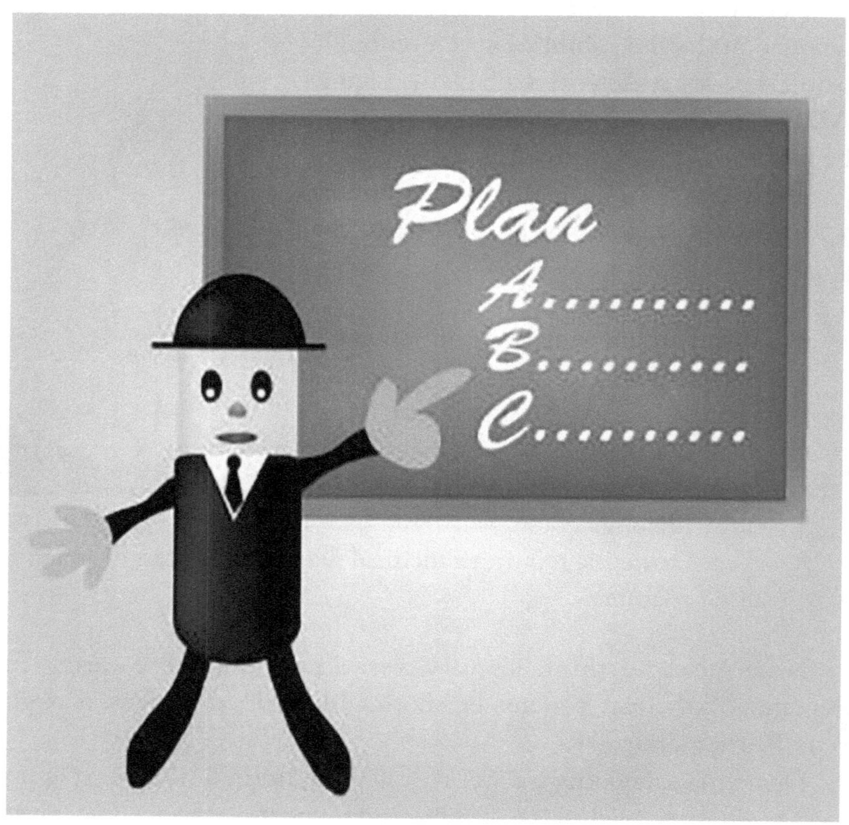

Always
Be
Caring

That's part of being an **"Excellent Caregiver,"** not only for the ones in need, but care for your coworkers too.

The ABC Care Plan is this: "Always Be Caring!"

Caregiver's Alphabet Soup

A loving spoonful to be taken **"EVERYDAY'**, doctor's orders!

A- Always be caring.

B- Be on time.

C- Culture awareness.

D- Dedication.

E- Ethics, get some.

F- Fundamentals "down pat"!

G- Give, Gratitude, and Grace.

H- Help Everybody, Everywhere!

I- Invest in Christ, spend time with him.

J- Judging others is a no, no!

K- Keep being kind, Keep being excellent! Keep this book!

L- Love one another like your sisters and brothers.

M- Maintain balance in your life; get plenty of sleep!

N- Nutrition adds more years to your life and looks good on you too!

O- Openness to forgive those who hurt and disappointed you.

P- Pray to God; read his word daily.

Q- Quitters never win; fight the good fight! Fix it; make it right!

R- Read, Read, Read! Turn the TV off and read God's Word.

S- Study to make thyself approved. Stay In School!

T- Teamwork makes the dream work, helping others don't hurt.

U- Universal law says you will reap what you sow—sow togetherness, unify, sow love and peace!

V- Versatility—learn different skills/trades, and be flexible too.

W- Wait on Christ, do not take matters in your own hands anymore.

X- X-rays, early detection saves lives; breast cancer awareness.

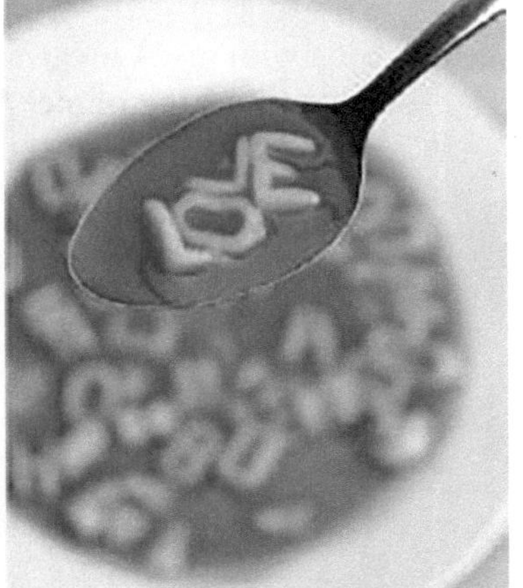

Y-   Yes, Lord! Send me, I will go! And start saying "Yes" to one another, Yes! I will help you, I'd love to!

Z-   Zebras can't change their stripes, but you are not a zebra you can, black or white, we all can change, no matter what you do, or whose who. 'ALL' are part of one body, and equal in God's sight. Give hatred and division up, get born again. Become a New Creature in Christ. zoom on, go for "Eternal Life"!

Sing with me "Caregivers!" Now I know my **ABC's,** tell me what you think of me? **ABCDEFG**...................!

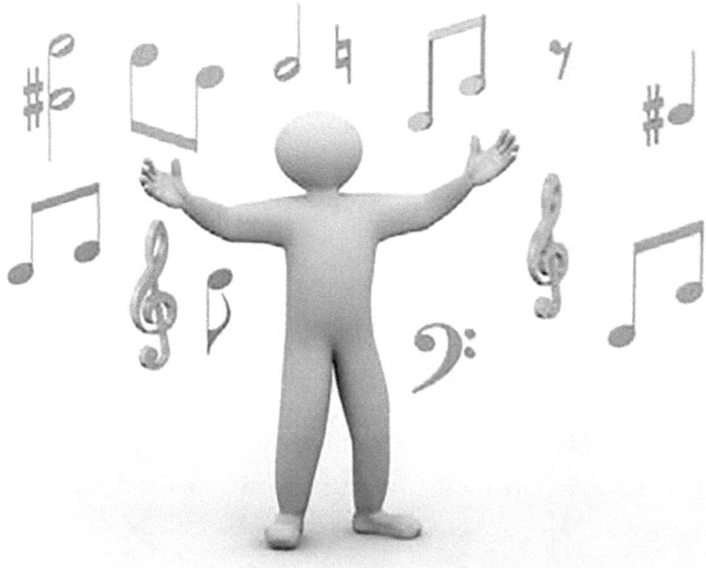

     MISS ASONDRA StarN'air

Daily Affirmations for CareGivers

I am a professional caregiver.

I am beautiful in every way.

I am successful; I love being a health-care provider.

I am learning new and useful skills.

I am a competent caregiver.

I am supportive of other caregivers.

I am a team player.

I am taking better care of myself.

I am making smarter food choices.

I am exercising more now.

I am starting to drink more water.

I am saying no to junk food.

I am always on time to work.

I am a positive person.

I am done with negativity.

I am minding my own business from now on.

I am done with gossiping.

I am welcoming change, growth, and development in every area of my life now.

I am a child of God, and it shows in my behavior.

I am happy.

I am full of gratitude.

I am starting to rest more. I realize getting a good night's sleep is very important.

I am changing in a great way. I have lots of love and respect for my bosses and coworkers.

I am finding more time to spend with God and his word now.

I am starting to read the Bible a lot more, and I see the difference in my life. I have more peace of mind. I feel like I can do all things in Christ, who strengthens me. **'I Feel Brand New!'**

Twenty-Five Affirmations for Caregivers

1. I am an excellent caregiver.
2. I am a professional.
3. I am smart and intelligent.
4. I am so blessed.
5. I am doing something about stress; I'm getting rid of it.
6. I am patient and kind.
7. I am prosperous.
8. I am faithful to God.
9. I am sorry for my sins, I shall repent and not do it again.
10. I am a child of the Most High.
11. I am developing into what God wants me to be.
12. I am thankful.
13. I am learning something new every day.
14. I am becoming a nicer, and a more loving person.
15. I am a team player.
16. I am staying away from strife from now on.
17. I am changing, getting closer and closer to God.
18. I am starting to read my Bible every day now.
19. I am going the extra mile. Love does not depend on two hearts; it depends on one (mine).
20. I love my ***Caregiver's Bible to Excellence*** book, and I'm telling everyone I know about it.
21. I am a empathetic, understanding, passionate, and a honest reliable loving caregiver, I deliver!
22. I am ready to do whatever God calls me to do without murmuring or complaining.
23. I am starting to seek God's will and purpose for my life.
24. I am dying to self so Jesus can come and live inside me.
25. I am giving my life to Christ; I want to follow him now.

Abuse Pledge for Caregivers

- I will not allow those in my care to hit me.
- I will tell them "It's wrong"!
- I will asks the individual to stop.
- I will not provide personal care until abuse stops, this is for my own protection and theirs.
- I will reassure the person that I am going to take excellent care of their needs and help provide a safe environment for both of us but abuse is not allowed.
- I will take the necessary breaks in between to help bring balance to the situation.
- I will ask management for instructions on how to handle the situation when those in my care are abusive.
- If the abuse does not stop, I will no longer care for that particular person. Abuse of any kind is **WRONG** and must be dealt with by the management team. Caregivers don't come to work to get punched, hit, kicked or spit on.
- My environment has to be a safe place for me to work in at all times.
- I will love and pray for those who hurt other people, but I will not be a victim anymore.

Bottom Line

'Abuse is Abuse' and anyone who does it must be stopped. No one should have to go to work and get abused, especially the caregiver, enough is enough!

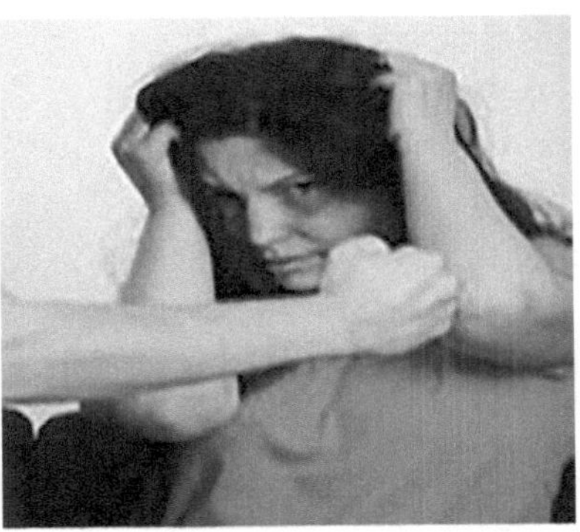

CAREGIVER ABUSE

1. Don't argue with the person.
2. Shift the conversation.
3. Ask, how can I please you?
4. Show me how you want things done.
5. Excuse, yourself if it's safe to do so, take a bathroom break and breathe, ask God to help, go back out and start again.
6. Wait, let them talk, you listen. Be humble.
7. Come up with something creative to do with them.
8. If nothing is working, just do your work, give them space and time to cool down.
9. Don't ever take abuse personal. but, **"REPORT IT"**
10. Ask for help from your company or if you are a family care provider, take a break, use respite care.
11. Document the behaviors times and dates.
12. If the caregiver abuse does not get resolved come off that assignment and contact your ombudsman.

"Caregivers Matter"!

Don't Go There!
Conversations Caregivers Should Avoid

1. **Your Personal Beliefs.** It can result in backlash if the other person doesn't agree.
2. **Private Information**—it can make things awkward moving forward for both you and the other person.
3. **Gossip of any kind.** Close your mouth!
4. **Discussing subjects like religion and politics is taboo.** Don't go there, period.
5. **Controversial Dialogue** can get ugly, don't go there either.
6. **Avoid "Office Grapevine"** with you as the primary focus. Shift the conversation quickly. "Oh, look at the time, I need to finish up my paperwork" would be a great exit.
7. **Avoid Disagreements;** call the office if you need profes-sional advice.
8. **'The Tongue'** talk less, listen more, do your chores!
9. **Avoid getting in lengthy conversations, period.** Aren't you supposed to be working? Hello!
10. **Leave your opinions out, you're asking for it!** Instead focus on caregiving and excellence!
11. **Avoid asking for food, drinks, etc.** Where is your lunch box? Bring it!
12. **Practice 'Professionalism'** don't give out your number.

Tame The Tongue!

Don't Let it Trap You!

 MISS ASONDRA STARN'AIR

Don't Cross the Line
It's a Thin Line Between Professionalism and Friendship!

What's crossing the line? "Glad you want to know" it means we are starting to behave in ways that are not socially acceptable. For the caregiver it means, we are not behaving like professionals. We are starting to mix things up a bit shall we say, for example, becoming too personally involved with the client.

Kissing and hugging on the way out the door, that's not professional, here's what is: "with a smile" say, 'it was a plea-sure taking care of you today, do you need anything else before I leave, if not, have a great evening, I'll see you tomorrow now that's a professional caregiver! The latter is crossing the line in my opinion. We should not be kissing our clients, ok, maybe after many, many years of service, but certainly not within weeks or months into the **WORKING** relationship. Again, I say it's unprofessional! But some may disagree. That's okay too.

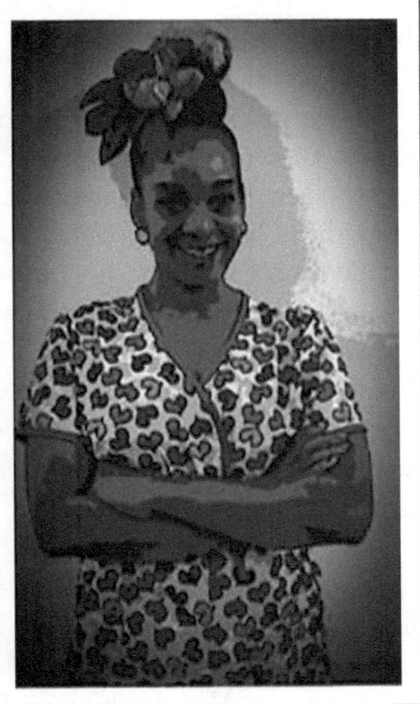

But, truth be told, we all want to be liked, but your work ethics is what's most important here. Our attitudes, hospitality, how well we give service, are we on time? Do we know want we're doing? Are we skilled, Competent? These kinds of Qualities are what individuals in our care really want.

Caregivers, listen to me, we do not have to manipulate other ways to be liked or become favorites. Stay Professionals, Be **EXCELLENT** at what you came there to do, and they'll keep calling back for you!

One more time, **'Don't Cross the Line!'**

Always Be Professional, Yet kind!

NO Dumping!

What is dumping? By definition it's the disposal of waste, garbage, unwanted material.

But by my definition it's anyone who brings their problems to work then dump them off on others. In this case, clients, or vice versa, the client does all the dumping.

As caregiver professionals we must be professional at all times. We must know when to shift conversations. Keep them bright and light, I say! Furthermore, we have no business discussing very personal matters with our clients in the first place; yes I call this dumping. Your business should stay your business! Talk to God about your problems, not to those in your care.

Our clients do not need to know about your lovers (God is not please at all about that one. read the scriptures!) your boy-friend or babies daddy drama. Nor do they need to know you are behind in your bills,

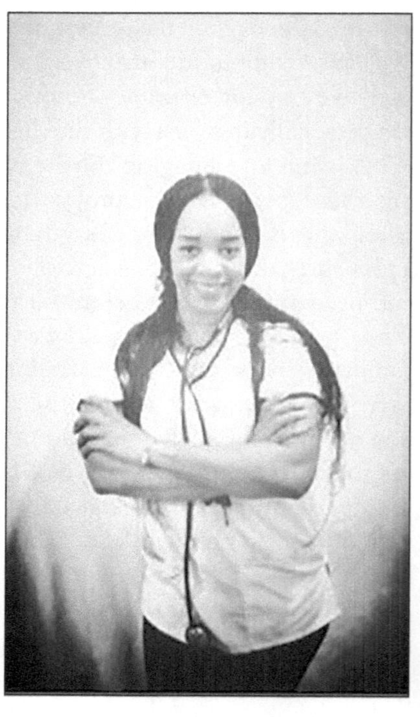

haven't you heard, "America's" behind in bills! Our everyday problems are not their problems, equally true, theirs are not ours.

Here's the thing, we always want to be a gentle ear, and have compassion for others, of course, but when it's turning into dumping, we must learn to shift the conversation quickly. Again, aren't you supposed to be working? Hey, if you can't find anything positive or interesting to talk about, then talk about weather, just get it together, don't be a drama queen, be a Caregiver for Christ queen/king!

Rock with me, enact a "No Dumping" policy right from the start, zone it, own it! If your mouth and behavior is not professional, you're not a professional! It's as simple as that! You have more training do.

        Miss Asondra StarN'air

Accepting What Is

Accepting what is, can be the new game changer in just about any persons life, especially for those growing older and older. Growing old does not have to be so rough or depressing.

With the help of family mem bers, friends and caregivers, life can still be full of adven ture and joy.

All it takes is a great attitude toward **"Accepting What Is"** and a willingness to be open to try new things.

That's where we come in, lets show them how to have fun again! All we have to do is come up with activities or something that engages their curiosity and gives them a reason to get out of bed everyday.

If that person is bedbound, yet alert and oriented, care-giver you are not off the hook. Get creative, stay creative too, find something you can do to-gether to make the day more enjoyable. look at some images together, watch a movie, play cards, share laughter!

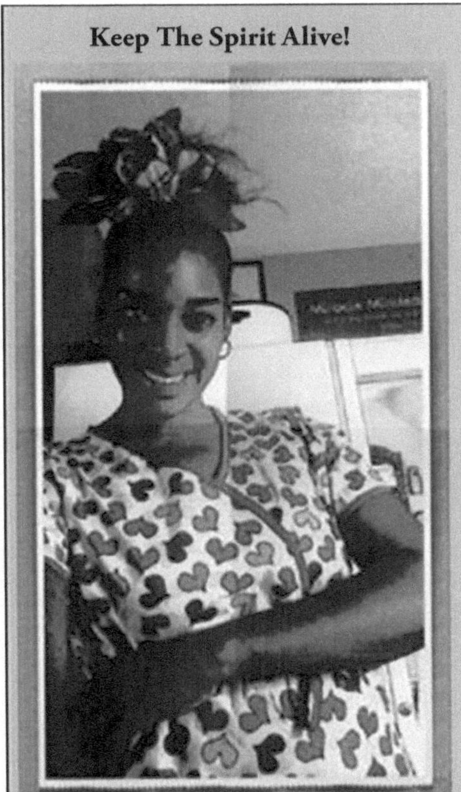

GETTING OLDER IS GETTING BOLDER!

Caregivers it is our responsibility to make sure those in our care especially seniors do not give up hope lets help them keep the spirit alive!

Sharing Laughter!

When we do things like this we are gradually aiding them into the mind set of **"Accepting What Is"** and when that happens, magic happens too.

Suddenly things start to come alive, like stars in the sky, no longer asking God why? You've helped then to go with the flow, relax, and "Accept What Is"! Fact of life, **"Everybody Gets Old"**, it is written, All go to the same place, all come from dust and to dust all returns. **Ecclesiastes 3:20**
But in the meantime, there is still a lot of living to do, caregivers we play a vital role in helping them to reach that state of mind. We should never let those in our care, especially seniors give up hope or fall into depression 'Ever'.

Remember this, **"LIFE"** isn't over because we're getting older oh no, on the contrary, **"Getting Older Is Getting Bolder!"**

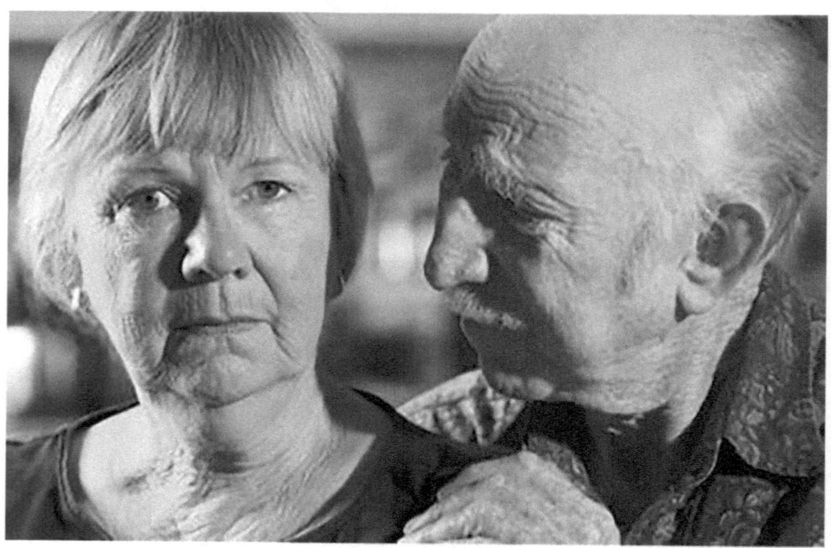

Come On, Lets Go Wheel Chair Bowling!

No matter what age or condition, we owe it to ourselves to live the best life possible. And with God all things are possible!

 MISS ASONDRA StarN'air

Caregiver's Closet

StarN'air's Closet

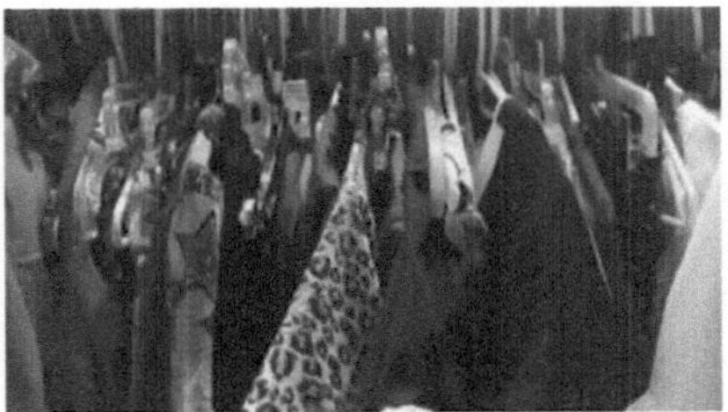

When it comes to Scrubs, I think having lots of variety makes going to work more fresh and exciting!

A Professional Caregiver

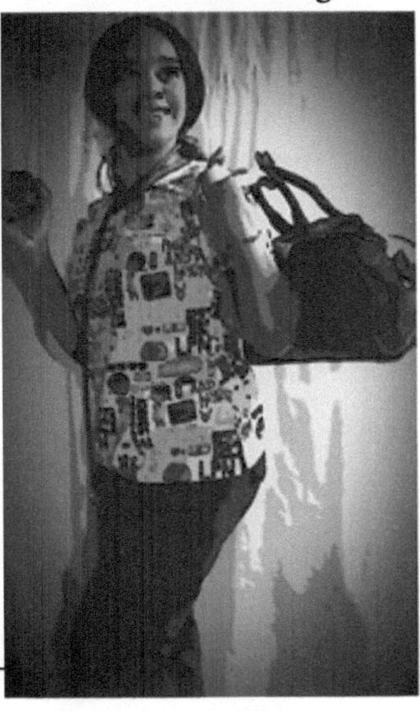

She's got the look, that says **"You're Hired"** What about you?

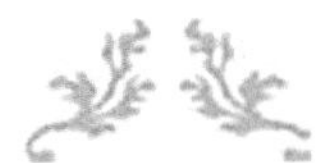

You Are What You Wear!

Make sure you are dress for success

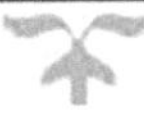

Tips

- Make sure your hair is pulled back, away from your face.
- do not over use make up, save that for a night out on the town.
- Limit jewelry, but caregivers work watch is okay!
- Keep a work supply bag with you.
- An apple a day wouldn't hurt either!
- Get to work fifteen minutes early, no matter weather conditions.
- Wear medium loose fitting work apparel, never wear spandex it's so not cool; mightiest well be naked! Body shaping pants and leggings are too revealing. They don't belong in any work place period.

Diabetes

Diabetes is a metabolic disease in which the body's inability to produce any or enough insulin causes elevated levels of glucose (sugar) in the blood.

Millions of Americans live with diabetes: **Type 1 and Type 2.**

Snapshot

Type 1: The body makes little or no insulin due to an overactive immune system; therefore, that individual MUST take insulin EVERY DAY.

Type 2: The body prevents the insulin from working right—meaning it may make some insulin, but not enough.

Our Part

As caregivers, we want to support those living with this disease by helping them enjoy the healthiest life possible. That means, too, preparing and serving them appropriate meals.

TEAMING UP WITH DIABETES

- Educate yourself about diabetes; share what you learned with client.
- Encourage them to stick with a healthy diet.
- Check sugar level regularly.
- Keep mealtimes consistent.
- For emergencies, keep honey, hard candy, and orange juice available at all times.
- Encourage movement, exercise, walking, range of motion, etc.
- Arts and crafts; find great recipes for diabetics.
- Help that individual set small goals.
- Make a poster board displaying their accomplishments.
- Keep them "active."
- Be a good support system. Again, keep encouraging physical activities and healthy lifestyles choices.
- Have fun, laugh and en-joy each other!

Caregivers, "We Rock!"

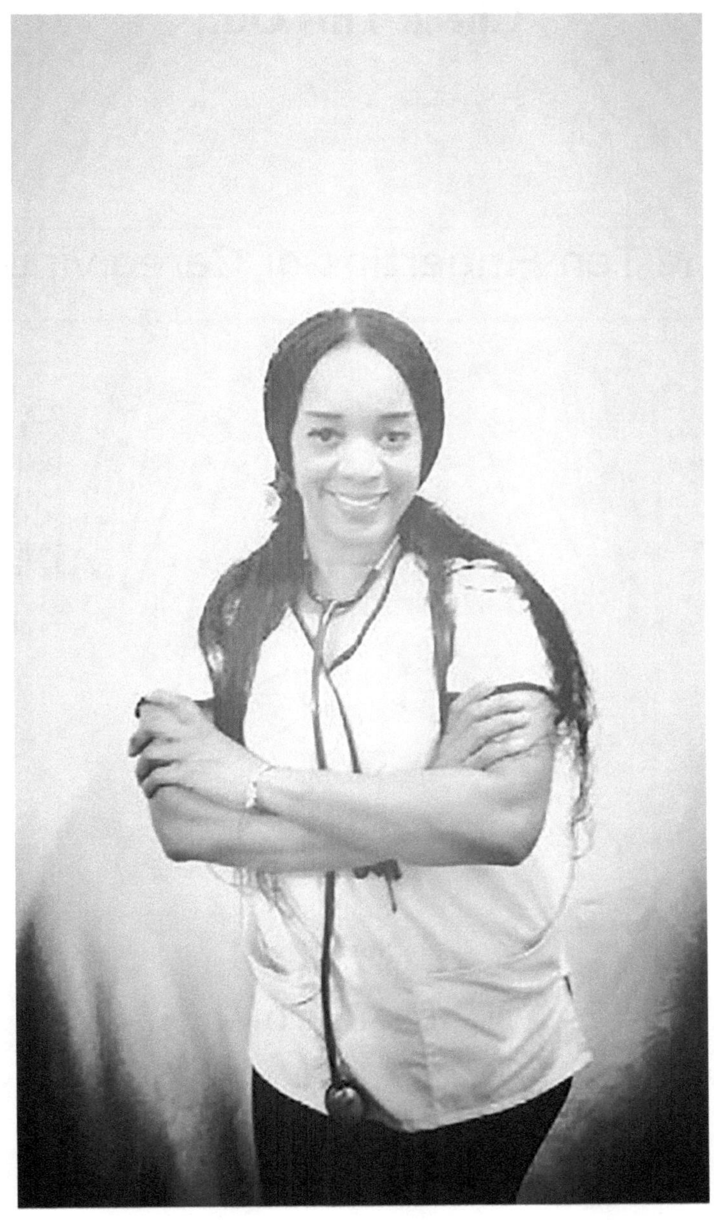

Check This Out!

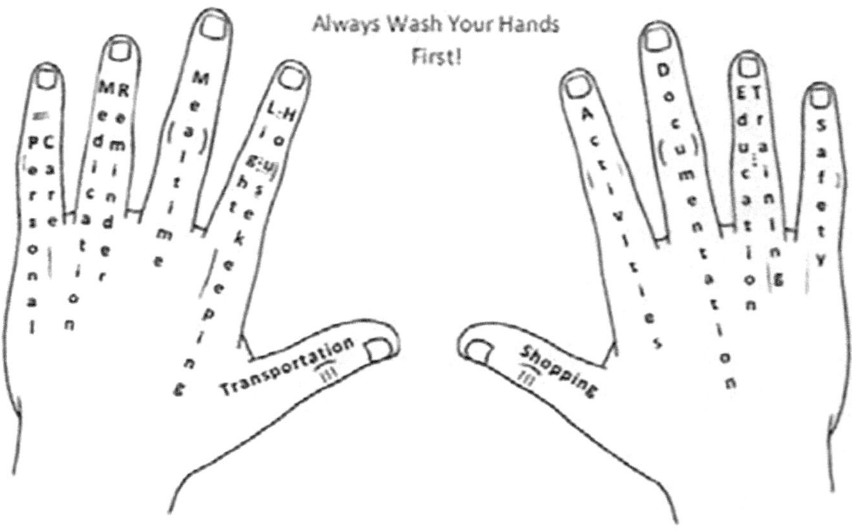

Now!

Flip Your Hands Over!

WOW!

Ten More Caregiving Tips Inside Your Hands

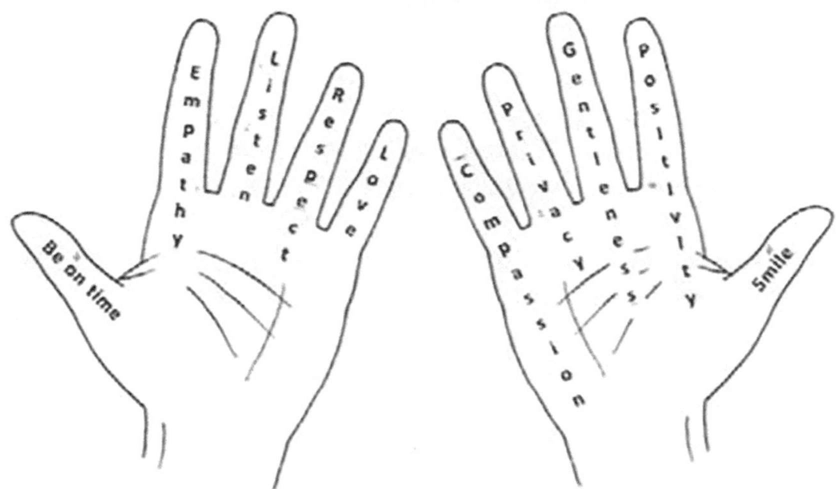

WOW!

Stay In The Know!

Signs and Symptoms to Report.

Evaluate the situation, is it safe? Do I call 911 or can I handle it within my scope?

Educate, tell the individual /family why you are doing what you are doing.

Keep records, make sure they are neat, accurate, concise and complete. Documentation is a must!

Help the person relax.

Eye and ears open, "Caregivers" watch out for changes in breathing, sounds of destress or pain.

Lay down slowly or sit up whichever is preferred and most comfortable to the person.

Position them comfortably and keep them warm, do not allow a chill to occur.

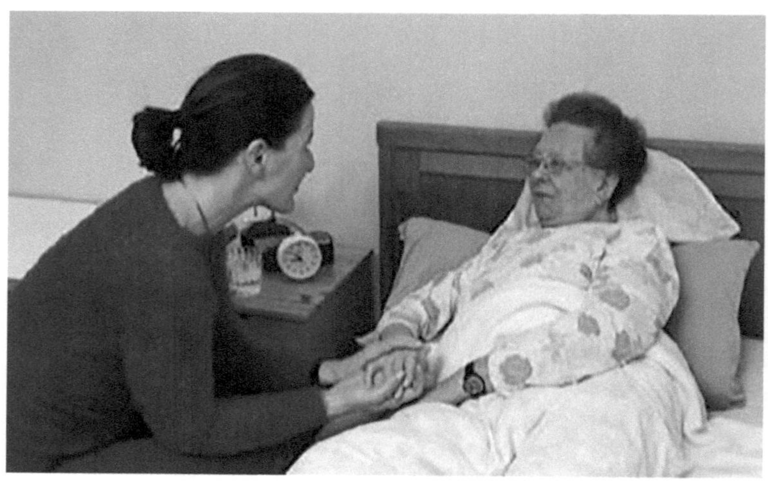

 Miss Asondra StarN'air

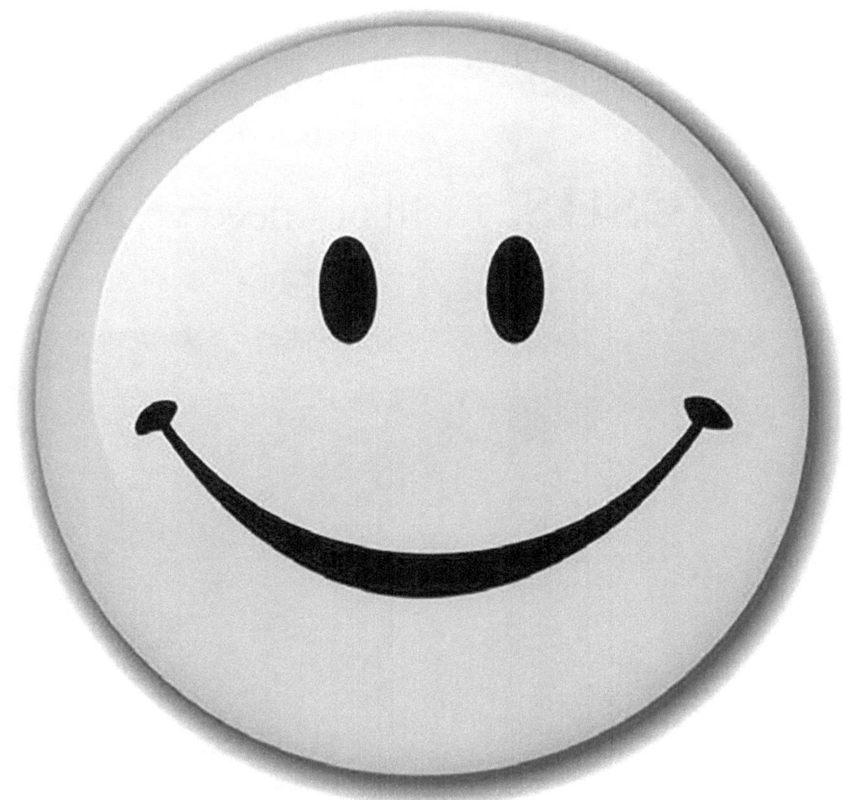

Keep smiling throughout the day. Act like you love what you do. Caregivers, you do love what you do, don't you? Then,

"SMILE"!

Hello, Caregivers

This is **Jesus!** I will not need your help today

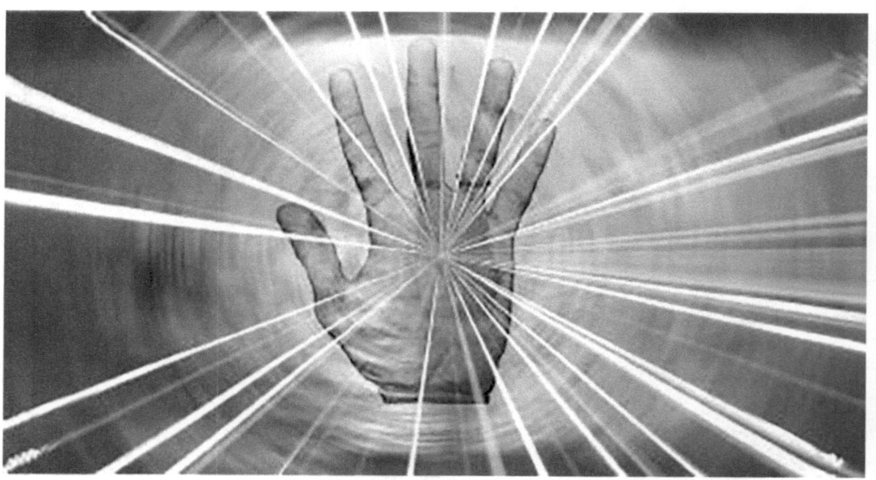

Just step aside and let **Me** lead the way.

The Lord nurses them when they are sick and eases their pain and discomfort. **Psalms 41:3**

First Day On The Job!

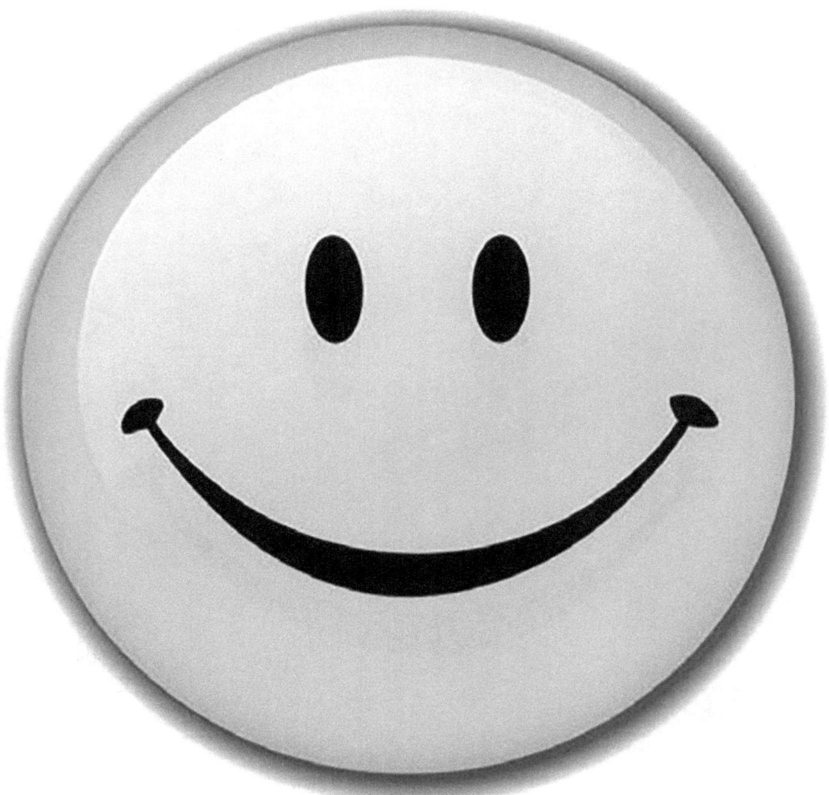

Okay, we're getting ready to go into a residence home. Are you ready? **Let's Go...**

Put on a Happy Face!

Hello, my name is _______________ I'm your "Caregiver" and how may I serve you today?

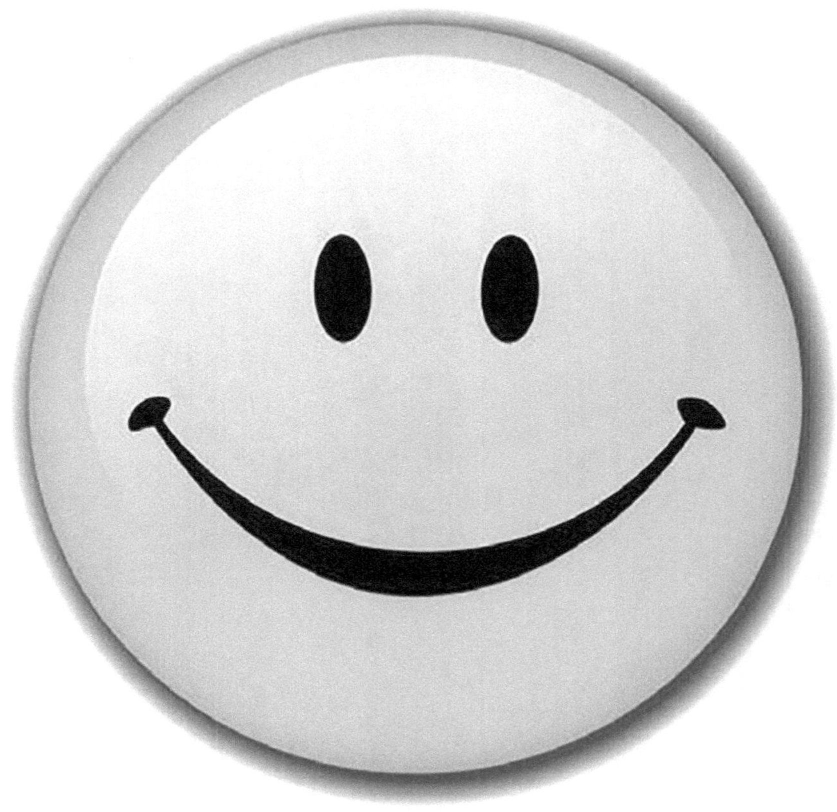

A Reminder

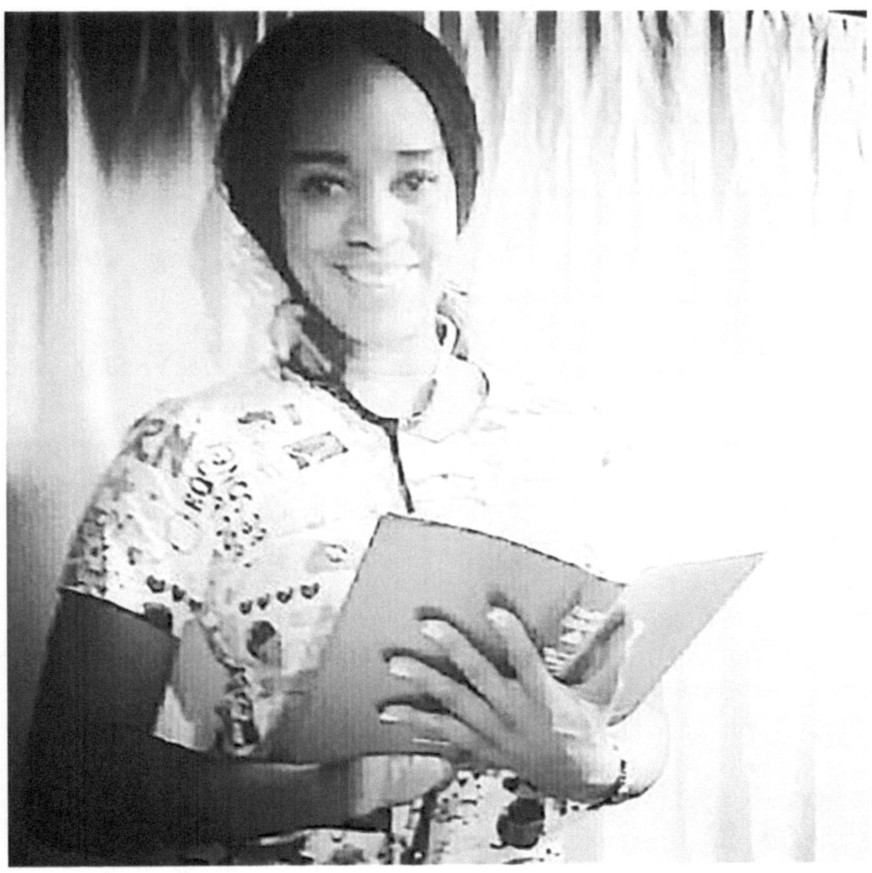

Don't forget to find the caregivers binder with the residence careplan in it. If you don't see it ask the resident for it. Make sure you follow it and docoument what you did after, not before. Check the box and go on to the next task, **'Get the Care Plan, Follow the Care Plan!'**

Good Morning!

Good morning, time to start the day!

---

6 a.m. to 10 a.m. Personal Care/ Hygiene/ ADLs

Breakfast/ Medication Reminders, etc.

10:00 a.m. to 12:00 p.m. Cleanup/ Light Housekeeping, Activities/ ROM Exercises/ Light Snacks/ Offer Water

Check and Change/ Incontinent Care/ transfers/ Vitals

Find something you both enjoy doing together; it makes caregiving and receiving care fun and bonding.

If you are caring for total-care patients or special needs keep in mind that everyone loves music, story time, and picture books, I don't know anyone who doesn't. Just be creative; do something wonderful with those in your care.

Don't forget **"Hand Hygiene."** Keep your hands clean and groomed. Standard and Universal Precaution must be executed to ensure the health of both you and the other person. Wash your hands throughout the day!

Keep this in mind always, today is all you both have, so make it a good one. Tomorrow is not promised to us, therefore, love and have fun!

Yet you do not know what tomorrow will bring. What is your life? For you are a mist that appears for a little time and then vanishes.
James 4:14

 Miss Asondra StarN'air

Good Afternoon!

It's lunchtime already; we were having so much fun!

12:00 p.m. to 2:00 p.m. Meal Preparation, set the table/tray.

If possible, bring out your lunch bag and have lunch with those in your care. Do not share your food; they may be allergic to some spices or ingredients. If you are at a facility, follow their protocol please.

Practice good nutrition, make sure everyone drinks plenty of water and eats fruits and vegetables. Remember our bodies belong to Christ, not us. **1 Corinthians 3:16**

Next, ease the moment into righteous loving conversations; avoid all gossip. Imagine you are at a fine restaurant; have fun and enjoy each other's company.

Again, if you are at a facility, it's about the residence, not about what you did last night. Make them the center of attention. Talk about you all you want, but do it on your own time, not theirs.

Okay, lunch is almost over. Clean up, collect trays, and start your check and changes/ transfers/ medication reminders, etc.

Incorporate hospitality; offer tea or coffee. Find out if there's something special they want to do, read or watch on TV, or do they require a light nap or time alone?

If so, finish up on your light housekeeping / facility protocol and such.

Remember, how a residence room/ house looks reflex's on us too. Straighten up a bit! Go the extra mile, Jesus will smile!

Midday Activities

From 2:00 PM to 4:00 PM

Rest Time (Optional)

But for those of you who want to have a good time, how about some arts and crafts, or maybe do some sing-alongs, maybe popcorn, and a movie. Oh, I got it! How about a glamour bazaar, we can do hair and makeup; Cooking with StarN'air has a flare too! There is so much one can do to make the day fun and memorable.

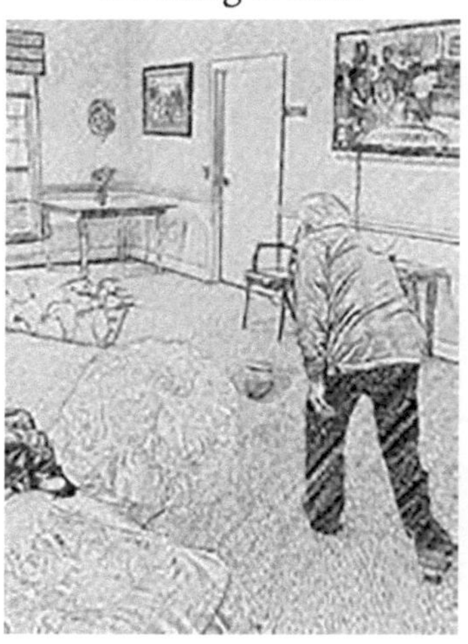

Bowling is Fun!

Caregivers, we must make every effort to get back to enjoying everyday life. Christian and Charismatic leader Joyce Meyers and I believe that we must make living for God a priory in our lives. But just because we are Christians doesn't mean we can't have fun and enjoy every day life with other too, I do.

We are becoming caregivers for Christ, so it is our duty to enhance the quality of life of those we are serving by making sure they continue to thrive and have fun that's what God would want his caregivers to do.

So stay proactive, offer daily activities that are appropriate and safe. Find out first from those in your care what they like or want to do, and try to make it happen; or you come up with something and don't forget to pass out lite refreshments. After that, do another check and change, make sure that person is still dry, if not, partial lower body wash, clean underwear/ depends. Freshness matters! Lastly, retake vitals, if instructed to do so. And another thing, make sure you document throughout the day and record your vitals if required. Now if all is well, clean up and start preparing for dinner, "Winner". Well done, well done!

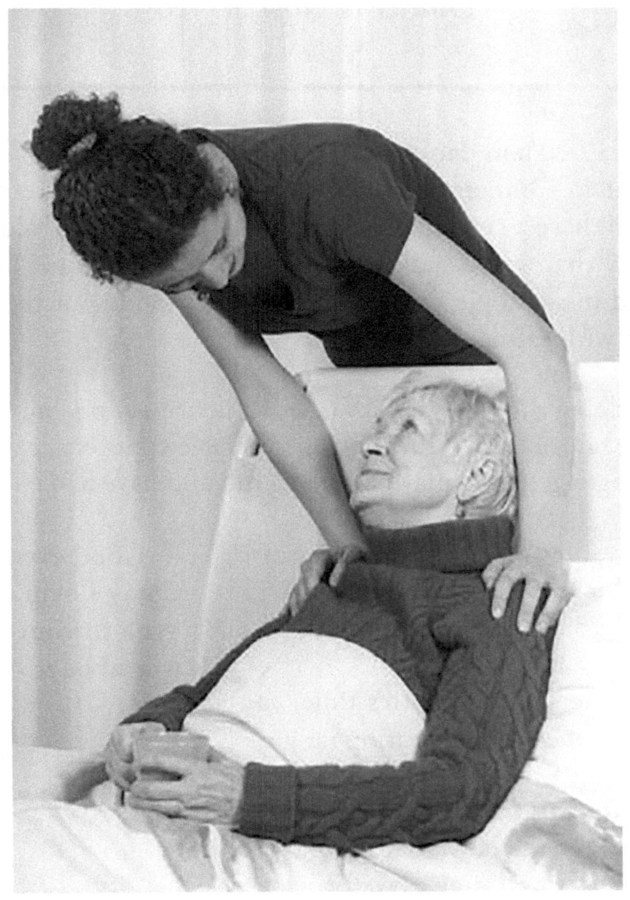

Good Evening!

Dinner Is Now Served

5:00 p.m. to 7:00 p.m. Hospitality is a key ingredient to becoming great at what you do. Dinner time should feel special; table or tray should, in my opinion, have a centerpiece. How about a 'Sunflower' along with a smile surely that would make a great impact on everyone! Next, offer to cut food in small pieces if you see they are too big or the person is struggling with eating utensils.

If you are doing a feed, feed with ease, without rushing. Smile like you love taking care of them. Offer liquids in between portions, pay attention to body language. They may be getting full and have had enough.

Get to know how much those in your care input percentages are—for example, 10%, 25%, 50%, 75%, 100%, or refused.

Chart/document. In a month's time, you should know their average eating range.

Remember too, do not rush dinner; it's the last full meal of the day. Most people use dinner time as social time as well.

Offer another cup of tea or coffee. Many look forward to dessert after every meal; So make the dining experience wonderful for that individual. Again, hospitality is key! Look over to the right **"Hi"** that's me!

After dinner, do your fundamentals again, bathroom 'Check and Change etc.

Good evening, may I help escort you to your table? It would be my pleasure!

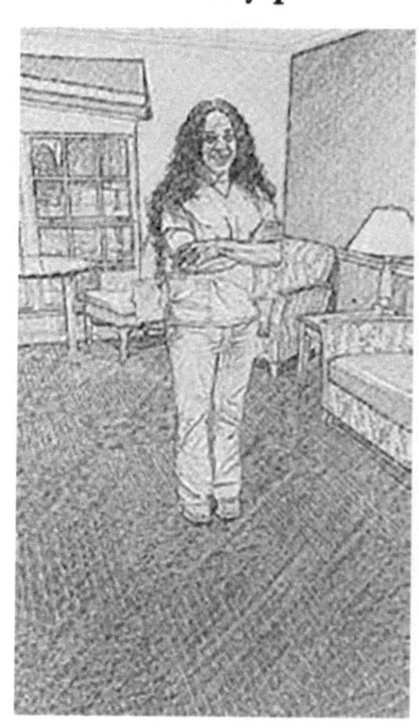

 Miss Asondra StarN'air

Evening Care Plan

Bedtime—Make it Special and Full of Comfort!

8:00 p.m. to 11:00 p.m. Many of our seniors are ready to get in bed shortly after dinner, so go prep the room. Make sure they've had all their medication reminders. Do your night-time check and change personal care routine; offer another light snack and place a cup of water on their night stand, unless they're restrictions put in place by the doctor.

Next, allow the person some quite time alone, to prayer or... just be on standby. If you are changing shifts, before you leave go and wish that person a good night's sleep; tell them when you'll be back.

Also, leave with this: Mr./Ms. ____________ it was a pleasure being here and I hope you were happy with the care and services I provided for you today. I look forward to seeing you again soon. (note if you know that date, tell them. If it's tomorrow, same time, say so. And if you are doing a twenty-four-hour case with multiple caregivers on the team don't just leave. introduce that caregiver. And too, give a verbal report to your team mate e.g. changes in conditions or FYI"s (For Your Information) things like that. Communication is key to a successful shift.
"Team Work Makes the Dream Work"!

After you've done all that, wash your hands, collect all your belongings. Leave nothing in the residence house or room **'PROFESSIONALS'** don't do that!

Follow your company's exit plan as well. Now go home and do the care plan I designed for special caregivers like you and if you haven't read it yet, it's in your caregivers back office I do believe. Again, **"Well Done!"**

You Took Excellent Care of Others, Now it's Time to **"Go Home"** and Take Excellent Care of **"YOU!"**

Have a Good Night!

"Smart Phones"
Here We Go Again ...

Is Your Smart Phone Really Smart? No it's not if you put it before your other important responsibilities, like work. Your personal calls and texting can wait!

Go tend to the customer, lets get our priorities straight!

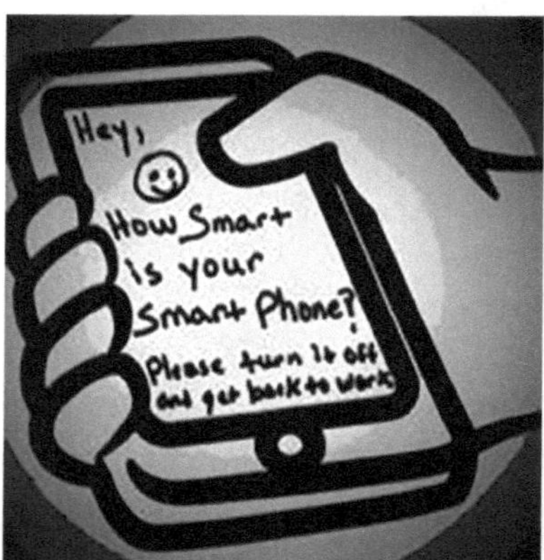

Stay Off Your Phones!

Hey, I'm just the messenger, don't get peeved off at me. However, I do agree, cell phones are becoming a nuisance in the work place. You can catch up on your calls and emails on your breaks. Come on, we must stay smart and professional.

'Our Phones Can Wait'.

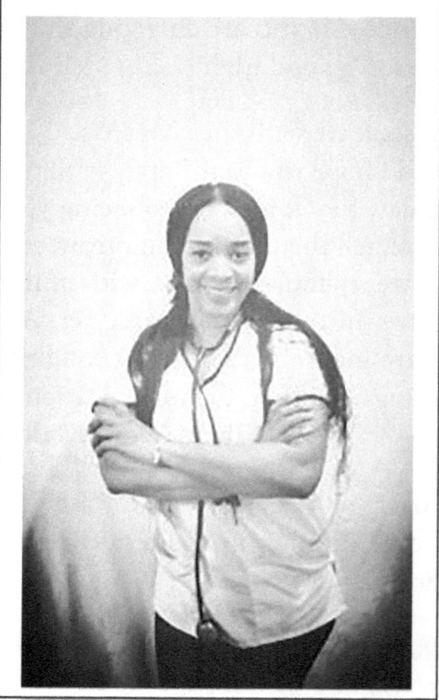

People, respect for the work place is all it takes!

Acrylic Long Nails

N- Not
A- Allowed
I- In
L- Long-Term Care or Facilities
S- Settings.

Clean hands are the single most important factor in preventing the spread of germs.

Wearing artificial fingernails increases the risk of germs because pathogens now have a place to hide—under the nails.

Professional Caregivers do not wear artificial nails and keep their real nails trimmed low.

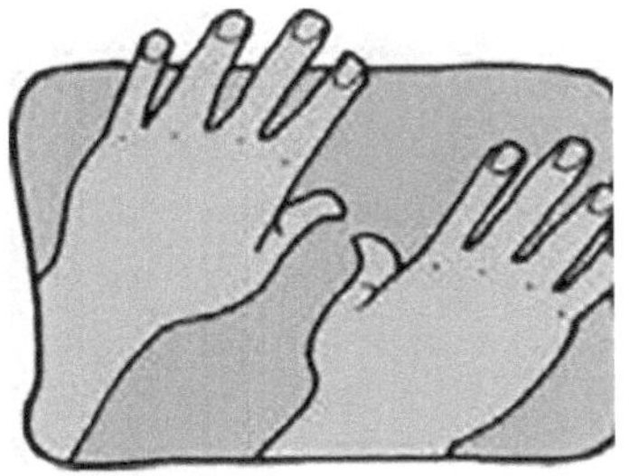

Good Nail Hygiene!

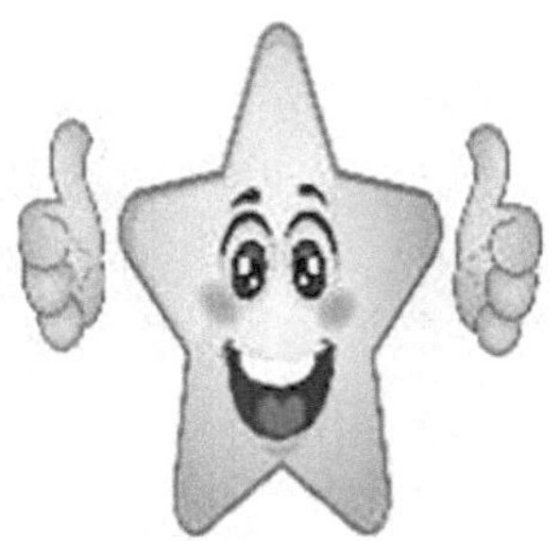

Way To Go!

How to Wash Your Hands

1. Make sure a clean towel or paper towels are there in advance.
2. Turn on the water; make sure it's warm.
3. Wet your hands.
4. Lather your hands with soap.
5. Rub your hands together.
6. Keep washing; rub both sides. Don't forget to rub between the fingers too and 3 to 4 inches up your wrist. Come on, wash those hands for about 20 seconds or more, sing a song, let that help you along!
7. Now rinse your hands, but don't touch the sink.
8. Dry your hand with your towel. Make sure you dry between the fingers and up the wrist too.
9. Use paper towel to turn water off.
10. Throw paper towel in trash and smile!

**Wow, "Good to Go"
Great Job!**

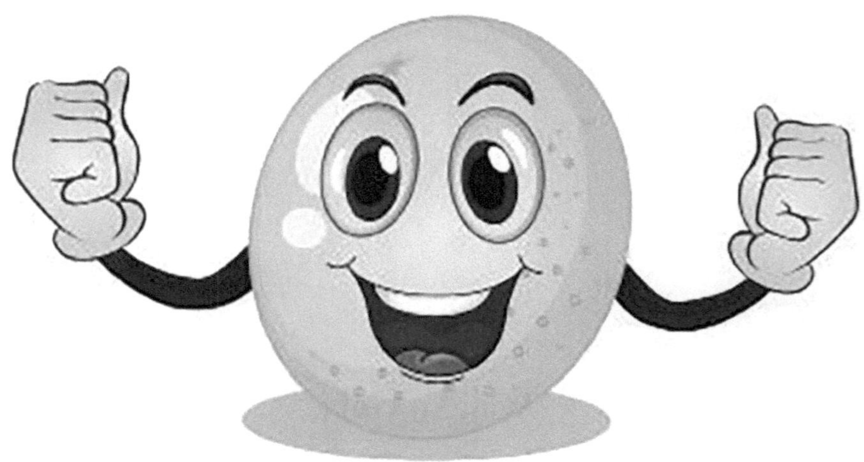

    Miss Asondra StarN'air

Don't Forget!

Wash Your Hands

Wash Your Hands

Wash Your Hands

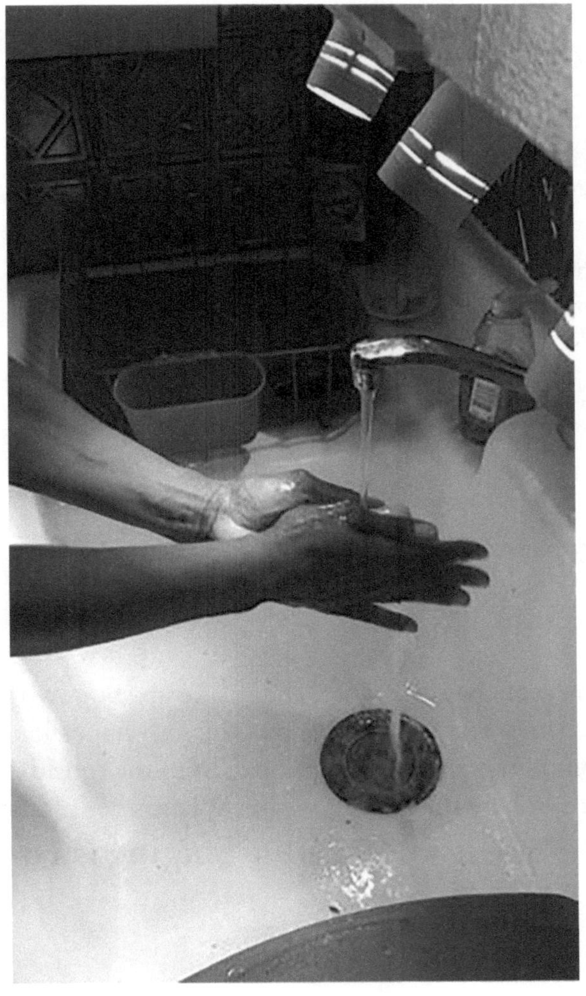

What don't you understand?

The Washing Hands Song

Washing my hands it keeps me free

From the spread of disease . . . es

For so many reason . . . es . . .

It protects me

It protects you

Yes, washing my hands keeps me free

From pathogens I can't see

From me to you

I know what to do

Washing my hands keeps me free

From the spread of diseases

Now you sing too! Use these words, but make up your own melody, and sing this one time. You would have washed your hands long enough to really get your hands super clean and free from the spread of disease. O come on, be a kid, be silly, sing it please. Where's your sense of humor? Sing it and be done, besides caregivers, **'Singing is Fun'!**

S.O.A.P

Serve Those in Need

Obey God's Word

Apply What You Read

Pray for Understanding

Once we do all that, "Our Hands" will really be clean!

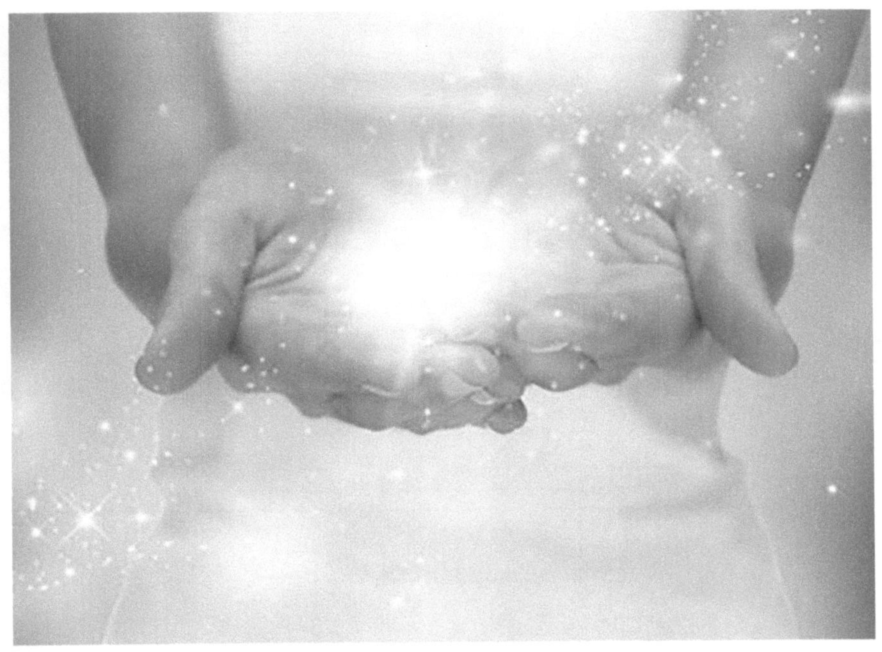

In Jesus name, Amen!

StarN'air's Sample Care Plan

Client's Name: ___________________________________

Name: ___________________________________

Week of _______/_______/_____39 _____/_______/_____

Wash your hands, Coming! Hello   **Homecare Provider**

Personal Care / Wash your hands	SUNDAY	MONDAY	TUESDAY	WEDNESDAY	THURSDAY	FRIDAY	SATURDAY
	DATES	DATES	DATES	DATES	DATES	DATES	DATES
Bed bath/Shower							
Skin care/shave							
Oral Hygiene/brush teeth							
Denture Care/cleaning							
Assist w/dressing & undressing							
Prepare for bed/transfers.							
Nutrition Wash your hands							
Prepare meals							
Breakfast							
Lunch							
Dinner							
Assist w/feeding							
Encourage Fluids							
Homemaking Wash your hands							
Make bed/change Linens							
Laundry/ put away							
Clean kitchen/bathroom/main room,							
vacuum /trash removal/disinfection/							
handwashing							
Elimination Wash your hands							
Incontinence care/barrier cream							
Reposes, report skin markings, sores							
Assist w/ toileting, standing, wiping							
Circle all that applies Wash your hands							
Other /specialties /pet and plant care							
Medication reminder, oxygen, vitals							
Grocery shopping, transportation							
Record, assist w/ making phone calls							
Emergency , 911, incident report							

Client's Signature_________________________________ Date_____________________

Caregiver's Signature_________________________________ Date_____________________

Wash Your Hands Going!

Caregiver's Note Pad & Mini Incident Report

Any incidents, circle Y or N. If yes, complete the following: Briefly describe, what happen?

____

____

____

____

____

____

____

____

____

____

____

____

Did you call the Office/Family/ 911? Circle Y or N

Write the full names of all involved and who you contacted below

(I) Involved	**(C) Contacted**
_________________	_________________
_________________	_________________
_________________	_________________
_________________	_________________

Were you injured? Circle Y or N   Did you follow to hospital? Y or N

Prepare to come to the office to fill out full incident report within Twenty-Four hours.

Thank You!

Documentation

CareGivers, I can't stress enough how important that we document. Documentation is a vital part of our professional job as caregivers. Not only does it provide clear and important information to the healthcare team, it protects us, you and me "The Caregiver".

When documenting, only document Factual and Actual Information, "nothing more, nothing less"

No Opinions or Assumptions. Write neat and use black ink if possible, in fact "Every Professional Caregiver "should keep a note pad and a black ink pen with them at all times.

And if you make a mistake, never scribble out, just initial and draw a straight line through it, and keep documenting.

Follow your Companies "Protocol" and summit documents in their allotted time.

DOCUMENTATION

Document The Following

- Time
- Date
- First name
- Last name
- Correct Spelling
- Your Full Name
- Your Title
- Location of Incident/or
- Brief Description
- Actual and Factual Info..
- Manager or Supervisor or person you contacted, First and Last Name.

Be ready to provide a 24 hour number you can be reached at, a working cell phone number is acceptable.

- Names and Contact information of witnesses if applicable.
- Give Information if 911 was called
- Where did they take them and did you follow?
- Private Caregivers, so what, document!
- Document what you were told to do and by whom.

Lastly, print your full name, sign and date.

__________ Thank You!

Caregiver's Don't Do It!

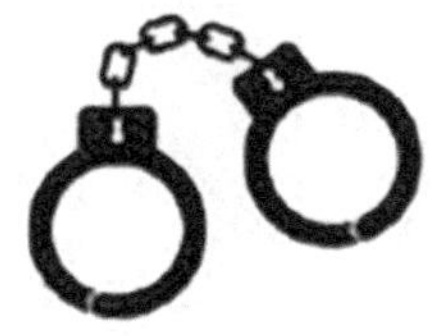

Everyday a number of individuals are caught engaged in some kind of theft and with disappointment, homecare is an area of great concern, so let's address it right now!

Homecare and private duty agencies face theft in clients homes by caregivers more often than reported. This is another form of elderly abuse that mustn't be tolerated.

The service of homecare requires a tremendous amount of trust, so when a caregiver breaks that trust by lying, cheating and stealing it hurts everyone. Yes everyone is affected, the client, the family, owners, management, and other care staff.

Because trust flows from the caregiver that business owner and management will follow through on the commitment made. When a caregiver steals, the company's reputation is damaged and some never recover.

That's why agencies now have a zero tolerance for stealing, anyone caught stealing will be prosecuted. But the good news is 95 to 99 % of Caregivers are honest and upstanding individuals according to my research and that's something to be proud of. And to the 1% that are not, I wrote a little something for you, check it out!

THEFT

Taking
Has
Eliminated
Future
Trust

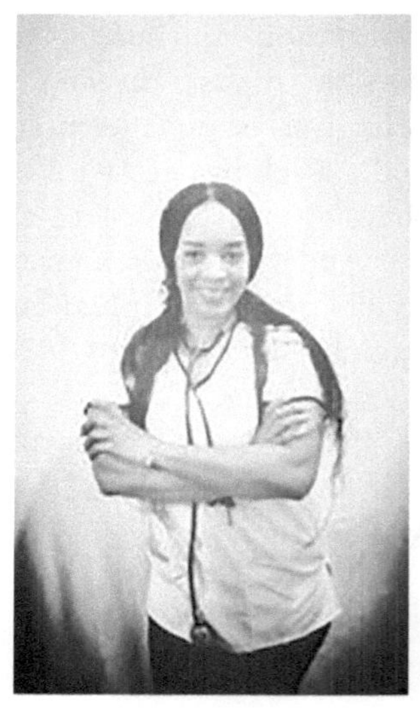

Don't Steal, Ask God and it Shall Be Given! Mark 7:7

'God Is Watching'

If someone seems to be getting away with doing something wrong,
trust me it won't be long before their gone
Maybe, God's just giving those a chance to make it all right
For his grace and mercy is new every day, and every night!
If you need something just humble thyself, get on your knees and
pray, trust him, he will surely bring it your way.
Stealing is wrong, it's never okay. Remember God knows and see's
everything but if you don't stop stealing your doorbell shall surely
ring. You are under arrest!
You have the right to remain
silent anything you say can be
used against you in a court of law,
you have a right to an attorney
"Warning, warning...no baloney!"

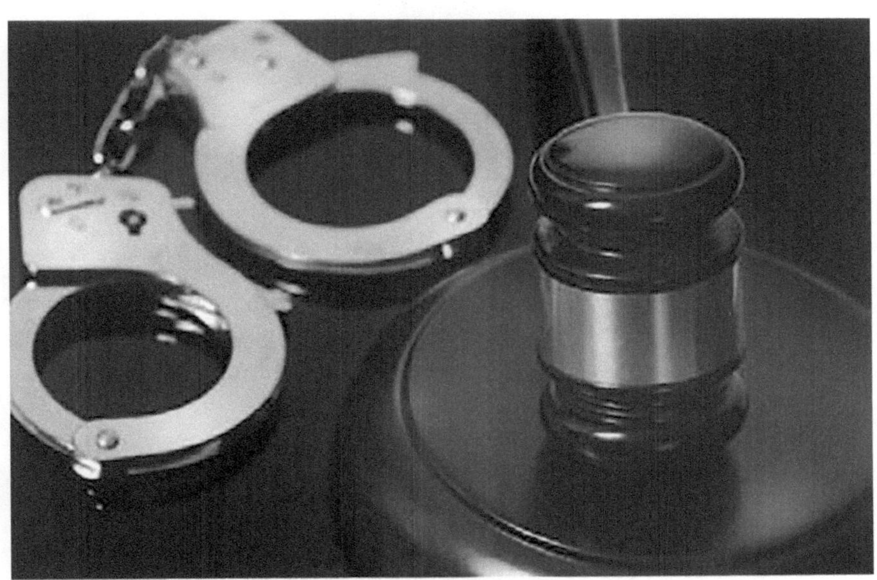

'Caregivers' Don't Do It!"

Taking is Theft!

Caregiver's Don't Do It, Don't Even Think About It!

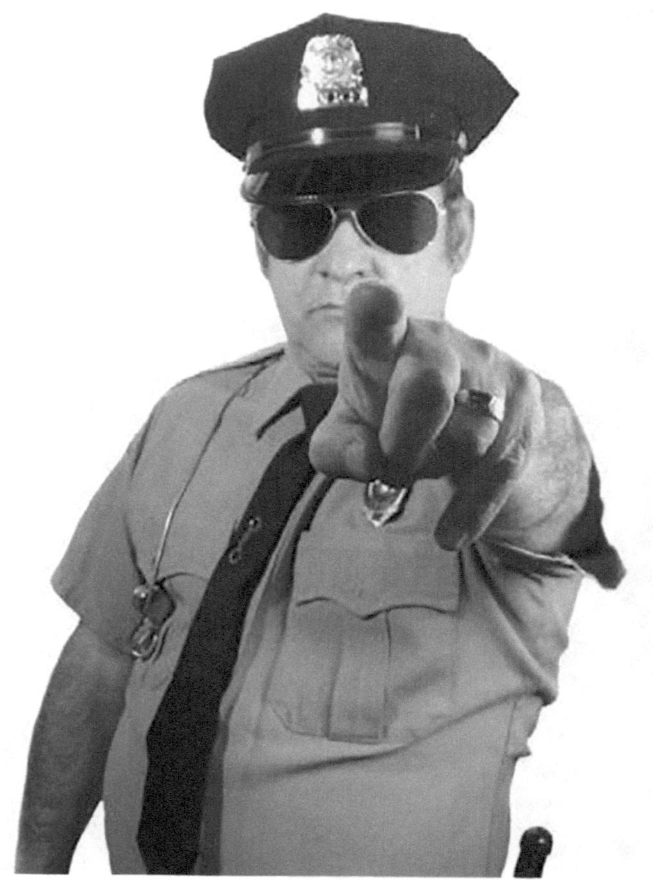

Stealing From Others, "Is WRONG!"

If You Do

"YOU" are going to jail, so long!

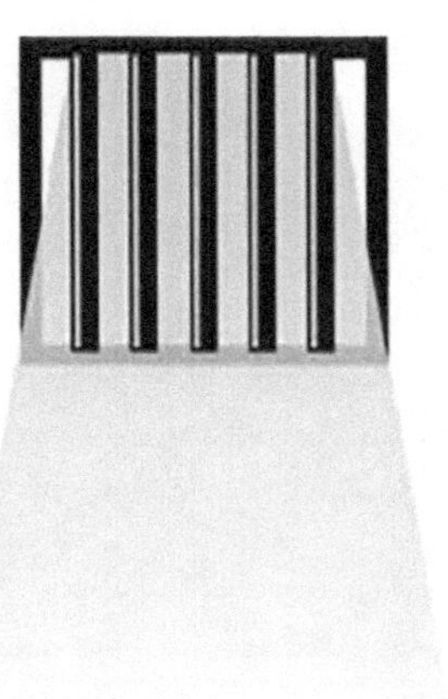

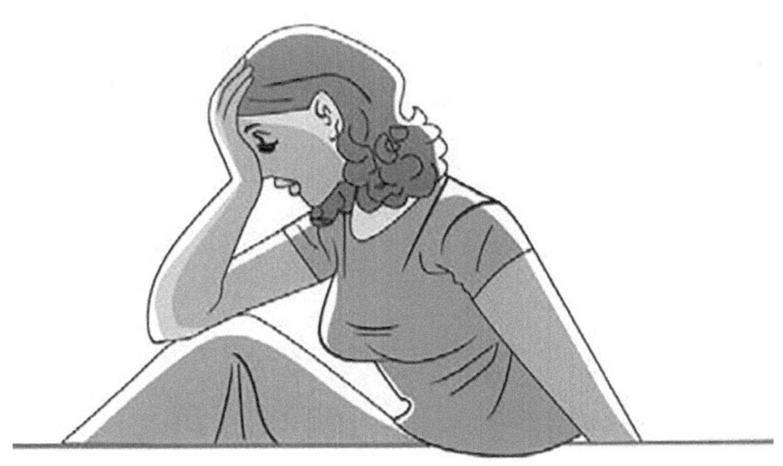

Told You Not To Do It!

Stand Up!

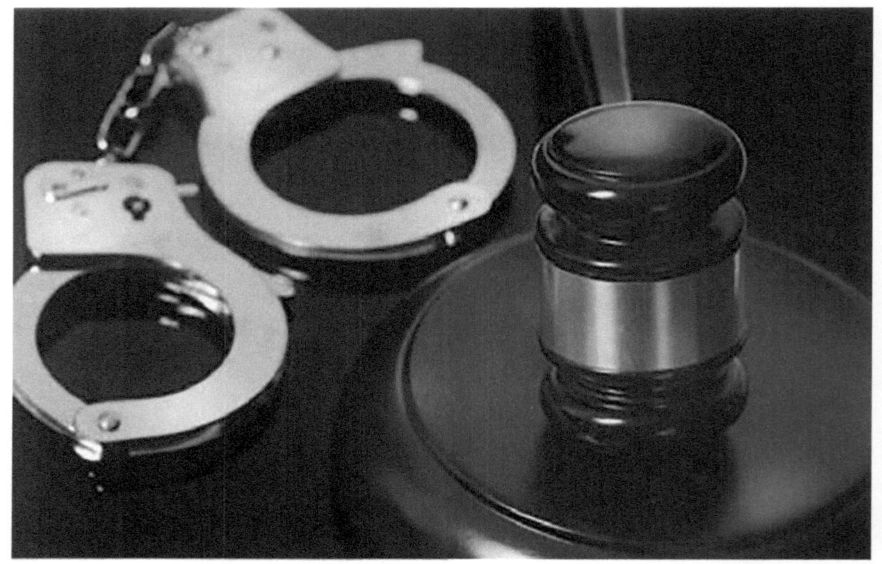

How Do You Plead?

"Guilty"!

Now you have plenty of time to read A Caregiver's Bible to Excellence!

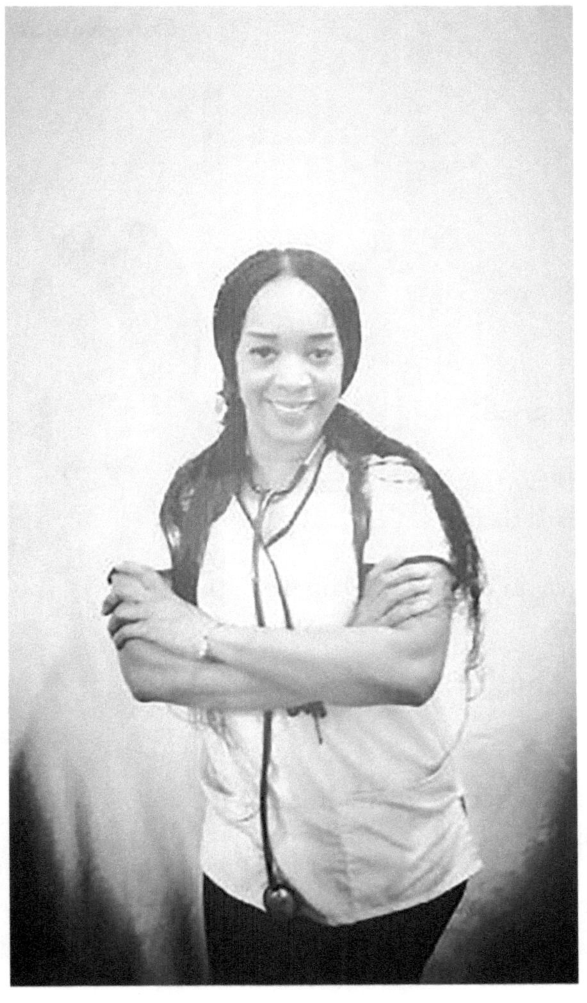

I Will Pray For Your Return!
Everyone Deserves A Second Chance.

Don't Do It! 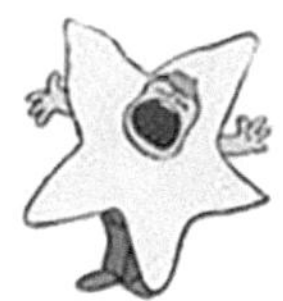

Don't
Open
No
Trap

Doors
Or

Initiate
Trouble for yourself!

- Don't falsify your hours in and out times, that's theft!

- Don't turn in sloppy or damaged timesheets.

- Don't pre–fill out your weekly care plan, ever!

- Don't use markers or nontraditional colors like red or green.

- Don't scribble out or use pencils.

- Don't eat your clients' food or drink their beverages.

- Don't lie, don't cheat, and don't be a thief. **Don't Do It!**

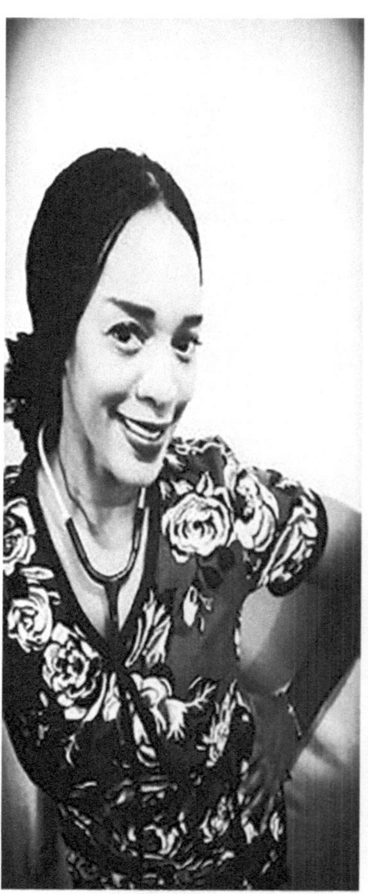

Caregivers Stay, Wise

Don't cheat, steal or tell lies!

Learn from Jesus, come out of the world, be wise!

  Miss Asondra StarN'air

Do's! 

Develop

Optimal

Skills and Service Attributes

Do always sign in and out using client's phone only.
Do write neatly and clearly before submitting to the office.
Do fill out your weekly care-plan notes daily.
Do use only black or blue ink.
Do draw a line through your mistakes; initial and date.
Do bring your own meals and drinks.
Do have integrity, do be honest, and all will go well with you.

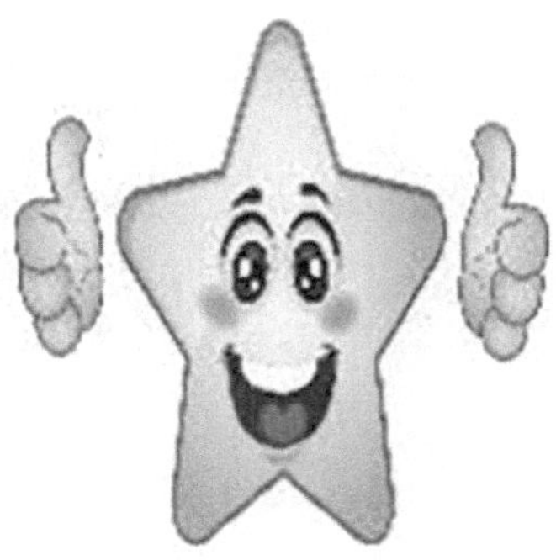

Way to Go!

**Here are some more
Do's For Ya!**

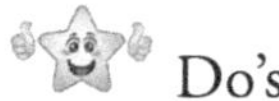 Do's

- Do show up to work on time every day you are scheduled.
- Do take pride in your work and the way you look on the job.
- Do great and noticeable work.

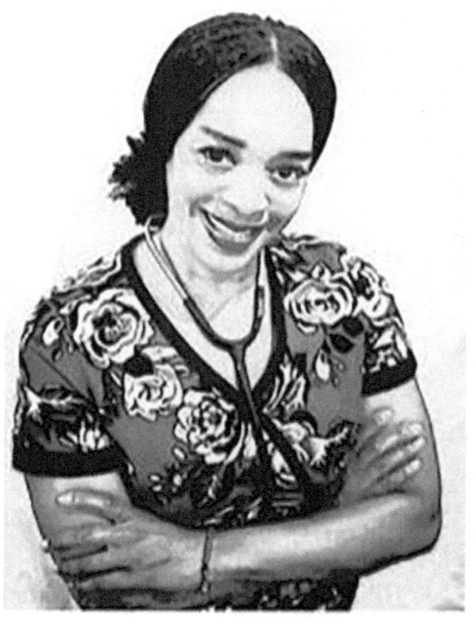

- Do love your enemies, pray for them too.
- Do what Jesus would do, when faced with a problem.
- Do Jesus, not 'YOU'!
- Do be an excellent team player!

- Do pray daily.
- Do call on the name of Jesus, if you are in trouble.
- Do respect authorities and yourself.
- Do get plenty of rest and sleep!
- Do come to work, but leave you problems at home, work it out with Jesus.
- Do A Caregivers Bible To Excellence, written by a caregiver, for caregivers!
- Do bless the Lord at all times, let his praise continually be in your mouth!

    Miss Asondra StarN'air

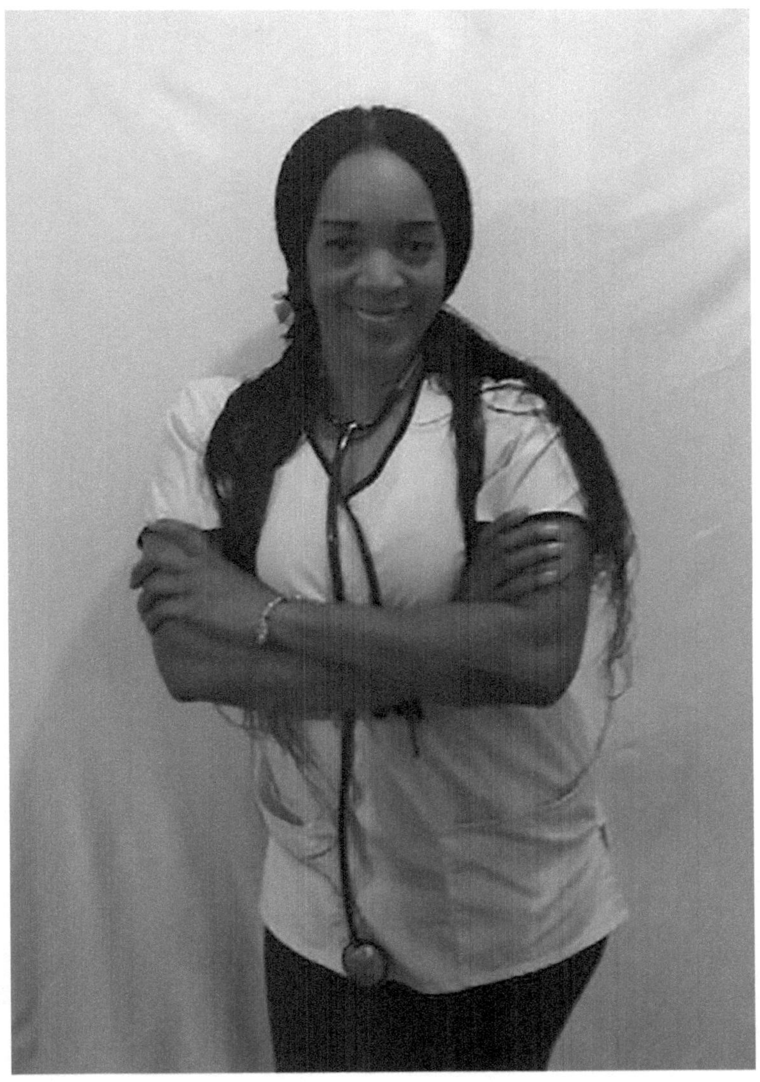

If you don't read and study, you won't become a pro or grow! So, let it flow, 'Learn', 'Grow'!

Stay Excellent, Stay in the Know!

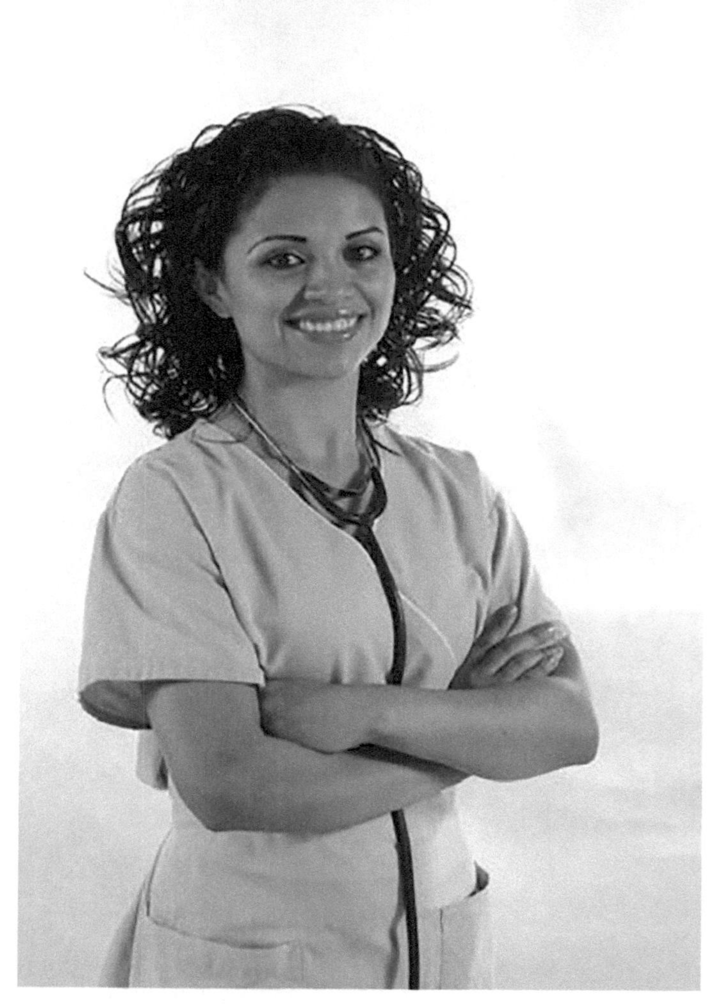

 Miss Asondra StarN'air

SECTION II

Nursing Home/Assistant Living

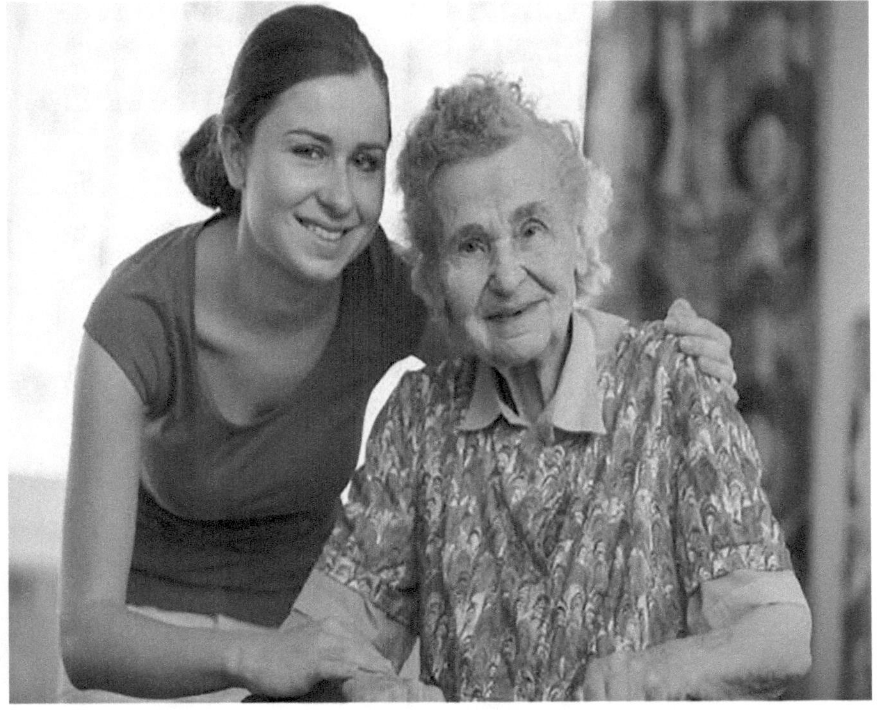

A career that just keeps on giving!

I am proud to say I am a caregiver, how about you?

It's a beautuful thing!

Long Term Care, Be There!

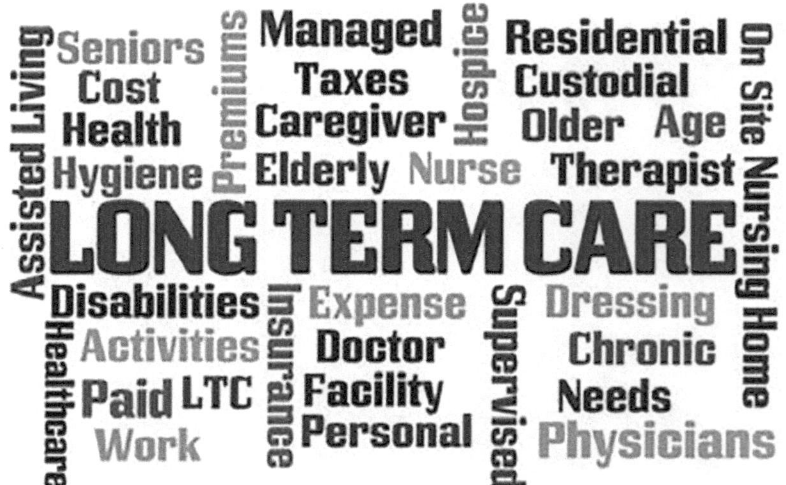

A Home Away From Home!

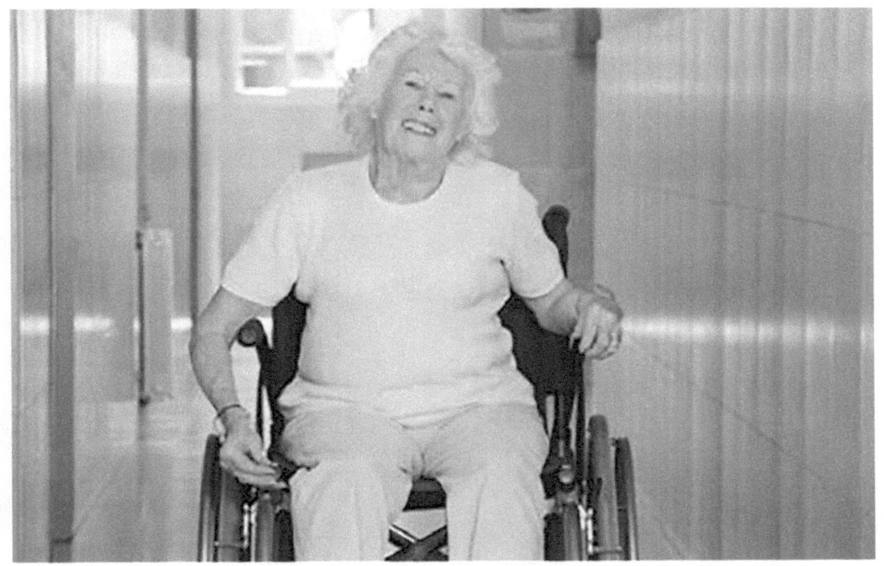

And A Nice Place To Roam!

Assistant Living

Christ 'Caregivers' are Loyal and Giving!

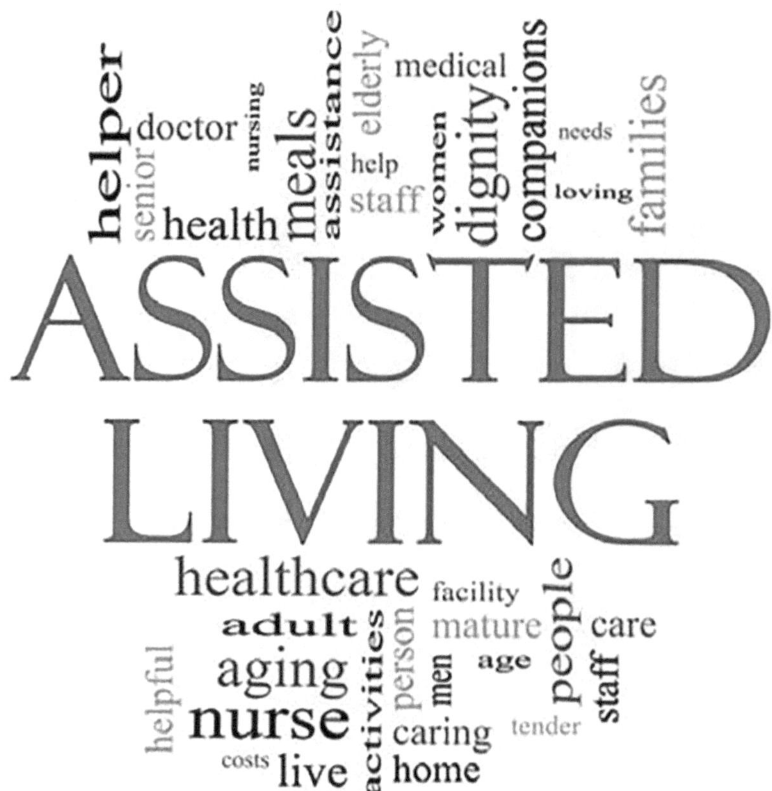

"SMILE"

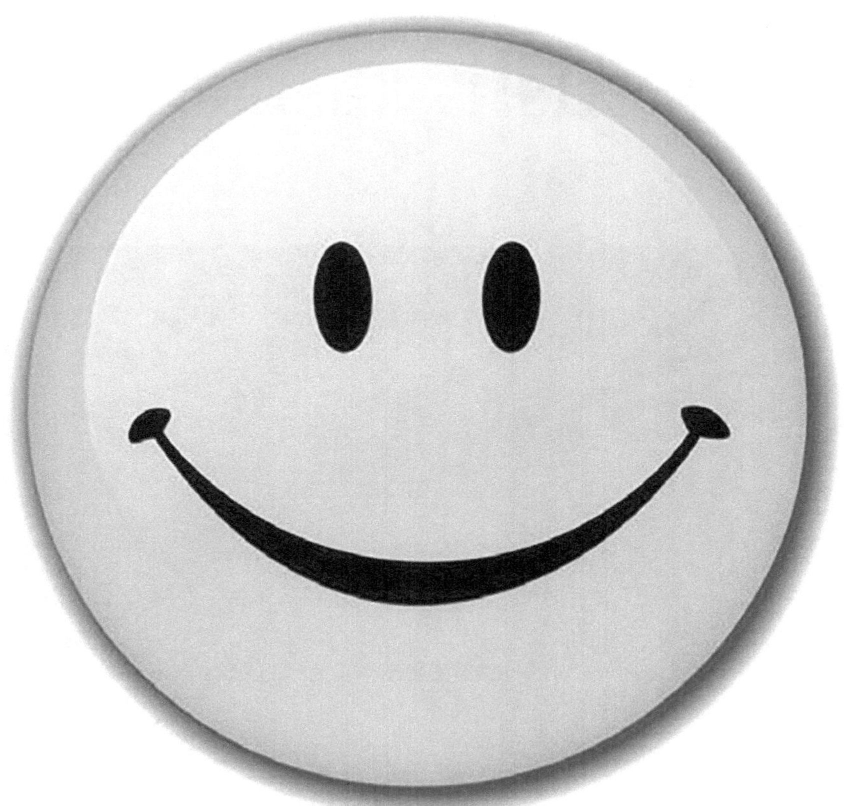

You're on Candid Camera!

Hello Caregivers

This is **Jesus!** I will not need your help today

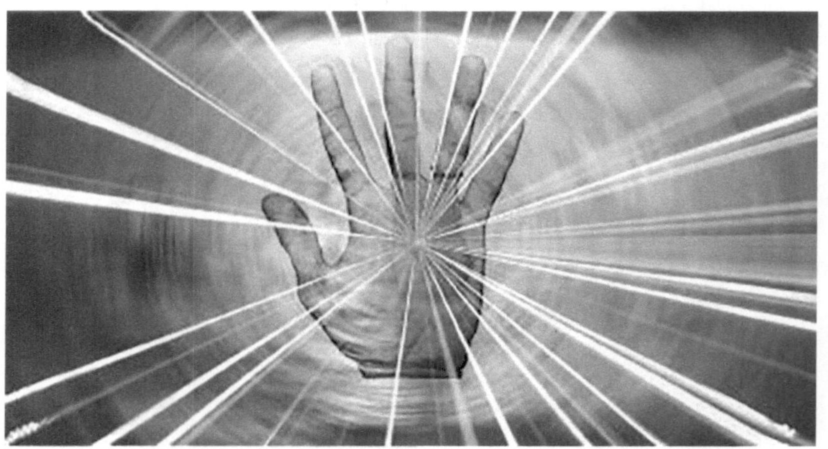

Just step aside and let **Me** lead the way.

The Lord nurses them when they are sick and eases their pain and discomfort. **Psalms 41:3**

Long-Term Care (LTC)

Long-term care is the care you need when you can no longer perform daily task, such as the following:

- Transferring
- Continence/Incontinence Care
- Dressing
- Eating
- Bathing
- Toileting
- Activities of daily living, such as housework, shopping, etc.

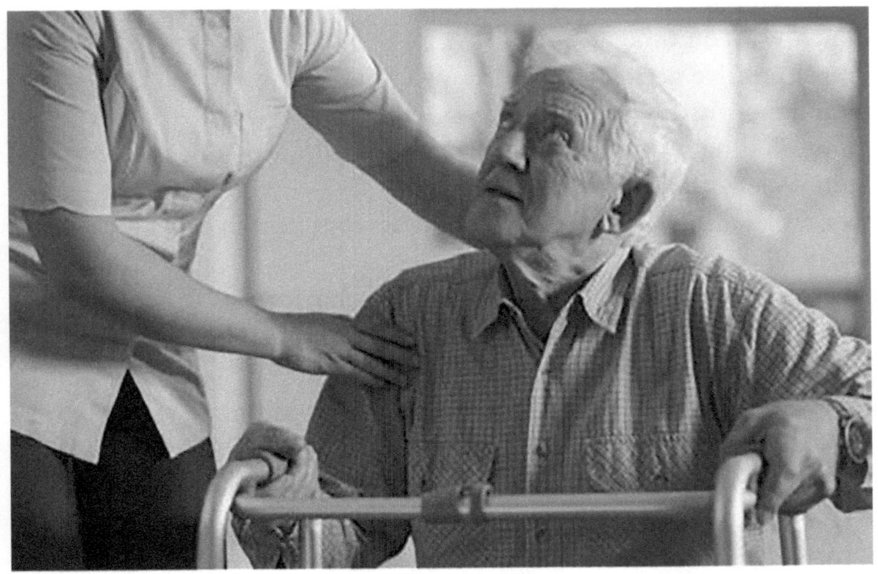

Daily Affirmations for CareGivers

I am a professional caregiver.
I am beautiful in every way.
I am successful; I love being a health-care provider.
I am learning new and useful skills.
I am a competent caregiver.
I am supportive of other caregivers.
I am a team player.
I am taking better care of myself.
I am making smarter food choices.
I am exercising more now.
I am starting to drink more water.
I am saying no to junk food.
I am always on time to work.
I am a positive person.
I am done with negativity.
I am minding my own business from now on.
I am done with gossiping.
I am welcoming change, growth, and development in every area of my life now.
I am a child of God, and it shows in my behavior.
I am happy.
I am full of gratitude.
I am starting to rest more. I realize getting a good night's sleep is very important.
I am changing in a great way. I have lots of love and respect for my bosses and coworkers.
I am finding more time to spend with God and his word now.
I am starting to read the Bible a lot more, and I see the difference in my life. I have more peace of mind. I feel like I can do all things in Christ, who strengthens me. **'I Feel Brand New!'**

 Miss Asondra StarN'air

Twenty-Five Affirmations for Caregivers

1. I am an excellent caregiver.
2. I am a professional.
3. I am smart and intelligent.
4. I am so blessed.
5. I am doing something about stress; I'm getting rid of it.
6. I am patient and kind.
7. I am prosperous.
8. I am faithful to God.
9. I am sorry for my sin. I shall repent and not do it again.
10. I am a child of the Most High.
11. I am developing into what God wants me to be.
12. I am thankful.
13. I am learning something new every day.
14. I am becoming a nicer, and a more loving person.
15. I am a team player.
16. I am staying away from strife from now on.
17. I am changing, getting closer and closer to God.
18. I am starting to read my Bible every day now.
19. I am going the extra mile. Love does not depend on two hearts; it depends on one (mine).
20. I love my *Caregiver's Bible to Excellence* book and I'm telling everyone I know about it.
21. I am a empathetic, understanding, passionate, and honest reliable loving caregiver, I deliver!
22. I am ready to do whatever God calls me to do without murmuring or complaining.
23. I am starting to seek God's will and purpose for my life.
24. I am dying to self so Jesus can come and live inside me.
25. I am giving my life to Christ; I want to follow him now.

Abuse Pledge for Caregivers

- I will not allow those in my care to hit me.
- I will tell them "It's wrong"!
- I will asks the individual to stop.
- I will not provide personal care until abuse stops, this is for my own protection and theirs.
- I will reassure the person that I am going to take excellent care of their needs and help provide a safe environment for both of us but abuse is not allowed.
- I will take the necessary breaks in between to help bring balance to the situation.
- I will ask management for instructions on how to handle the situation when those in my care are abusive.
- If the abuse does not stop, I will no longer care for that particular person. Abuse of any kind is WRONG and must be dealt with specialist by the management team. Caregivers don't come to work to get punched, hit, kicked or spit on.
- My environment has to be a safe place for me to work in at all times.
- I will love and pray for those who hurt other people, but I will not be a victim anymore.

Bottom Line

'Abuse is Abuse' and anyone who does it must be stopped. No one should have to go to work and get abused, especially the caregiver, enough is enough!

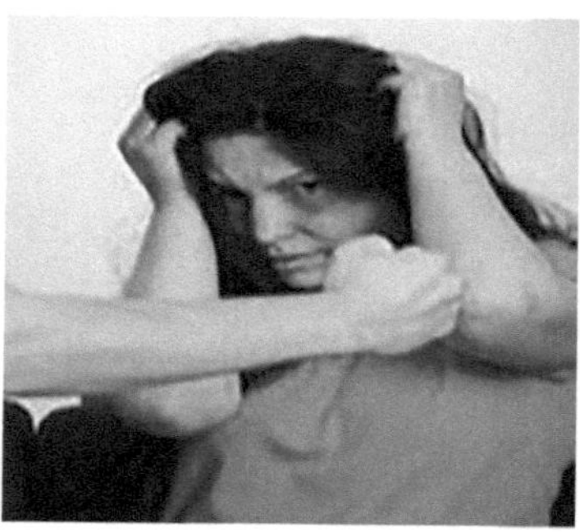

CAREGIVER ABUSE

1. Don't argue with the person.
2. Shift the conversation.
3. Ask, how can I please you?
4. Show me how you want things done.
5. Excuse, yourself if it's safe to do so, take a bathroom break and breathe, ask God to help, go back out and start again.
6. Wait, let them talk, you listen. Be humble.
7. Come up with something creative to do with them.
8. If nothing is working, just do your work, give them space and time to cool down.
9. Don't ever take abuse personal, But
10. **"REPORT IT"**.
11. Ask for help from your company or if you are a family care provider, take a break, use respite care.
12. Document the behaviors times and dates.
13. If the caregiver abuse does not get resolved come off that assign-ment and contact your ombudsman.

"Caregivers Matter"!

Nursing Homes

The nursing home is normally the highest level of care for older adults outside of a hospital. Nursing homes provide what is called custodial care, including getting in and out of bed, **ADLs**, and round-the-clock nursing care. Caregivers must be **STNAs**, State Tested Nurse Assistants to work in this type of facilities.

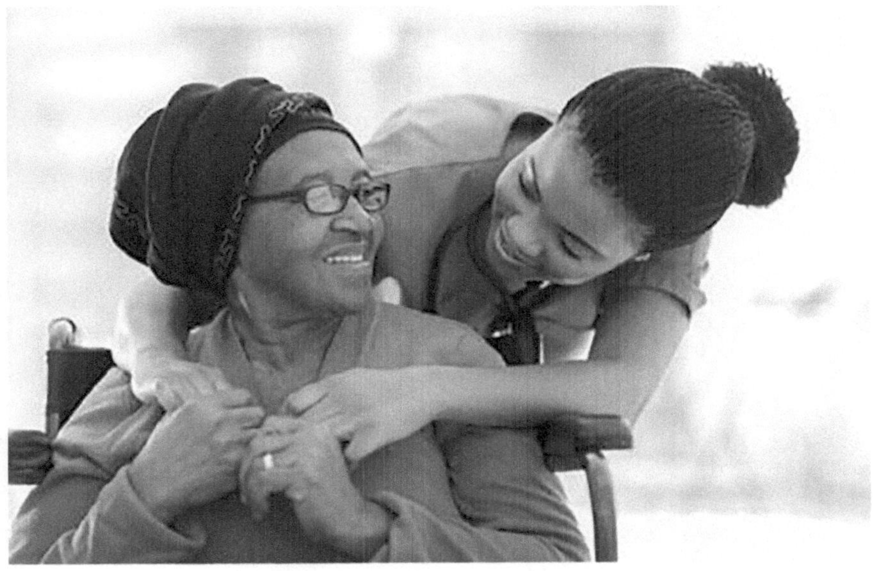

When You Need Us, We're Be There!

Become A Caregiver For Christ!

How is it going so far, remember, we are working for Jesus, not man, let's look to him for excellence!

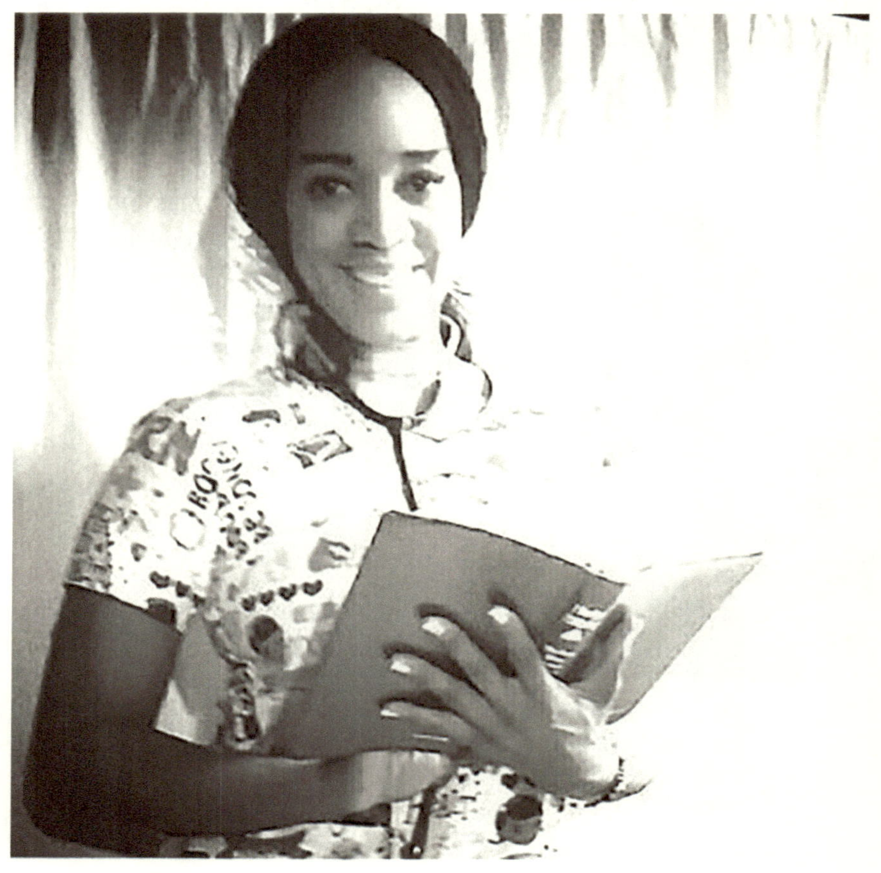

For it is written, Very truly I tell you whoever believes in me will do the works I have been doing and they will do even greater things than these... **John 14:12**

"Stop And Notice"

**Have you noticed any changes today with
the persons you are caring for?**

Seems different than usual
Talks less, than usual, "quite"
Overall, just not with it, some confusion
Puts off doing activities, use to love it

Ate and drank very little or not at all
No interest in anything, food, activities or socializing etc.
Don't seem to have any enthusiasm or energy or care anymore

Note: caregivers, are there any bruises, rashes, bed soars or skin tears
On and off their daily routine, unable to get up or remember things
Tract infection (**UTI**) urine cloudy, dark, bloody, strange smelling etc.
Is weak and disoriented
Calling out for help more often than usual or not calling for help at all
Elimination: off a bit, diarrhea, constipation, not voiding at all

"Tell Your Nurse!"

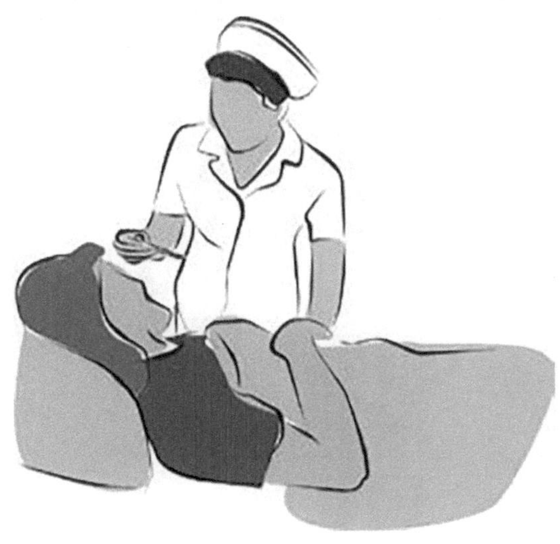

Warning, Warning, Stop!

Don't Go In There By Yourself Rooms.

Caregivers did you know that some facilities have these kinds of rooms, known too as two persons rooms? Well they do, but many won't tell you, until it's too late. In these rooms are individuals who love to falsely accuse and set up unsuspecting workers, caregivers and nurses too, doesn't matter. These individual have nothing to lose so they shake the place up, cause trouble, threaten lawsuits, whatever.

Therefore, you must protect yourself and your license, so here's what you do, ask the facility are there any rooms that are **'Don't Go In There By Yourself Rooms?'** Or you could say, two person rooms, your choice. **'Red Flag'** don't go in there by yourself! You've been warned!

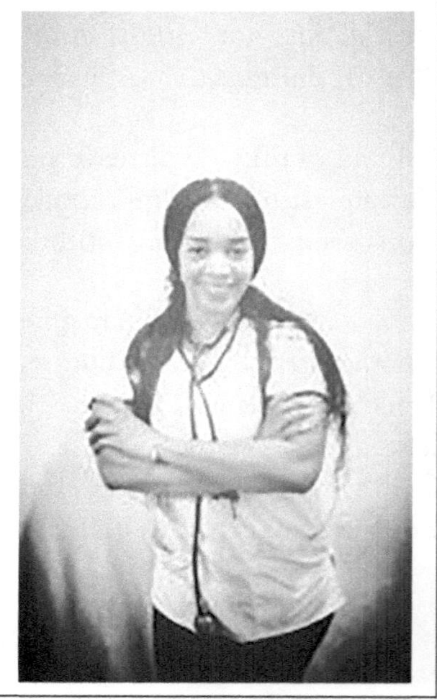

 Miss Asondra StarN'air

Two Person Transfers

Caregivers, two person transfers are just that, two person transfers. I don't care if you can do it by yourself, you are risking everything when you don't follow the care plan. Too many caregiver have lost their license or jobs, because they can do it by themselves. I know some of your co-workers do two person transfer by themselves, especially when short staffed, and nurses let them do it. Nobody says anything, right? Right!

No, of course they don't, until something happens, drop or injure that residence and see what that nurse has to say, the one whose been letting you do it, (while she/he looks away), I'll tell you exactly what they'll say: **Did you read the care plan? It says in your notes and in the charting that they're a two person transfer.** (they've just thrown you under the bus) tip, the care plan is the only thing you can trust! Look, when it comes to professional care don't let co-workers take you there, don't follow them, follow the care plan. Today we have *STNA,'s* in jail because they fail to listen, **"I Can do it by my self"** yeah and you can do time by yourself too!

Now stop, be quiet and listen, in order to ensure the safety of you, and that person don't go chasing waterfalls, because we have some people out there who don't care if you lose it all!

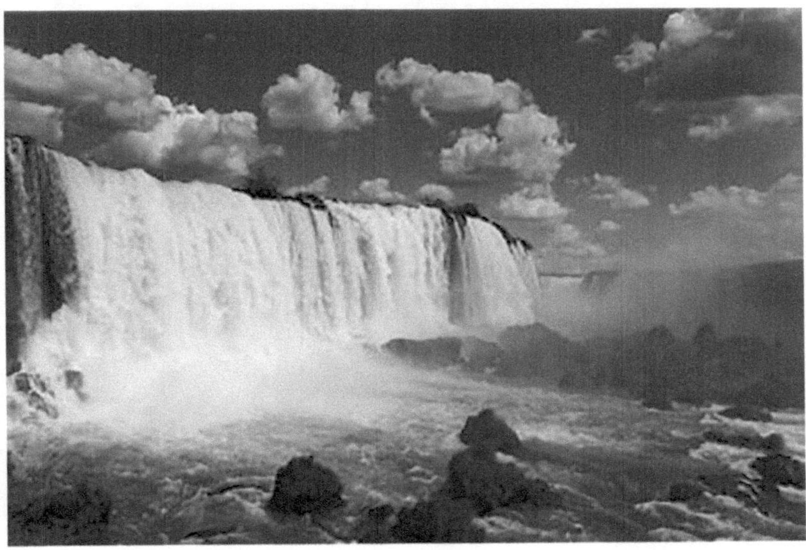

Lifting Devices

Caregivers, if the care plan says use a lift, use a lift! Don't take it upon yourself and transfer that person any other way, unless there's an emergence e.g. "a fire" or you were given written permission with the nurses' signature to do so, protect yourself. **Hoyer lifts require two caregivers at all times.**

Now make sure you are using the correct lifting device. A Hoyer is a Hoyer, and a Sara Lift is not, therefore know your lifting devices because there are a lot of them out there. They seems to be coming up with something new all the time, so stay **In The Know!**

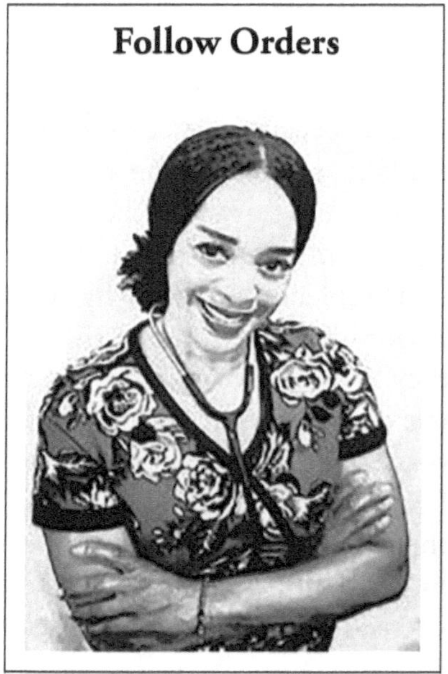

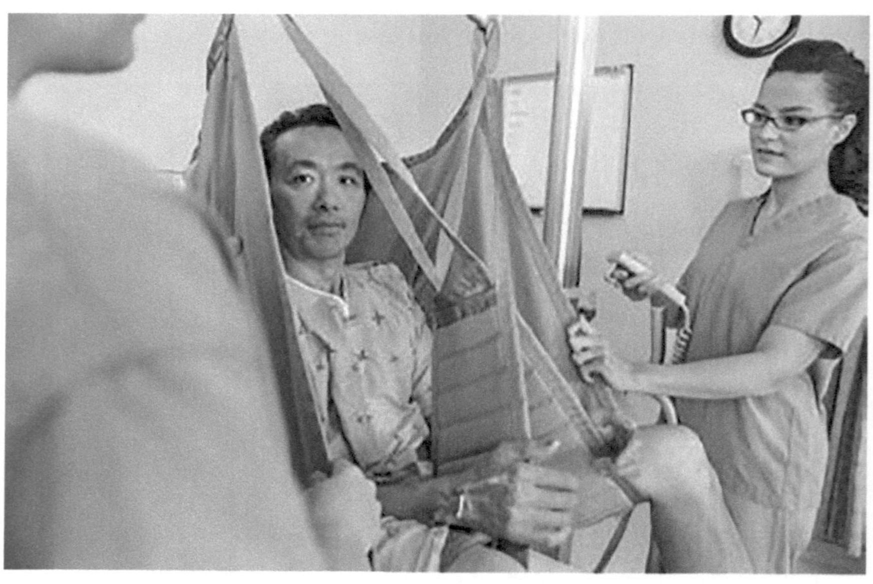

 MISS ASONDRA STARN'AIR

Dementia

Dementia is a general term for loss of memory and other abilities severe enough to interfere with Activities of Daily Living (ADL's) it is caused by physical changes in the brain.

Alzheimer's disease is the most common type of dementia, accounts for 60-80 percent of cases.

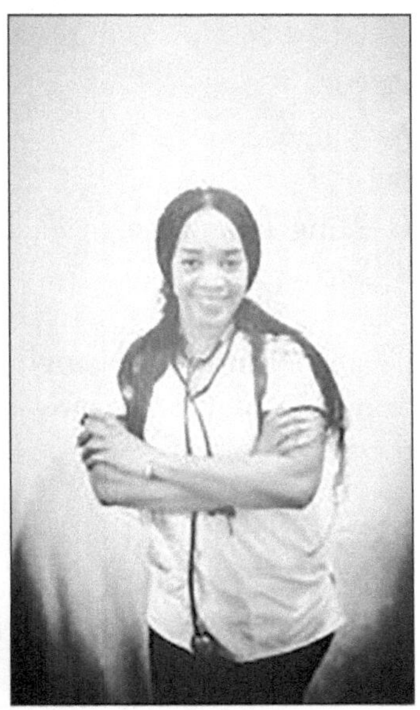

- There are more than 3 million cases per year and growing.
- Dementia can't be cured but treatment may help.
- Dementia is chronic can last for years or be lifelong.
- Also, Dementia requires a medical diagnosis, lab test or imaging often required.

Nevertheless, I think it's very, very important those caring for Dementia/Alzheimer patients be thoroughly trained, in fact, it ought to be 100% mandatory.

Dementia caregiving is a world of its own, normal rules don't apply.

Therefore we need all the training and support we can get. Caregivers **WE** will be the ones to motivate and help keep them safe. Family Caregivers and Professional Caregivers alike, must master working with memory care individuals if you are going to be effective.

We must stay informed, competent, and professional at all times.

Welcome to the world of Caregiving, we are not the caregiver's of our parents' generation. Today we are truly "Healthcare Professionals". Stay Educated!

Acrylic Long Nails

N- Not
A- Allowed
I- In
L- Long-Term Care or Facilities
S- Settings.

Clean hands are the single most important factor in preventing the spread of germs.

Wearing artificial fingernails increases the risk of germs because pathogens now have a place to hide—under the nails.

Professional Caregivers do not wear artificial nails and keep their real nails trimmed low.

Good Nail Hygiene!

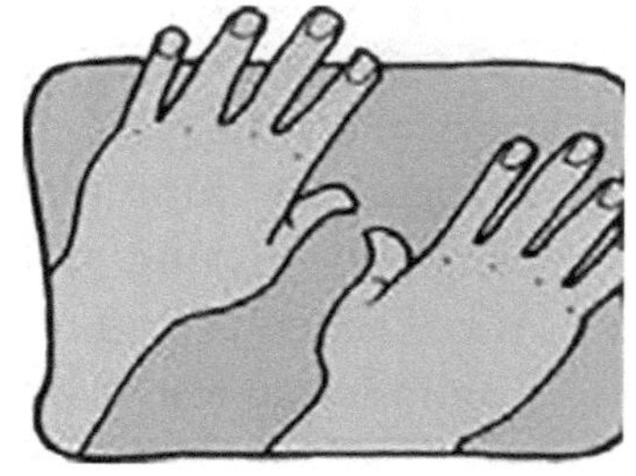

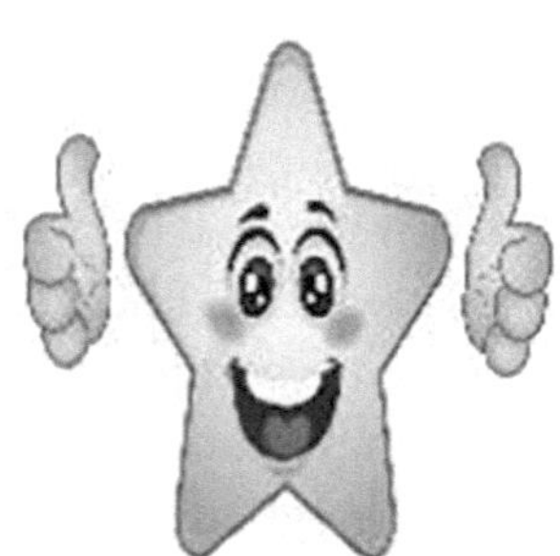

Way To Go!

Standard Precaution

Standard precautions are for everyone. It's not just for health-care workers. It's good practice for children and adults. Everyone around the world should be washing their hands several times a day. Practicing good hand hygiene is very important. It helps reduce the spread of germs that can cause us to get sick; and the sooner we start, the better.

Clean hands save lives—yours and mine!

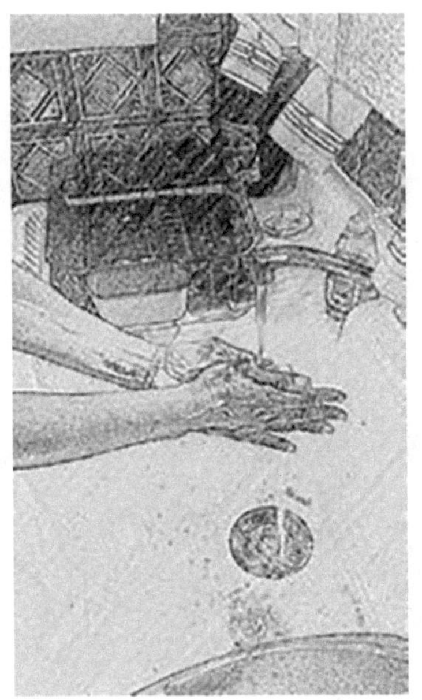

Wash those germs right out of your hands and send them on their way.

When to Wash Your Hands:

1. After arriving and leaving.
2. After sneezing or coughing.
3. Before making or eating food.
4. After playing with animals.
5. Before and after toileting.
6. After being outdoors, gardening, etc.
7. Before changing contact lenses.
8. Before and after patient care.
9. After shopping.
10. During and after social and entertainment events.
11. After intimacy.
12. Before and after personal grooming.
13. Before and after using office and computer/machinery.
14. Before and after child care.
15. After public exposure to elevator buttons and doors knobs.
16. Wash your hands several times throughout the day! And anytime there's gathering or public interaction. "Wash Your Hands!"
17. Hey, don't forget about your smart phones too! "Wipe Clean".
18. Wash hands after all meals.
19. Wash hands after physical contact.
20. Wash your hands when you forgot to wash your hands.

Wash Your Hands Everyday!

S.O.A.P

Serve Those in Need

Obey God's Word

Apply What You Read

Pray for Understanding

Once we do all that, "Our Hands" will really be clean!

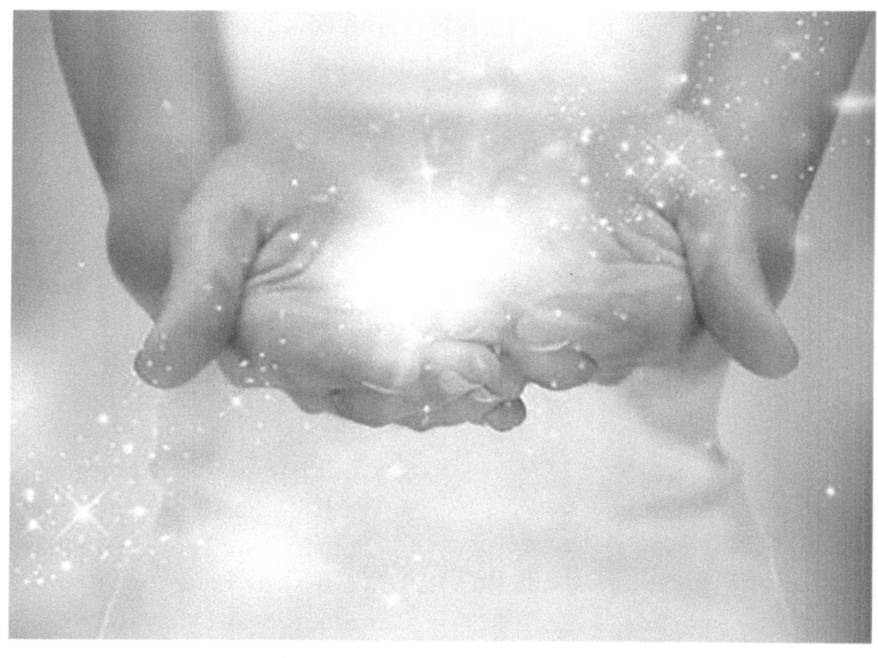

In Jesus name, Amen!

 Miss Asondra StarN'air

Don't Go There!
Conversations Caregivers Should Avoid

1. **Your Personal Beliefs.** It can result in backlash if the other person doesn't agree.
2. **Private Information**—it can make things awkward moving forward for both you and the other person.
3. **Gossip of any kind.** Close your mouth!
4. **Discussing subjects like religion and politics is taboo.** Don't go there, period.
5. **Controversial Dialogue** can get ugly, don't go there either.
6. **Avoid "Office Grapevine"** with you as the primary focus. Shift the conversation quickly. "Oh, look at the time, I need to finish up my paperwork" would be a great exit.
7. **Avoid Disagreements;** call the office if you need profes-sional advice.
8. **'The Tongue'** talk less, listen more, do your chores!
9. **Avoid getting in lengthy conversations, period.** Aren't you supposed to be working? Hello!
10. **Leave your opinions out, you're asking for it!** Instead focus on caregiving and excellence!
11. **Avoid asking for food, drinks, etc.** Where is your lunch box? Bring it!
12. **Practice 'Professionalism'** don't give out your number.

Tame The Tongue!

Don't Let it Trap You!

Caregivers On The Run
It's Not My Job!

This is a story about four Caregivers on a Team, named **Everybody, Somebody, Anybody** and **Nobody**. There was an important Job to be done and **Everybody** was sure that **Somebody** would do it.

Anybody could have done it, including **RN's** and **LPN's** but **Nobody** did it. **Somebody** got angry, wasn't me, I wasn't there, I heard about it. They got angry because they felt, it was beneath them, it was not their job, (sounds like a snob) They said, "oh no", "Really"! "I don't think so", "it's not my Job! Oh yes it is says the **LORD!** He's involved now! **Anybody** could have done it! But this particular person, just sat there, drinking red

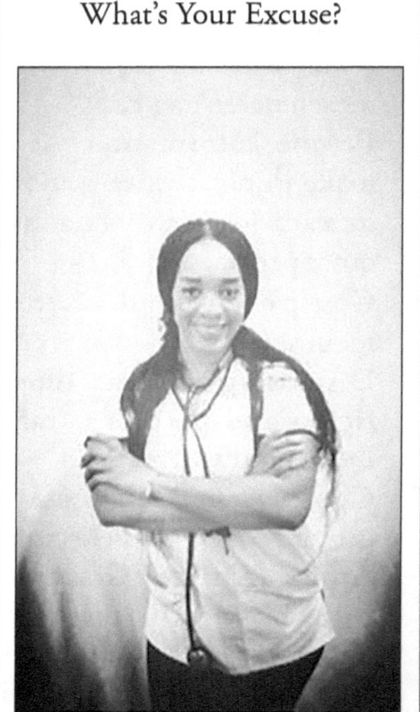

bull to stay awake, "please"! What ah headache, and they take too many breaks! "Wait" I know some of you out there are laughing, because you know I'm telling the truth, but I don't find it funny. We need individuals who come to work to make a difference and are ready to help in time of need. Maybe we ought to ask ourselves are we really there to work or is it greed? Please read: If you are in the health care field and work closely with seniors then STNA's, LPN's and RN's alike must began work together to get the job done! Those residence are all of our responsibility.

Nevertheless, **Everybody** thought **Anybody** could do it, but **Nobody** realized that **Everybody** wouldn't do it, Nope, **Everybody** was chilling.

Check this out, it ended up that **Everybody** blamed **Somebody** when **Nobody** did what **Anybody** could have done. So God got a call, and was told, (by the way, it wasn't me) that the crew, all of you, neglected the residence. So now, **Everybody, Somebody, Nobody** "Hello" **Anybody** all of yawl got some explaining to do? I would have done it but like I said, I wasn't there. Question, were **YOU?**

We're listening, what's your excuse?
"Team Work Makes The Dream Work"!

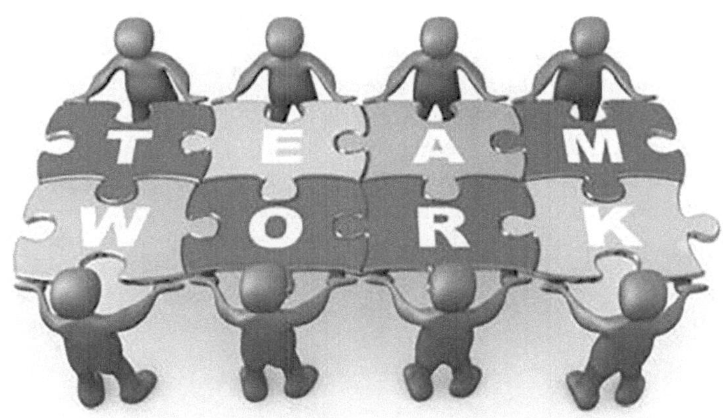

Being there for others should never
make you mad, or hurt!

Answer Your Call Lights!

Nothing is worse than working on a floor with caregivers who don't answer their call lights until they get good and ready. If you are not servicing another resident, stop what you are doing and **"Answer Your Call Lights!"**

Caregivers, let's get our priorities straight, shall we. Understand this, the residence **MUST** be our first priority, not chat-ting with co –workers or charting, that can all wait; Jesus is calling! That's my mind-set when I hit the unit or floor. It is written in the bible in two places I know for sure, first in **Ephesians 6:7**, which says "Serve wholeheartedly, as if you were serving the Lord." Next in **Colossians 3:23–24**, and it says, "Whatever you do, work at it with all your heart, as working for the Lord, not for a human master, since you know that you will receive an inheritance from the Lord as a reward. It is the Lord Christ you are serving."

I never forgot that, and I never will. So when my call lights goes off, I stop what I'm doing and go care for Christ! Bottom line, we are with these residence a lot so much so that we have become their extended family so let's not neglect them or let them down. And here's a big "GIANT" problem, **"Cell Phones"** stop talking and texting on your not so smart phones **"THAT CAN WAIT"**, Jesus is calling.. go... **"Answer Your Call Lights!"**

What to be Excellent?
"Answer Your Call Lights!"

12 Tips on Excellence

1. "SMILE" leave your problems at home.
2. Do a walk-through, make sure everyone is OK.
3. Introduce and greet each resident.
4. Stock materials needed for your shift and the next shift.
5. Smile, speak and say hi to your co-workers.
6. Upon your arrival, ask for report, upon leaving, give report!
7. Extend a helping hand to other co-workers. Always be willing to work as a team. Remember the dream, "Excellence" in Jesus name! Amen
8. Keep washing your hands in between patient to patient care and wear and change gloves constantly.
9. Check back in on your residence throughout your shift.
10. Try to come up with something creative to do or say to each one of those in your care that will make them happy—smile! Love on them, show them, that you care and glad to be there.
11. Keep a sunflower smile on your face and help brighten up the place!
12. Finally, thank God for allowing you to be his servant!

If you are going for excellence, get ready, set, grow!
Learn to do things more "Professionally!"

Jesus Is The Light!

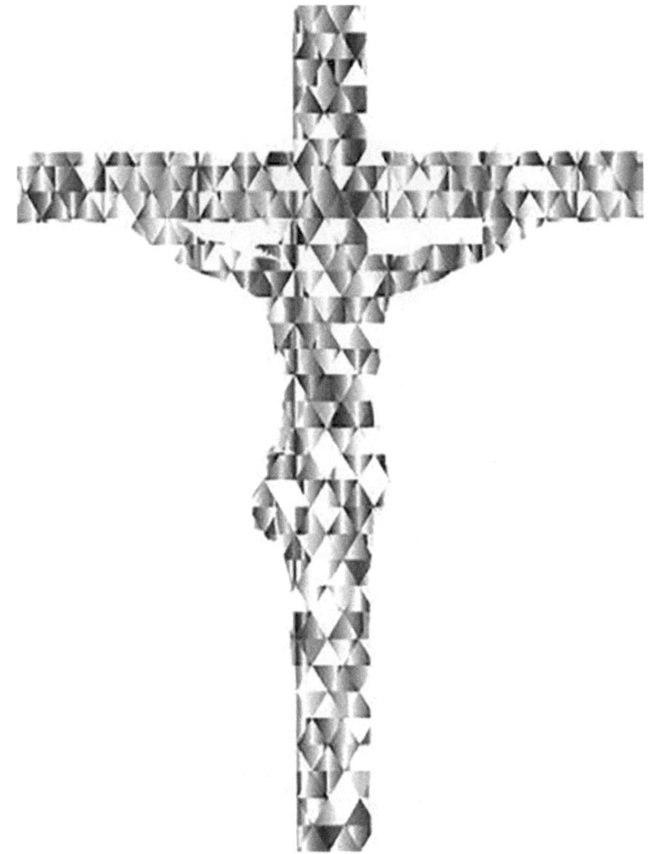

Through Believers, He "Shines Bright!"

Miss Asondra StarN'air

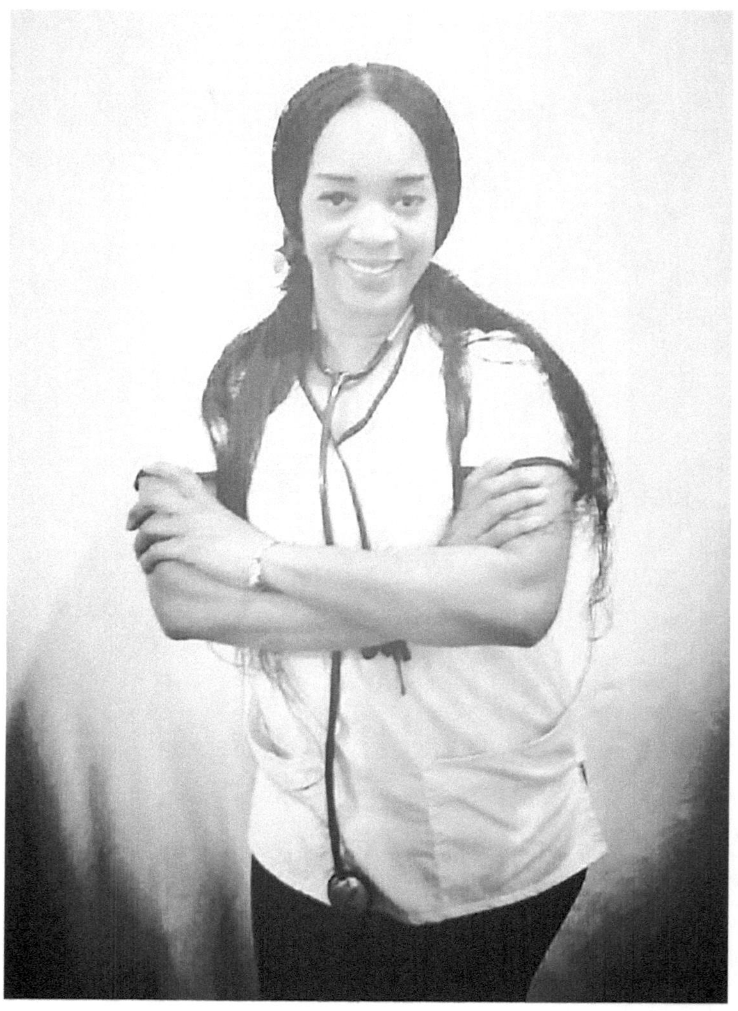

If You Are Going To Do It, Do It Right!

Stay In The Know!

Signs and Symptoms to Report.

Evaluate the situation, is it safe? Do I call 911 or can I handle it within my scope?

Educate, tell the individual /family why you are doing what you are doing.

Keep records, make sure they are neat, accurate, concise and complete. Documentation is a must!

Help the person relax.

Eye and ears open, "Caregivers" watch out for changes in breathing, sounds of destress or pain.

Lay down slowly or sit up whichever is preferred and most comfortable to the person.

Position them comfortably and keep them warm, do not allow a chill to occur.

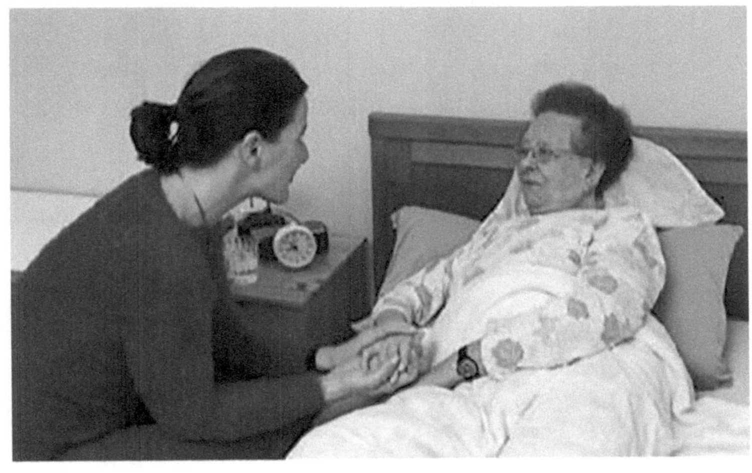

A Caregiver's Bible To Excellence!

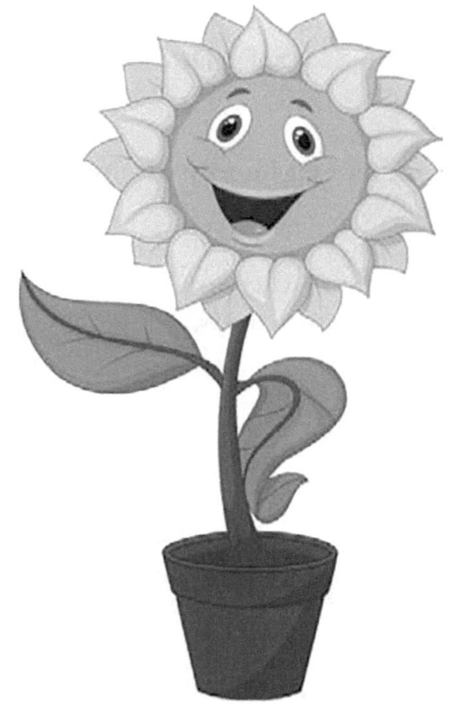

Where is that "Sunflower Smile"?

Don't bring your problems to work, leave them at home, ask God to help you work it all out, and he will. But make sure you are not the real problem, pehaps *He's* teaching you a lesson, I'm just sayin'!

Get your house in order, and keep your house in order! Righteous living is the key, to a big bright future and ah **"SMILE"**!

As for me and my house we shall serve the **LORD!**
Join Us, "Get On Board"!

Hello Caregivers!
Put On A Happy Face!

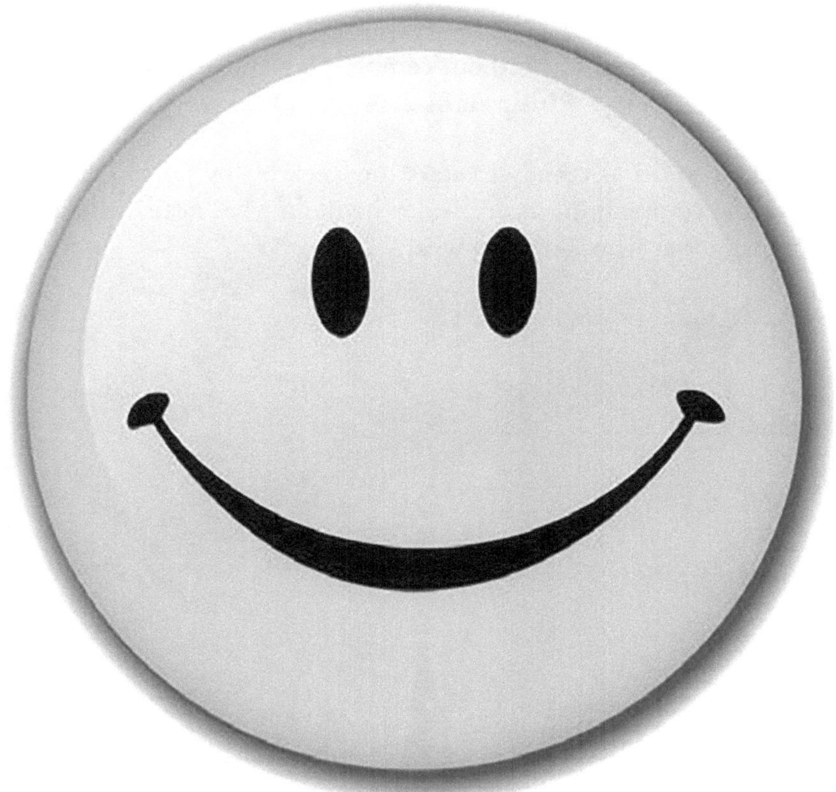

It's Time To Serve and Shine
and You Must Be On Time!

Are you ready, let's go......

7 Days a Week: Be Loving, Kind and Sweet!

Monday

Do everything without complaining and arguing
Philippians 2:14 (NIV)

It's Monday and I am ready to start the week off by putting all murmuring and complaining aside. Today I will do what needs to be done, not caring about who didn't do what.

Yes it's Monday and today I will:

Maintain

Optimism

No complaining.

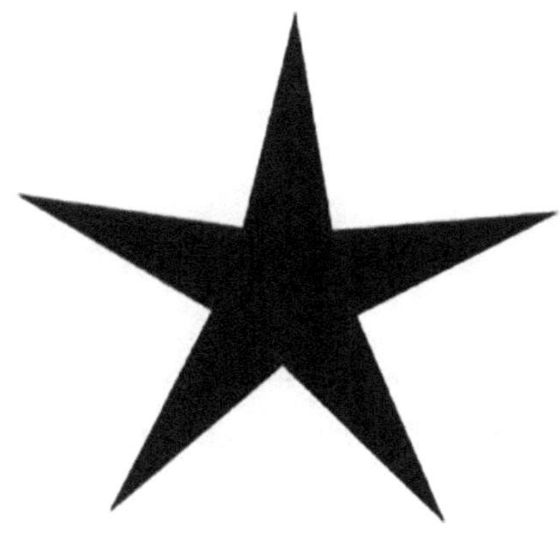

Day of Peace!

A Great Attitude Is Everything!

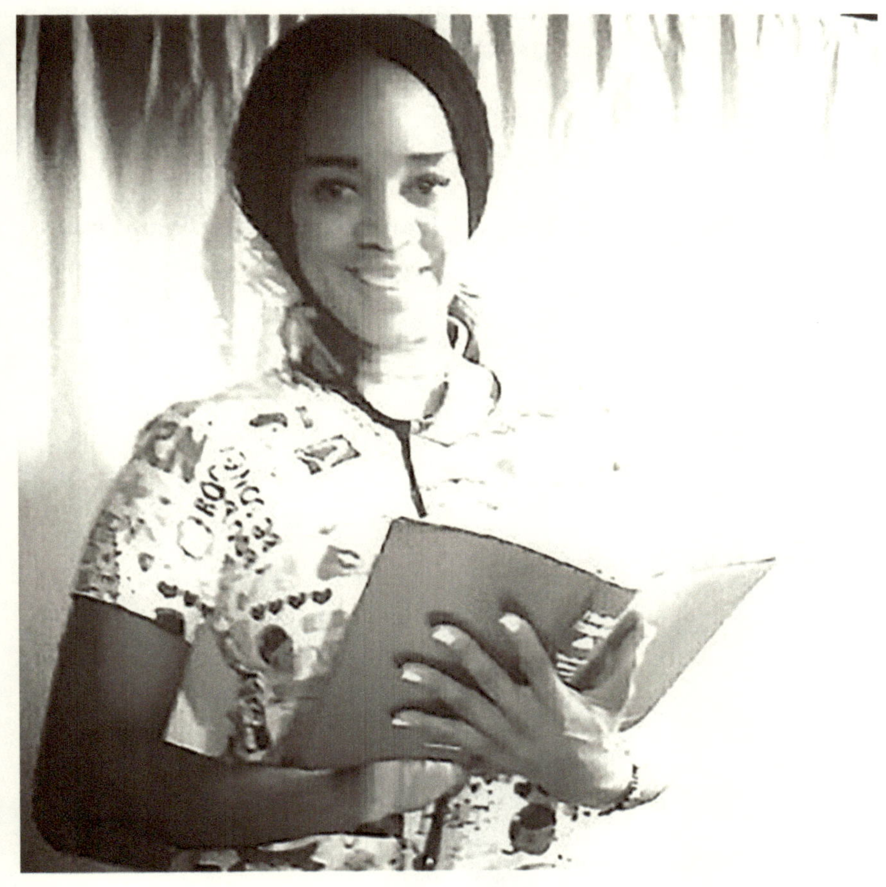

Especially When You Are Serving *"The King"*

Tuesday

And we know that in all things work together for the good to them that love God, to them that are called according to his purpose.
—Romans 8:28 (KJV)

Today I will accept the things I can't change. I will do whatever is necessary to make the day go smooth for everyone.

Whatever I'm called to do, I will do it. Because I realize teamwork gets the job done faster and makes everybody's job a lot easier.

"Two (or More) Heads/Helping Hands Are Better Than One!"

To

Unite in

Every

Situation and help out!

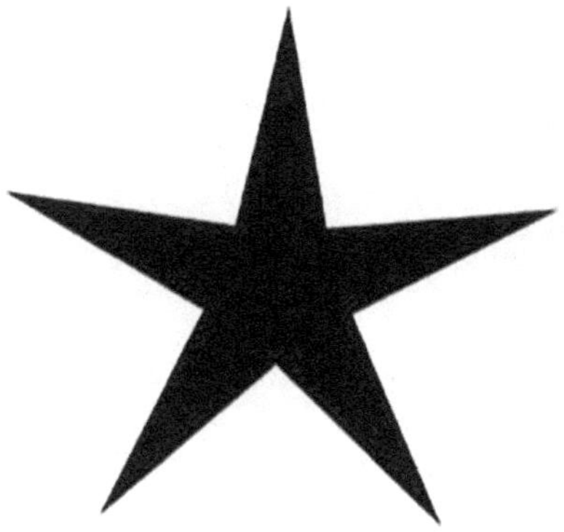

Day of Togetherness!

Unity, that's what I'm talking about!
You and me, working as a team!

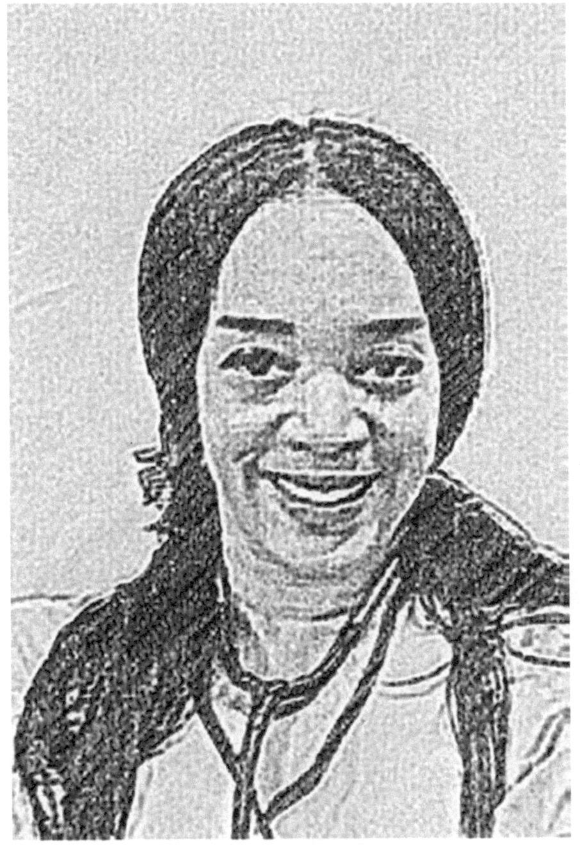

Don't make things hard, help out, don't be cruel
or mean, work like a winning team!

Wednesday

This is the day the Lord has made. We will rejoice and be glad in it.
—Psalm 118:24 (NLT)

The world calls Wednesday "Hump Day"—we shall call it a day of peace, love, and joy.

We've made it halfway through the week! But we're not done yet. Today we will celebrate caregiving and how wonderful it is to be a professional caregiver. Today we will do or bring something to one of our co-workers to show fellowship and appreciation for one another.

**We will love one another like sisters and
brothers today and always.**

We

Enjoy

Diversity; we celebrate our differences by coming together in love.

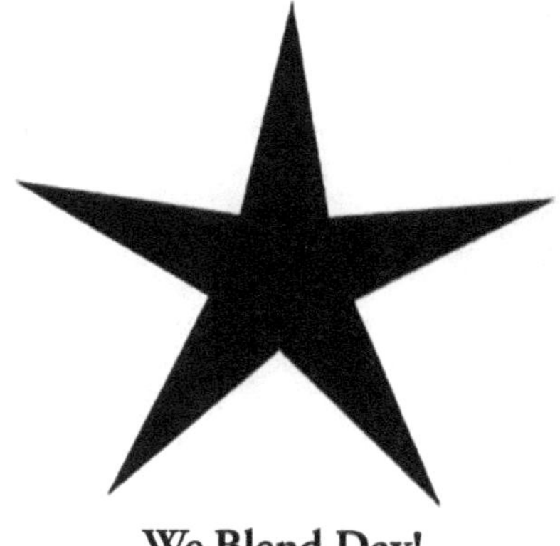

We Blend Day!

Diversity, "Works For Me!"

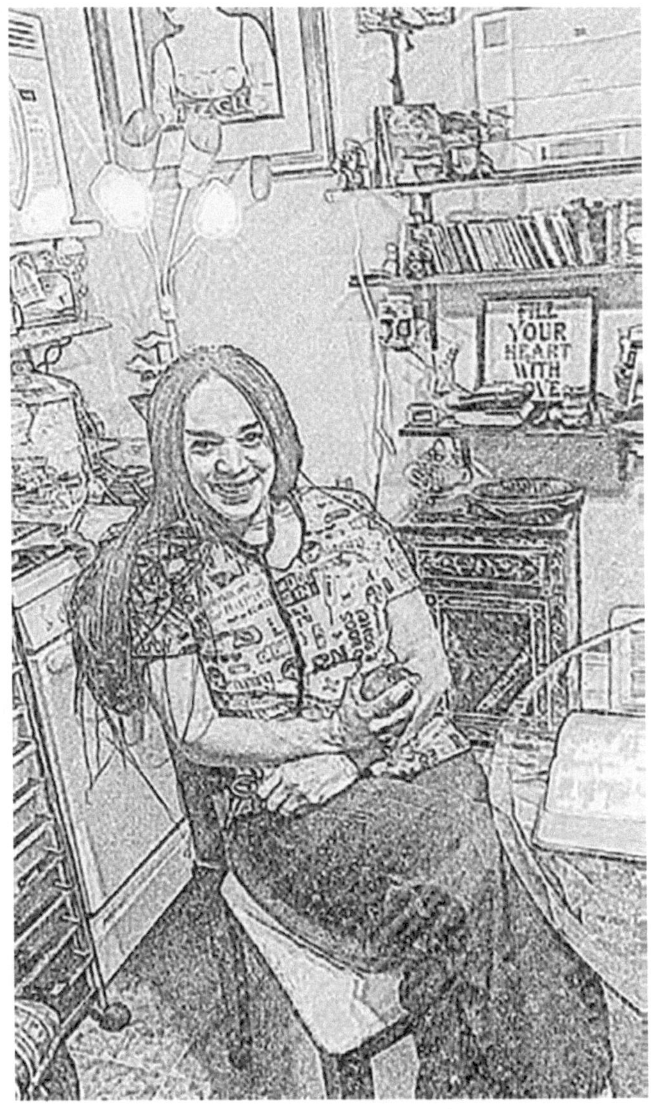

Welcome, and remember "Love" is the Key!

Thursday

Repent ye therefore, and be converted, that your sins may be wiped away in order that times of refreshing shall come from the presence of the Lord.
—Acts 3:19 (KJV)

Today is almost Friday! But it's Thursday, and we need to make sure our house is in order today. Get your mind, body, and soul together.

Think only positive thoughts, and love and forgive one another.

Catch up on some **'Bible Study'** today, it's going to develop you in ways you never imagined. Also too, today is a good day to make that change, especially before the weekend arrives. Wear your full armor! Be prepared, "Satan thrives" so be smart,don't drink and drive!

Trust in the Lord, and be wise!

Hold thyself accountable.

Uplift His Holy Name!

Refuse to give into temptation.

Salvation is for anyone who wants to be saved from this dark and evil world, be it woman, man, boy or girl. "Come out of the world!"

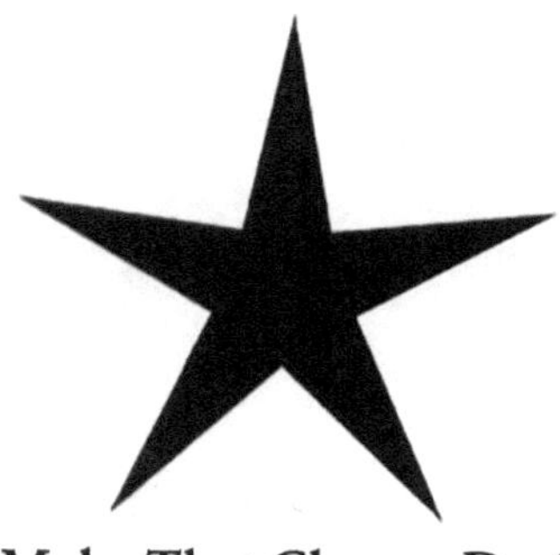

Make That Change Day!

   Miss Asondra StarN'air

"I'm Glad I'm Saved!"

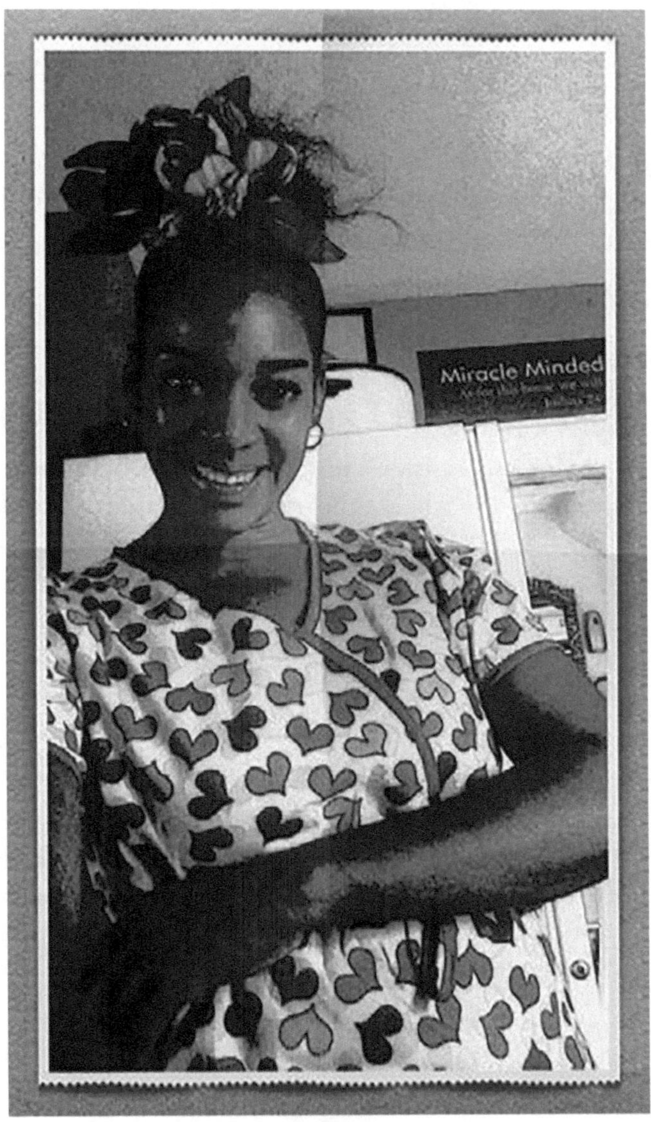

God has changed my life in so many wonderful
ways, again glad I'm saved!

Friday

For many, 'Friday' is payday! But for us **'Trusting True Christians',** it's a day of gratitude, thankfulness, and loyalty to God. For it is God who allows us to work, prosper, and receive those blessings.

The world says **TGIF: "Thank God It's Friday."**

But those who follow 'Christ', we say,

TGIFF: "Thank God I'm Fruitful and Faithful!"

Today if it's payday, we set aside a tenth, to give to God what belongs to him. God said, bring the whole tithe into the storehouse that there may be food. We are fruitful, and we are a faithful people. **TGIFF!**

First Fruits

Received

Instantly goes to **GOD, A tenth to God is** all He's asking for, that act alone on your part is worth more than you could ever imagine, just do it! **Mal.3:10** Bring the whole tithe into the store house, that there may be food in my house. Test me in this "says the **LORD Almighty."** and see if I will not throw open the floodgate of heaven and pour out so much blessing that there is no room to store it.

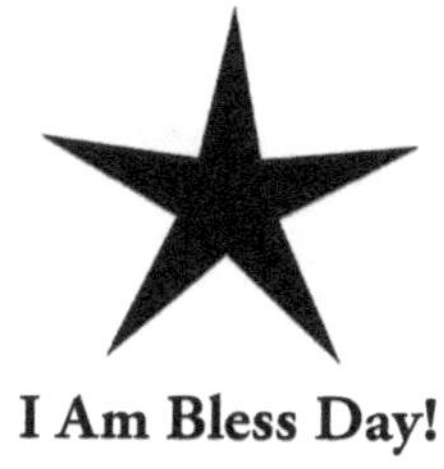

I Am Bless Day!

Be A Giver, Fill Your Heart With Love!

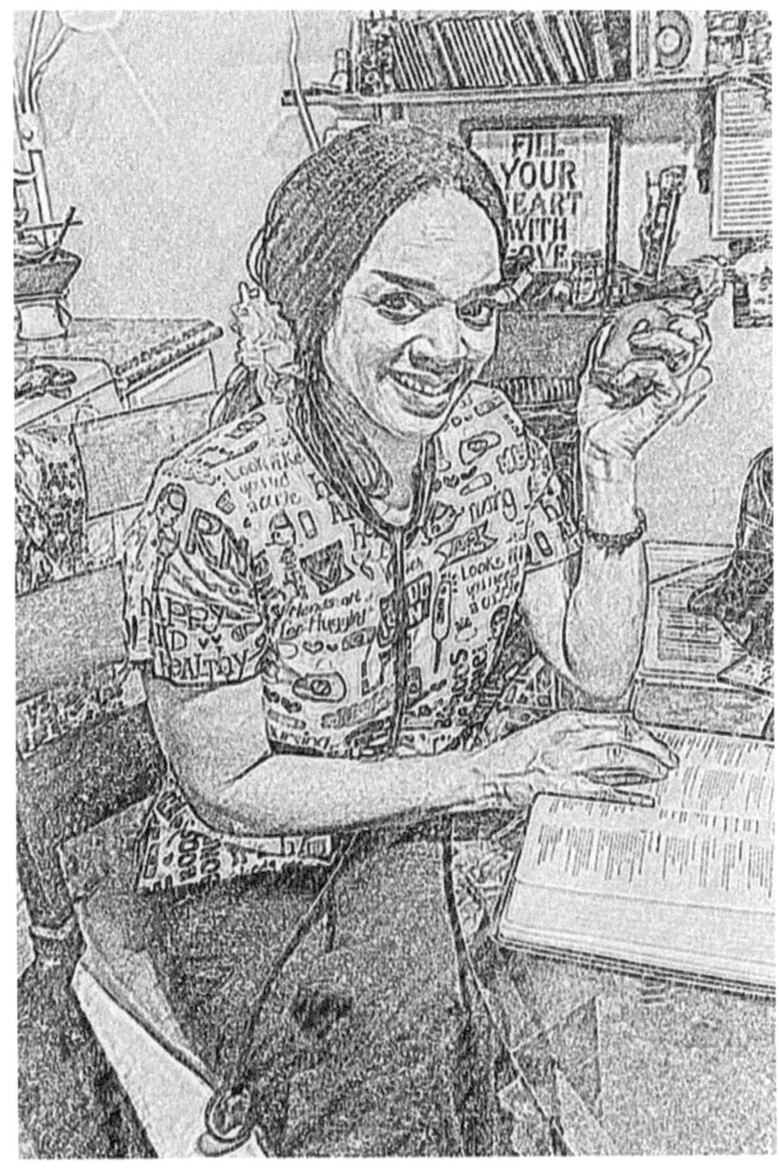

Saturday

Make a joyful noise unto the Lord, all ye lands. Serve the Lord with gladness: come before his presence with singing. **Psalms 100**

It's Saturday, hope you can sleep in—if not, treat yourself to something good.

Be silly today, have fun! Spend time with someone you love. If you're working, get creative. Think of something new to do.

Sing Something It's Saturday!

Sing like no one is listening

Activities

Today is your day to have fun, I know exactly what I'm going to do, I'm going karaoking tonight, that's right!

O 'this little light of mine, I'm going to let it shine, this little light of mine I'm going to let it shine, let it shine, let it shine, let it shine... "Hey, D J, Mellie Mel," give me the Mic, it's my turn!

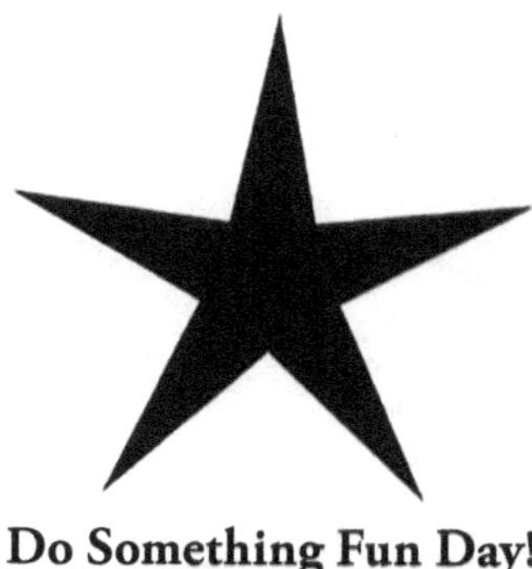

Do Something Fun Day!
At Work or At Play!

All Work and No Play, Makes You Gray!

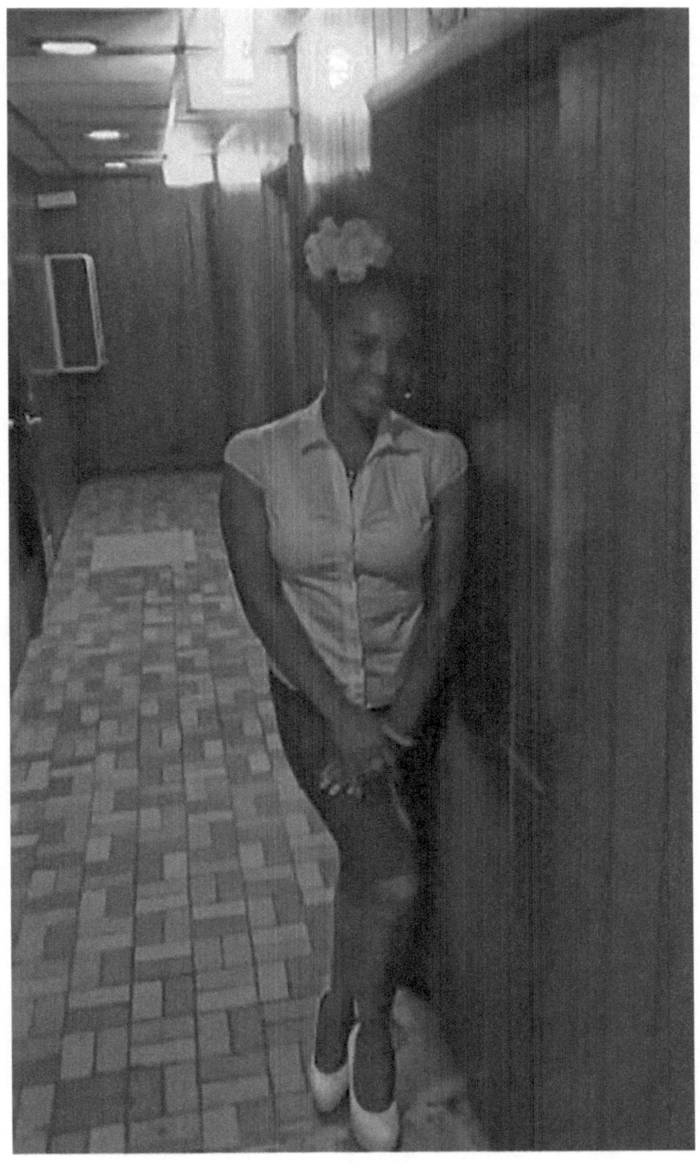

Coming To The Mic....

Sunday

Remember the Sabbath day, to keep it holy,
six days you shall labor, and do all your work,
but on the seventh day is the Sabbath of the Lord your God.
Exodus 20:8-10

For those in the health-care industry, caregivers often have to work on Sundays; but working seven days a week is forbidden, no matter what. Please use one of your days off and make it holy unto God. No work. Rest, spend quality time with God, and develop a personal relationship with him.

Spend

Uninterrupted

Nourished quality time with God and his word, Taste and see that the Lord is Good!

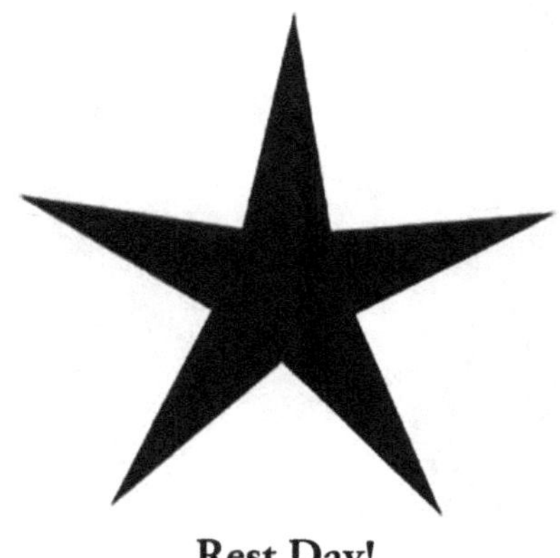

Rest Day!

 Miss Asondra StarN'air

The Importance of Sleep

It is in vain that you rise up early and go late to rest, eating the bread of anxious toil; for he gives the beloved sleep. **Psalms 127:2**

Caregivers, I know working overtime allows you to catch up on some of your financial responsibilities or provides a way to enjoy the finer things in life—nothing wrong with that.

Here's the problem, you can't stop working overtime all you do is work! **What about Jesus?**

When are you going to spend time with him?

When are you going to rest and get a good night's sleep?

Lack of sleep or skimping on sleep can wreak havoc from head to toe; many of you do not get the recommended eight or more hours of shut-eye a night. And pretty soon, it's going to catch up with you; you are risking your health and don't even know it. There are nightmare-inducing truths on what can happen to a person who lack, rest or sleep.

One article I read recently put it like this:

"Lose Sleep, Lose Your Mind and Health."

I absolutely think there's something to all of this, and that caregivers really need to be careful when it comes to working so much overtime. Seriously, take a minute and really think about it. Is it really worth it in the end? No it is not, I say, because you are risking way too much, your health, future plans, dreams and such, look, too much is, too much!

Furthermore, this may also help explain all the workplace rivalries among co-workers and poor care of our residence. Listen up, **"Sleep matters!"**

Energy drinks such as Red Bull and other brands are not the natural order of things. People we need sleep. God created us to rest and sleep for a reason. So we can perform well, think well and do well. What I am trying to say to some of you over-timers out there, is this, others suffer when we don't respect a goodnight of sleep.

Lack of sleep as I have witnessed, contributes to a lot of ugly and negative behaviors for example, Sleep deprived individuals can become short-tempered, moody, and irritated easily making it almost impossible to work with them. Too, they lack teamwork, they're too tire to help out. In facilities these overworked and sleep deprived individuals will sometimes hide off in empty rooms, away from every-body, they don't want to be bothered. This is happening everywhere, and it's sad. Everybody suffers the whole entire team and especially the one that needs the care. Because when a person don't get enough sleep physically and mentally they're not all there, and nor is **'Quality Care'.** Lets be fair! People deserve professional care. And our co -workers expect us to do our share. Hello is anybody there? Now lets listen to what our creator says about sleep: *it is vain that you rise up early and go late to rest, eating the bread of anxious toil, for he gives his beloved sleep.* **Psalms 127:2**

Somebody, gimme the Mic, time for the remix: 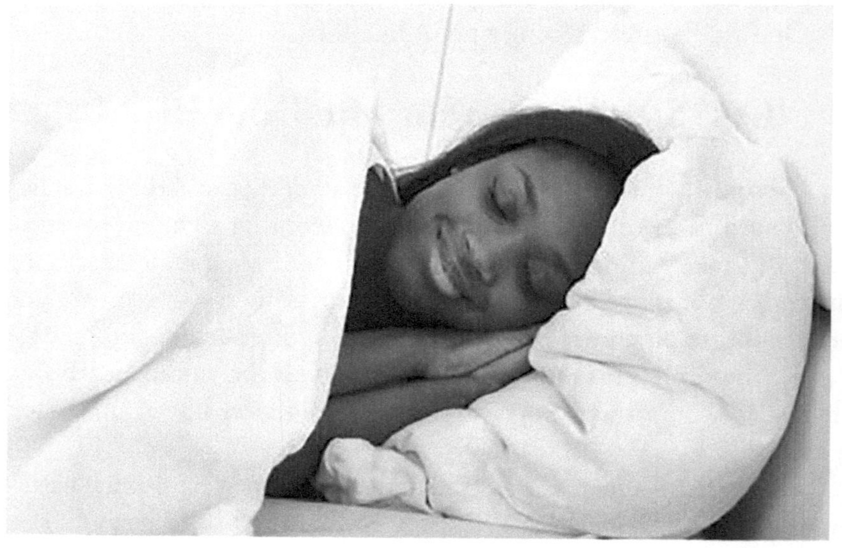 It is vain and unprofessional humans not to sleep, if we don't start to respect sleep, we'll reap; that means advanced aging, bad health and worn out feet! So if you feel me, **"SLEEP!"**

Sleep Is A Gift From God, Don't Be Robbed!

Caregiver's Closet

     MISS ASONDRA STARN'AIR

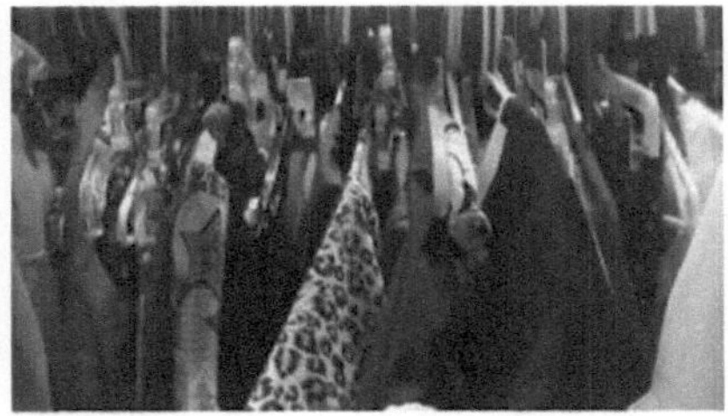

When it comes to Scrubs, I think having lots of variety makes going to work more fresh and exciting!

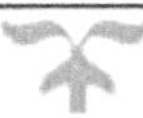

You Are What You Wear!

Make sure you are dress for success

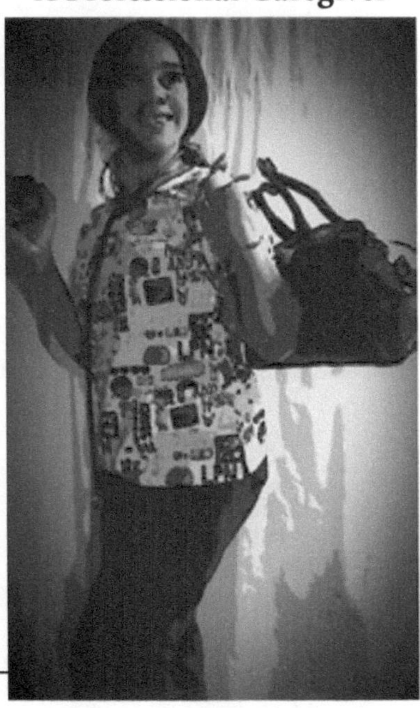

She's got the look, that says **"You're Hired"** What about you?

Tips

- Make sure your hair is pulled back, away from your face.
- do not over use make up, save that for a night out on the town.
- Limit jewelry, but caregivers work watch is okay!
- Keep a work supply bag with you.
- An apple a day wouldn't hurt either!
- Get to work fifteen minutes early, no matter weather conditions.
- Wear medium loose fitting work apparel, never wear spandex it's so not cool; mightiest well be naked! Body shaping pants and leggings are too revealing. They don't belong in any work place period.

"Smart Phones"
Here We Go Again ...

Is Your Smart Phone Really Smart? No it's not if you put it before your other important responsibilities, like work. Your personal calls and texting can wait!

Go tend to the customer, lets get our priorities straight!

Stay Off Your Phones!

Hey, I'm just the messenger, don't get peeved off at me. However, I do agree, cell phones are becoming a nuisance in the work place. Catch up on your calls and emails on your breaks. Come on, we must stay smart and professional.

'Our Phones Can Wait'.

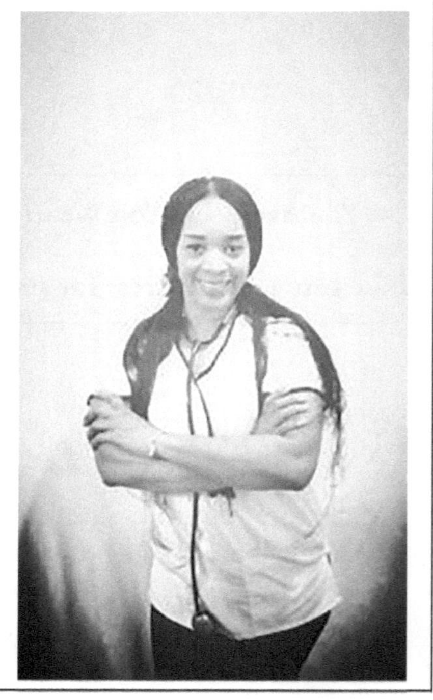

People, respect for the work place is all it takes!

Foot Care for Caregivers

Being on your feet all day can be harmful to your feet. When your feet hurt, you hurt!

Caregivers we need to be mindful of good foot care and make it a priority as part of a daily routine to take better care of our feet.

By addressing the problem early we can decrease the chances of a more serious condition that sometime require injections or surgery.

Caring for the feet is relatively simple, it starts with wearing the right shoe and foot care on a regular bases.

TLC FOOT CARE

1. Don't wear cheap shoes.
2. Avoid wearing flat shoes.
3. Wear special work shoes designed for comfort and arch elevation.
4. Sit while you chart, if possible.
5. Sit on your breaks, take a load off
6. Pray over your feet ask God to heal them.
7. Soak and pamper your feet at least three times a week.
8. Relax on your off days, Keep your feet elevated, feet up, read your bibles. have a cup of tea!
9. Wiggle your toes and feet daily for stretching and circulation.
10. Keep toenail cut low.
11. Do foot massages regularly.
12. See a Podiatrist, to find out the underlying problems if these tips are not helping.

In your tool box over to the right, I have provided you with some tips on how to tender love and care for your feet, something we don't do enough of, until we are in pain, or hurting and forced to see a doctor.

We don't have to let it get that far, if we began now, early, our feet can do what Jesus did, walked! Jesus Walked and So Must We!

God Bless You!

Don't Put a Price on a Good Shoe and it Won't Put a Price on 'YOU"!

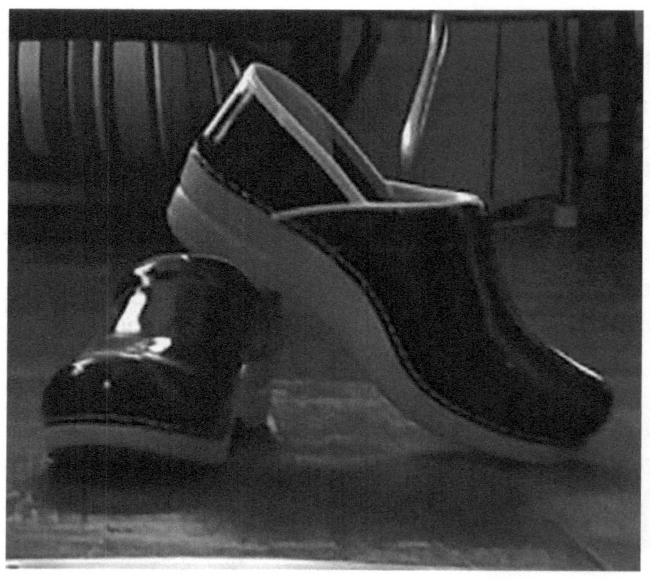

Comfort Matters, You Get What You Pay For!

 Miss Asondra StarN'air

'10 Types Of Caregivers'
Which One Are You?

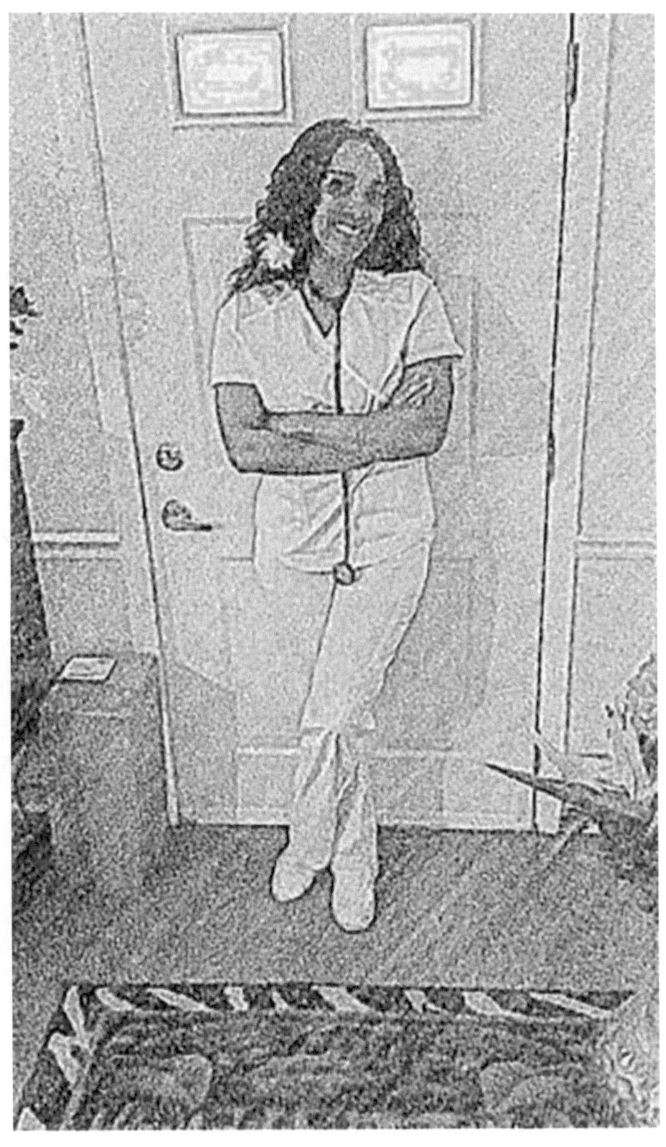

Caregiver Number One

This particular caregiver has been at the same location or facility for a very long time, they think they own the place. And if you don't do things their way, they go and make trouble for you. And let me warn you, this person has lots of wicked friends that will help this caregiver do whatever it wants them to do so they'll come after you too; whatever gets the job done!

This caregiver also maybe very 'Old Schooled', they like things just the way they've always been. They refuse to let new wineskin in. People who read their bibles know exactly what I'm talking about. And if "YOU" want to know more about new wineskin and how that ties in, then get a bible and go to **Matthew 9:17** and you'll know what I mean. **Caregiver One** is so use to the old ways of doing things, they reject individuals like you and me who may do things slightly different from how they think it ought to be done. Our creativity and sophistication and confidence many times makes **'Caregiver One'** feels threatened and uneasy. So they get busy, plotting and scheming; they want you out, or want to make you so miserable that after they're done lying and scheming on you, you'll want in to quit, but don't quit. Employees like what I'm describing are bloodhounds, they came after me, they'll come after you. But here's what you do, always keep your bible with you. Stay in the word and allow the holy spirit to guide you. And watch your back! Too, start keeping a running record of the harassment along with names, dates and times the behavior began and remember **Jesus is your only friend!**, burned.

How do we handle this one? Keep feeding them kindness but with a long handed spoon watch your back and stay on track, focus on Jesus, focus on excellence. Maybe one day they'll come around and began to change their evil and wicked ways, and realize that old and new can learn from each other, and that times are changing. Things can't always stay the same. And no matter what always remember this: ***"Light Is Powerful Than Darkness!"*** Do Your Job and Do it Well, Live to Tell!

 Miss Asondra StarN'air

Caregiver Number Two

Caregiver Two **'The Follower'** this caregiver doesn't care if co-work-ers are right or wrong, they just want to fit in, 'tag along'. They are what the bible refers to as **"Luke Warm"** they are neither **"Cold or Hot"** from my experience this one is the most pitiful kind of caregiver out there.

And they're two faced, yelp, two faced like ah **'Two Faced Clock'** and their sucking up never stops. Sometimes they're a work buddy friend other times they're your foes, depends on whose running the show!

Yeah, this one just goes with the flow, for example, if a group of caregivers and nurses don't like you, although you've done nothing to anyone, plus you do your job well but so what, now Caregiver Two decides to join the rest of the crew, they don't like you now, and they're starting to put you down. But hang in there, wear your Jesus crown! *Hang Onto Christ, Hang Onto Light, Keep Smiling and Shining Bright!*

Caregiver Two, do what they do, they're not going to look out for you, if you can, stay far away from this one. This one just might be the one trying to set you up, while they're are laughing and smiling in your face.

How to handle this one?

Pray for all those who have turned their backs on God, and refuse to get to know him like you have, and keep it movin; Take my advice, don't get into it with them, keep your mouth shut! Just stay focus on giving **'High Quality Care'**. And if you can, avoid haters, liars, gossipers, and employees like number Two, communicate only if you have to and concentrate on your work. And remember this: when persecuted and mistreated we must forgive them and say what Jesus said: Father forgive them for they know not what they do. *Luke 23:34* Remain loving and kind, stay true to you. But still, protect yourself, you might want to keep a running record, with names, times and dates with this one as well. Because when you have several people hating on you like that, there's nothing they won't do. They'll even go in and brain wash your resident and try to get them to turn on you or complain about your performance. Oh, if only you knew what I've been through you'd want to warn as many caregivers too! I do pray to God that this book do what it's suppose to do and that's to inform, lookout and protect you! **"Stay Excellent"** *'No Worries!'* What was meant for evil, God uses for ***"GOOD"!*** Gen. 50:20

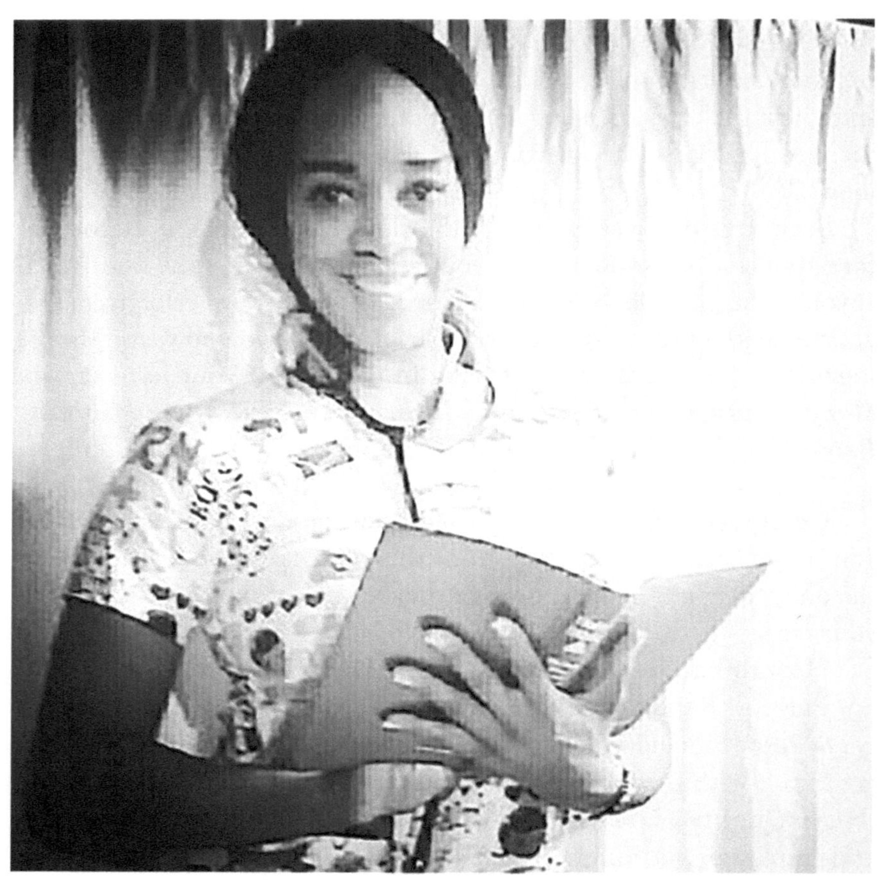

Miss Asondra StarN'air

You Are Not Alone!

Sometime life can be so stressful and unfair and it seems like nobodies there, but you are not alone, **GOD** is here with you!

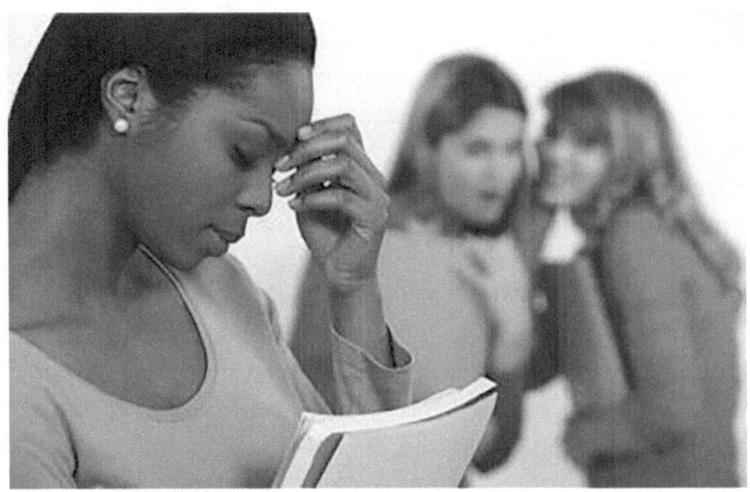

Red, White or Black we got to stay on track.
Jesus Christ our savior has always got our backs!

For our present troubles are small and won't last very long. Yet they produce for us a glory that vastly outweighs them and will last forever! So we don't look at the troubles we can see now; rather, we fix our gaze on things that cannot be seen. For the things we see now will soon be gone, but the things we cannot see will last forever.
2 Corinthians 4:7-18

So Lets Keep it Together!

Caregiver Number Three

This Caregivers, we'll call this one **'The Complainer'** all she/he does is murmur and complain, this one goes and find other caregivers to complain to. Yet stays on the same job for 20 years and ain't going nowhere. They're actually poisonous to the company and other caregivers too. They smear and slander the company and other staff members and anyone they don't agree with. **'Caregiver Three'** may be skilled and reliable, they usually are, that's why they have been there so long, but that does not change the fact that sometimes they're poisonous individuals to be around. Again, they seem to be looking for a reason to complain and drop names. It's always something with them, can't please them at all and they're noisy. **"No Peace"** they just won't let things be, they're not happy!

With all the murmuring, complaining and negative talk, this one can be quite contagious and I'm afraid, they can influence a whole new set of crop. And that crop if it gets trained by this one can turn into a bunch of crap like this one has become over the years. In my professional opinion, and I am a professional, **Caregiver Three** should not be asked to help train new employees. If they hate the company they work for and lets it be known secretly to newbies, I don't care how much they know, let someone else train the caregivers coming in, not this one. Furthermore, **'Caregiver Three'** here's a question for ya, Oh, you know who you are, isn't it about time to retire? If you hate the place so much now, why don't you retire early, take the money and Go! Because right now, as we speak, God is raising up and new set of crop and they're called: **'The New Day Caregivers'** and they will deliver! Therefore, number three, mightiest well stop all that negative talk, if you are not happy there, **"Take a walk"**!

How to handle this one: If they ask you if you want to have lunch with them? Say no thank you, unless of course you're going to introduce them to Jesus! Meanwhile stay your distance if you can unless you're working hand in hand! The bible warns us to stay away from individuals who Gossip and to guard our words when we speak about others. I do think that includes the company we work for. **Proverbs 20:19** Stay stay focus on **"Excellence"**, Stay Focus on **"Christ"**, Heed this advice!

1 Corinthians 5:11

 Miss Asondra StarN'air

Caregiver Number Four

This one is Obnoxious, they don't like nobody, they are unpleasant, hardly ever smiles and don't like helping other caregivers out with care -giving task like, physical transfers and such. **'Caregiver Four'** attitudes sucks! Oops, Lord can I say that? Yes! It sucks! Example, this is how some of them think, "If I can lift and do it by myself, so can you". But, that's not true. Everybody's skeleton and muscular strength is different, that residence is 265 pounds, I'm 130 pounds, come on, really! Yet, because they have this awful attitude toward other caregivers and don't support teamwork, caregivers like caregiver number four, like I said earlier, **"Attitude Sucks"** and how ironic, is this, there's usually four of them, and yes, I'm naming names. **Somebody, Anybody, Everybody and Nobody.** I tell you the truth, one really dread asking or going anywhere near one of these caregivers and that's exactly what they want, to be left alone.

Tell me please, how in the world did they get the job of caregiving in the first place, we don't know. **Somebody** in human resources got some explaining to do. Was it you? Oh my, not funny!

How to handle this one: Let me show you, "excuse me please, I need your help"... go to this caregiver for help as much as you can, until they realize they are there not only for the residents /patients but also for co-workers too. That person may have a negative aura about themselves, even intimidating, (oh my God, help me please, I've been there) but I tell ya, don't be intimidated, don't let them force you into lifting or transferring a bed bound person on your own just because they are intimidating or giving off a don't bother me vibe. On the contrary, go to them anyway and ask for help if you need help, if they refuse, follow the chain of command they don't want that I assure you.

I need to add this too and it won't take long, seriously, hear me on this, too many caregivers suffer today with back problems that could have been avoided if they had just asked for help and waited for help. Co-workers like 'Four' they don't have the final say, when it comes to safety, nor do the nurses or employers. Safety is a right of all Americans, including caregivers. If you work in long term care facilities and other staff members refuse to help you with rooms that a difficult for you to do a safe and thorough job,"including transfers". Don't do it "STOP" forget the clock! Wait for help, say to yourself, **"No Help", "No Move"**. Because if you **"Move"** that person and they fall, you'll have much more to lose, don't be fool! Look out for yourself and others. **No Help, No Move!** Get into the groove!!!!

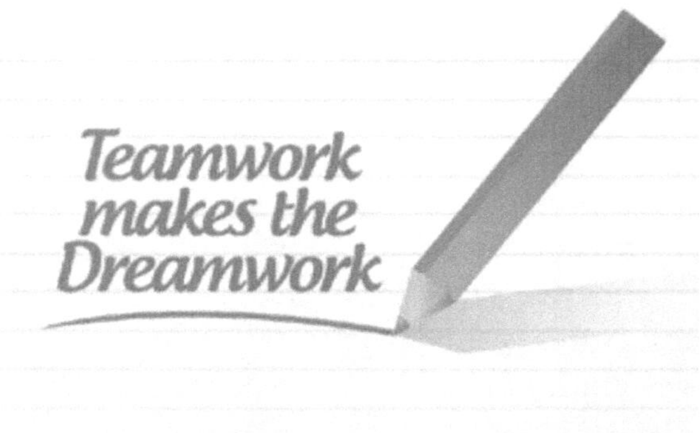

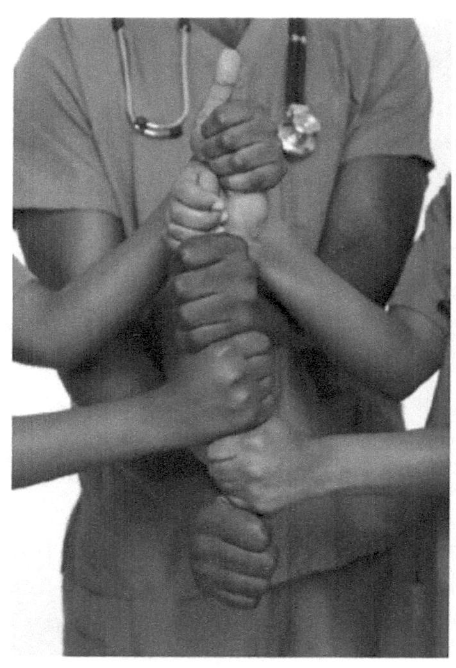

   Miss Asondra StarN'air

Caregiver Number Five

Caregiver Number **'Five Delivers!'** This one is going places, they're sharp, their future looks bright! These types of individuals tend to be very reliable, prompt, always on time; they're organized, and very efficient.

This caregiver is a professional, no doubt about it, they have no time for foolishness. The top priority here is the one needing the care.

And too, they're loving and kind to other co-workers as well and are always willing to help out when asked.

"Oh, yes this is what I'm talking about", 'Caregiving' at it's finest!

But sometimes and this happened to me, we become targets for abuse by mediocre caregivers and their clicks. **The bible says in this world good is bad and bad is good.** Isaiah 5:20.

Caregiver 'Five' gets a five star, because they got it going on and because they are so noticeably great, that may piss a lot of co-workers off, especially the ones who don't take their jobs seriously. And don't be good lookin' with a great body. Caregiver number Five if this is you, you are in trouble, you're in real big trouble! You're going to be hated by some, unfortunately, women have been known to be very jealous creatures, especially women of the world. With that being said, caregiver 'Five' must watch their backs constantly. I've already been through it and still go though it. Unfortunately, and sad too, today we live in a world were hatred and jealousy abounds. Around and around, envy's everywhere! Today in healthcare setting we have rivalry's go-ing on all the time. Female drama and the all the jealousy among each other has to stop. No one should ever have to apologize for having a nice physique, their beauty or the fact they got it going on or whatever you mad and envious about; besides Jesus is the only one with the real clout! In all sincerity, I feel that jealousy has become a cancer in itself, there are so many insecure and envious souls out there, *and if you are guilty of this kind of behavior **Jesus wants to help!** You do not have to keep mistreating people.* **"Change"** make mends with yourself. **"You Are Beautiful"** God created all of us in his own image. From now on people, can't we just learn to love the human race. **Everybody has the right to live in this place, called planet Earth and not get hurt!** Caregiver five, We love you, stay on the rise, if some don't like the way you look, let them close their eyes!

How to handle this one: Caregivers if you see something, say something! Don't standby and watch innocent caregivers be harassed or handled recklessly, (bullied) by jealous co-workers, Get to know this person, look out for them, be a true and loyal friend, God will bless you in the end!

High Five, To All You **"Five's"** Out There!

Beautiful Looking People Matters!
Jealousy and Hatred Don't!
Keep Going, Give It No Thought
Love Is The Boss!

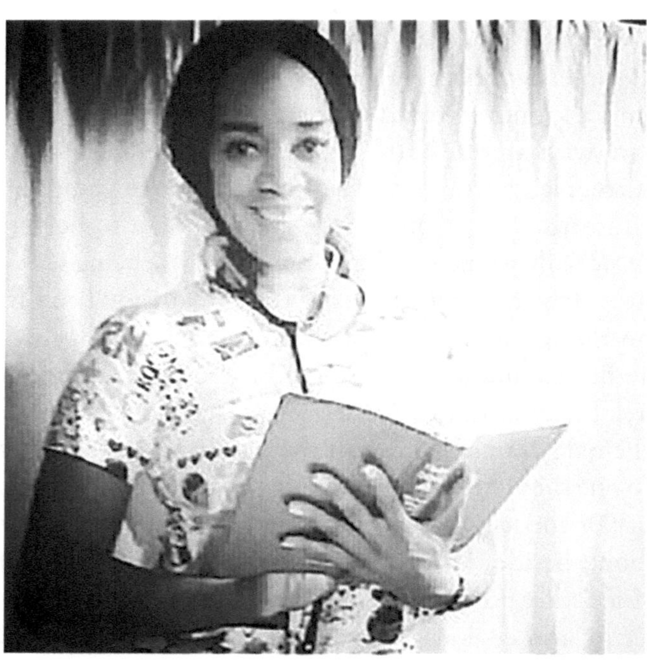

  Miss Asondra StarN'air

Caregiver Number Six

Here's a caregiver that's sweet and quite. They don't talk much and when they do it's positive talk. They seems to be of an introvert nature yet always willing to help out. This person is quiet and reserved, but know their stuff. You won't find them hanging around the water cooler, or involved in grapevine gossip. No, this caregiver is wise and very careful about who they talk to or hang out with. This is a sharp and smart caregiver, if I were you, I'd make friends with this one but be a real friend yourself. And let me warn you, **'Caregiver Six'** is not down with gossip, so be careful in your conversations with this one, there's a reason why that person stays off to themselves. They know what I know and it's this: words spoken can never be recalled, it's your word against mines, that's all! Now with that being said, take the work friendship slow, grow into it, prove to them over time that, you're going to be a loyal true work buddy!

How to handle this one: With respect, do not impose on that individual, by asking that person too many questions. Why? Because if that individual wants you to know something about them, they will tell you. Don't be too nosy either; they will open up once they sees it is safe to do so.

Don't get me wrong, some questions like are you married? Do you have children? Are okay to ask because those kinds of questions help bond us as people, I totally understand, I get that. Some curiosity, fine, cool no harm done. But still, don't ask too many questions and when they share that information with you please don't run off and tell others their business. Respect their privacy otherwise they will not trust you and I don't blame them either.

Lastly, realize this, it is wonderful when we have the opportunity to turn a work friend into a real friend! It makes caregiving all the more enjoyable. Everybody could benefit from having a good friend in their life especially at work! Caregiver Six, is it!

Caregiver Number Seven

Well there's just something very special and unique about this person, 'Number Seven', not only are they very skilled and professional, they're good role models.

This caregiver has leadership abilities and would be great leader and good boss. They work very well with people and they aren't arrogant or unkind nor do they show favoritism. You can tell they have what it takes to run or managed an organization. They are positive and bright! I tell you the truth, caregivers "YOU" want to hang around this kind of person. My advice is, meet up for lunch, learn all you can from them, let them mentor you too if they have time. Find out what their secret is for being so wonderful. I bet it's Jesus! Ask them what church they belong to, maybe start a bible study group together or something, stay in that person life if you can, they're going places!

How to you handle this one: Encouragement is what that caregiver needs. Yelp, keep right on encouraging them to go back to school, or go after their dreams, and you do the same. Great caregivers can do anything! Many times that's all some of us need is for others to believe in us; your kind words and en-couragement just might be the nudge they need to help caterpillar them on to higher success. And don't stagnate them in any way, envy and jealousy is never okay. If you stay around positive people like this, soon you'll be up and on your way! You become what you hang out with!

Keep going, keep learning, keep trusting God, **"YOUR"** call will come someday!

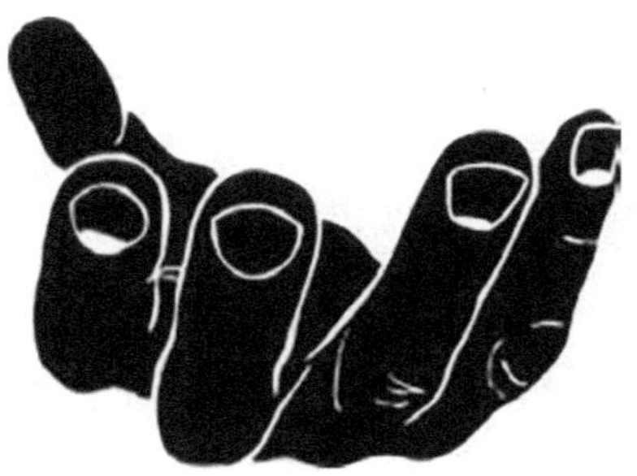

 Miss Asondra StarN'air

Caregiver Number Eight

"The Bully" these caregivers have always hurt and bullied people, they did it in school and now the workplace. Bullies are everywhere!

You don't have to do anything, if they don't like you or the way you look you are in trouble. Bullies tend to be quite popular, they don't work alone.

They'll make your life a living hell, and leave no evidence. It's your word against theirs and their friends all back them. Oh yeah, this type, schemes, will sabotage, and comes with an entourage! But, don't worry, they'll reap what they sow. And too, the bible says in Proverbs 26:27 *"Whoever digs a pit will fall into it"*.

Can I tell you this, caregivers that bully, has hurt me a lot emotionally and financially too. Have a heart, because this is a very painful topic for me to discuss. Listen, I have been a victim of number **'Eight'** The Bully, for most of my care giving years on the job. I endured a lot and lost a lot of time, money and opportunities that I can't get back. "Persecution", "Hardship", I have suffered greatly.

I know how they operate, these individuals thrive on darkness and hate. They are also very dangerous people, their hearts are evil, minds twisted and tongue full of lies. And they set out to destroy as many lives as they can, doesn't stop with yours or mine. Bullying others is powerful and fun for them, they get off on destroying people lives. They set out to ruin people's lives so much so, they hope you don't want to live anymore. How do I know this, because I been there before, I almost lost it, I know longer wanted to live, that's how bad it was for me for so many, many years. I was hated on sight, everywhere I went nurses and aides came after me.

Bullies MUST Be Stopped! I think there should be more stricter laws in place that says "Bully Means Jail Time" or something along those lines. Bullying is dangerous, it's a crime, people are killing themselves today. Innocent people who can't handle it anymore are suiciding, taking their own life, dying. Have you read the newspaper lately, or seen your local news? Bulling Kills! No one has the right to trample on someone and injure them inside, or lie and slander, destroy that persons good name and reputation and worst, scheme and cause that person to lose their jobs, their livelihood. All the while, sending that person into deep depression, no longer wanting to live. I tell you the truth, if it hadn't been for my love and my deep rooted relationship with Christ I'd be DEAD too, Yes I too, would have taken my own life. As I see it, bullying is another form of murder.

Today bullies are everywhere, not just in the work place, they're in our schools too. For the first time in history, kids are killing themselves. They are committing suicide, I repeat, **"Bullies MUST Be Stopped!"** World we have to get involved, we can no longer pretend it's not happening, "NO MORE"! "NO" we cannot just sit back and do nothing anymore. We have to get bullies removed from the workplaces and out of our schools. Together you and me as a country, we have to find a way to catch them, so they can't hide. World listen to me, bullies are killing and destroying lives, like Satan, they are becoming the 'New Hitler's' full of evil, corruption and genocide.

Sorry I went on and on, but bullying has become an epidemic, all over the world. A lot of people out there are suffering in silence and that can be psychologically dangerous. If you are being bullies, tell someone. Document too, try to get their first and last names, times and dates of the attacks. And write down exactly what's happening to you. Back to the nursing home, and caregiver number Eight, Unfortunately, working in nursing home care facilities bullying has become common place. Today it's become so easy to hurt others and get away with it, it's your word against theirs. **"No Witnesses"** or **"False Witnesses** just waiting to set you up see bullies rarely work alone. These kinds of workplace environments are filled with so many insecure, jealous and troubles women/men **'Eight'** is one of them. So put the full armor of God on each day you are there. Also, watch your back, watch your front too, watch those who says, oh, I'm on your side, watch them closely because bullies are on all levels: STNA's, Nurses, DON's, Housekeeping, Administrators and the list goes on. And please be careful because some will try to get close to you so that they can take back information to the trouble makers. Listen, in these places the only real friend you have is **JESUS!** Put all your trust and faith in him, he will take what was meant for your harm and use it for his good, but you have to be strong, stay scripture and prayed up. Don't try to take your life or give up, instead, be still and trust God, he will protect you from all evil doers and raise you up! You will triumph, you will drink from the *"Victory Cup!"*

Last thing, remember, Jesus was bullied too! But Jesus overcame the world and so will God's people. I'll end with this, bully's will have their day; woe unto them! God's wrath is no joke! Be not deceived; God is not mocked: for as you sow, so shall you reap. **Galatians 6:7**

How do you handle this one: You go to God, ask him to protect you, next you stay prayed up and scriptures up too; read the book of Job, read all the promises of God, know that, he will never leave or forsake you, He will take care of bullies in his own time and way. **"Everyday Pray!"** Stay rooted in Christ, help is on its way! Do not take revenge, my dear friends, but leave room for God's wrath.

To the **"Bullies"** out there, **"Vengeance is Mine,
I Will Repay, Says the Lord!"
Romans 12:19-20**

'Bullying Is A Crime and Deserves Jail Time!'

 MISS ASONDRA StarN'air

Caregiver Number Nine

"The Bystander" this caregivers stands back and watch co-workers bully and set up other unsuspecting caregivers and say nothing. They are cowards! How can a person witness mistreatment of another person and say nothing? But it happens all the time, Co-workers like this one sees what's happening but looks the other way. Ears are death and eyes are blind. They act as if they know nothing but that's not true, they do. But just like I told you, they're cowards, they watch other people do, what's in them to do. Truth be told, this caregiver may not have been the one who plotted or schemed, but they are just as guilty. They knew something, or saw something, yet, said nothing or did nothing. "Cowards!"

How to handle this one: You don't! This caregiver is weak, has no courage to help fight for others. Listen, when you know something is wrong and you don't speak up, you become part of the problem. On the flip side of things, perhaps the thought is this, "I'm not the one whose doing it", "it's none of my business" "I just don't want to get involved." If this is you, **"Question"** whatever happened to compassion and love? Jesus said that we are to look out and love one another like sister and brothers. Therefore, we must to get involved! "Yes, yes yes! "We are our sister and brothers keepers!" **If You See Something, Say Something!** If you don't, shame on you bystander! God will deal with each one of us in his own time and place. Meanwhile, I say to those who are being persecuted, lied on and handle unfairly by others hang in there, pray, help is on it's way. "Focus on Excellence", keep on keeping on!

Caregiver Number Ten

YOU

Finally we made it to **YOU** and "YOU" are most certainly a "Ten", in every way and here's why I say this, caregiver, you have seen many caregivers, come and go yet you still remain true to the call of caregiving.

Rarely do you complain and if you do it's for the betterment of the entire organization, but you do it the right way and for the right reasons.

You are a 10 because not only do you possess skills and know-how but you are a great team player too. This book solutes you! You refuse to be part of a click, you hate gossip, you mind your own business and you don't take sides and you will gladly help anyone who ask. Caregivers like you are becoming harder and harder to find. However I do believe

A Caregivers Bible To Excellence is getting ready to help change all that, "The New Day" Caregivers are about to emerge and with Caregivers like you on God's side, we will be a force to reckon with. Together we will help bring forth a much needed change. We are not the aides of the past, we reject such a low class name. Today we have become healthcare professionals, what we want is simple, **"R-E-S-P-E-C-T"** that means treat us like the professionals we are and pay us well! **'Number Ten'** all I can say is with caregivers like you on the team, we can't fail, all we can do is win. And win we shall because God rewards good stewards like **"YOU"** all I can say is get ready for more and more blessing. Don't be surprise when new opportunities comes your way!

How to handle this one: Let them spread their wings and help change the world, let'm **"Fly"**

say, if **Florence Nightingale** can leave a mark,

So Can I!

What a Journey!

So, there you have it, **Ten Types of Caregivers,** you decide your number. Some of you may be a combination of more than one number.

It is my hope that each one of us will take a look in the mirror and make that change. Let us be done with all foolishness, gossip, jealousy and strife. Right now, today, It's time to start working together as a team again. Remember, **"Teamwork Makes the Dream Work."**! Effective teamwork is key to attaining growth and success and that's what God want for us, "The Best!"

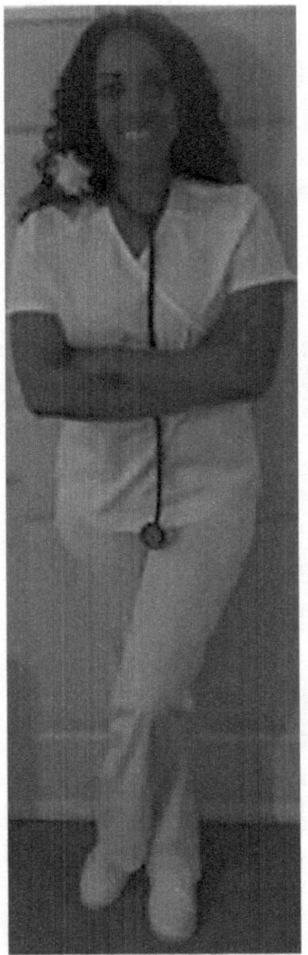

I Believe I Can Fly!

Forgiveness

Forgiveness, let's talk about this, I know it's easy said than done! But if we are followers of Jesus Christ then we **MUST** stay full of forgiveness always. **Jesus Cross, Is Our Cross!** If we live for Christ we are going to be mistreated. Haters hated Christ first! Jesus was mistreated and faultlessly accused all the time. But he forgave them all. On the last day of his human life he uttered these heart drenching words: **"Father forgive them for they know not what they do."** Those words spoken right there have kept me alive and although the attacks still continues today like others before me, I press on.... I keep my eyes on the prize. **"Eternal life with Christ"** is how I rise!

Therefore, I hold nothing against anyone, nor should you. The Bible teaches in Matthew 10:22 that following Jesus has a price; we will be hated by everyone, lied on, slandered, and mistreated. So get use to it! Do what I do, when that happens, go, quickly, grab your bibles immerse yourself in his word. It will strengthen you, plus make you stable and very, very strong. Meanwhile, saints be at peace, you've done nothing wrong.

Reality, this is the cross we must all bear and no matter how unfair and painful it may be, we must forgive those who hate us. In fact, the Bible tells us to count it all joy when we meet trials of various kinds. Again, remember what I told you, they hated Jesus first; and because we love and follow him, we will be hated and mistreated also.

But still, got to forgive! Our God will heal us too, he will also comfort us when we are wounded; but we must get back up, press on, and keep serving our Lord no matter what! Yes, press on, keep serving God, and love him with all your heart, mind, body and soul! And keep reading your bibles, do what you're told.

"Forgive 'Them For They Know Not What They Do' now let that become way of life for you. Furthermore, let us not take any of these attacks personally, because Satan the devil is behind all of it, I assure you. So Be strong and wise don't fight like the world fight, let it go, don't hold on to unforgiveness. Unforgiveness opens the door to resentment, resentment opens the door to retaliation, retaliation opens the door to destruction, destruction opens the door to war, and war opens the door to all kinds of things, including killings catastrophes.

So, please, don't hold on to Unforgiveness, instead, *FORGIVE!* In closing, forgiveness is the only way to love, peace, and joy—and the only way to God's heart. God is a loving and forgiving God! But he expects us to forgive one another like he forgave us; no matter whose right or wrong. Eph. 4:32 So you see, **'In Order To Live, We "MUST" Forgive!**

'Forgiveness Sets Us Free!'

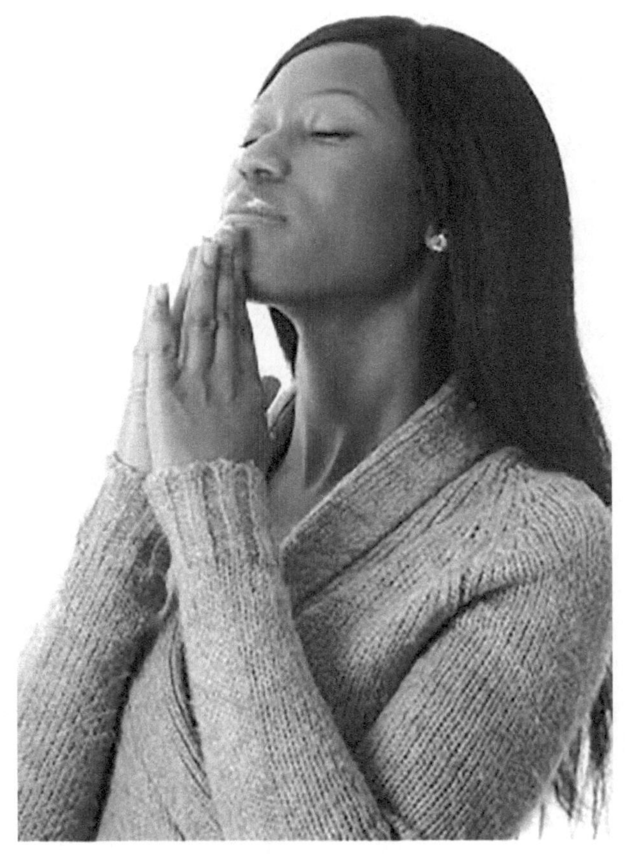

"Forgive Them For They Know Not What They Do'.
Luke 23:34

Daily Affirmations for Caregivers

I am a professional caregiver.

I am beautiful in every way.

I am successful; I love being a health-care provider.

I am learning new and useful skills.

I am a competent caregiver.

I am supportive of other caregivers.

I am a team player.

I am taking better care of myself.

I am making smarter food choices.

I am exercising more now.

I am starting to drink more water.

I am saying no to junk food.

I am always on time to work.

I am a positive person.

I am done with negativity.

I am minding my own business from now on.

I am done with gossiping.

I am welcoming change, growth, and development in every area of my life now.

I am a child of God, and it shows in my behavior.

I am happy.

I am full of gratitude.

I am starting to rest more. I realize getting a good night's sleep is very important.

I am changing in a great way. I have lots of love and respect for my bosses and coworkers.

I am finding more time to spend with God and his word now.

I am starting to read the Bible a lot more, and I see the difference in my life. I have more peace of mind. I feel like I can do all things in Christ, who strengthens me. **'I Feel Brand New!'**

Twenty-Five Affirmations for Caregivers

1. I am an excellent caregiver.
2. I am a professional.
3. I am smart and intelligent.
4. I am so blessed.
5. I am doing something about stress; I'm getting rid of it.
6. I am patient and kind.
7. I am prosperous.
8. I am faithful to God.
9. I am sorry for my sin. I shall repent and not do it again.
10. I am a child of the Most High.
11. I am developing into what God wants me to be.
12. I am thankful.
13. I am learning something new every day.
14. I am becoming a nicer, and a more loving person.
15. I am a team player.
16. I am staying away from strife from now on.
17. I am changing, getting closer and closer to God.
18. I am starting to read my Bible every day now.
19. I am going the extra mile. Love does not depend on two hearts; it depends on one (mine).
20. I love my ***Caregiver's Bible to Excellence*** book, I'm telling everyone I know about it.
21. I am a empathetic, understanding, passionate, and honest reliable loving caregiver, I deliver!
22. I am ready to do whatever God calls me to do without murmuring or complaining.
23. I am starting to seek God's will and purpose for my life.
24. I am dying to self so Jesus can come and live inside me.
25. I am giving my life to Christ; I want to follow him now.

Caregiver's Judgment Day

1. **Matthew 12:34-37** You snakes! You are evil people, so how can you say anything good? The mouth speaks the things that are in the heart. Good people have good things in their hearts, and so they say good things. But evil people have evil in their hearts, so they say evil things. And I tell you that on the Judgment Day people will be responsible for every careless thing they have said. The words you have said will be used to judge you. Some of your words will prove you right, but some of your words will prove you guilty."

2. **Ephesians 5:3-6** But there must be no sexual sin among you, or any kind of evil or greed. Those things are not right for God's holy people. Also, there must be no evil talk among you, and you must not speak foolishly or tell evil jokes. These things are not right for you. Instead, you should be giving thanks to God. You can be sure of this: No one will have a place in the kingdom of Christ and of God who sins sexually, or does evil things, or is greedy. Anyone who is greedy is serving a false god. Do not let anyone fool you by telling you things that are not true, because these things will bring God's anger on those who do not obey him.

3. **Ecclesiastes 10:11-14** If a <u>serpent strikes</u> despite being charmed, there's no point in being a snake charmer. The words spoken by the wise are gracious, but the lips of a fool will devour him. He begins his speech with foolishness, and concludes it with evil madness. The fool overflows with words, and no one can predict what will happen. As to what will happen after him, who can explain it?

4. **Proverbs 10:30-32** The godly will never be disturbed, but the wicked will be removed from the land. The mouth of the godly person gives wise advice, but the tongue that deceives will be cut off. The lips of the godly speak <u>helpful words</u>, but the mouth of the wicked speaks perverse words.

5. **1 Peter 3:10-11** If you want a happy, good life, keep control of your tongue, and guard your lips from telling lies. Turn away from evil and do good. Try to live in peace even if you must run after it to catch and hold it!

 Miss Asondra StarN'air

6. **Zechariah 8:16-17** These are the things that ye shall do; Speak ye every man the truth to his neighbour; execute the judgment of truth and peace in your gates: And let none of you imagine evil in your hearts against his neighbour; and love no false oath: for all these are things that I hate, saith the Lord.

Choose The Latter, Get To Know God Better!

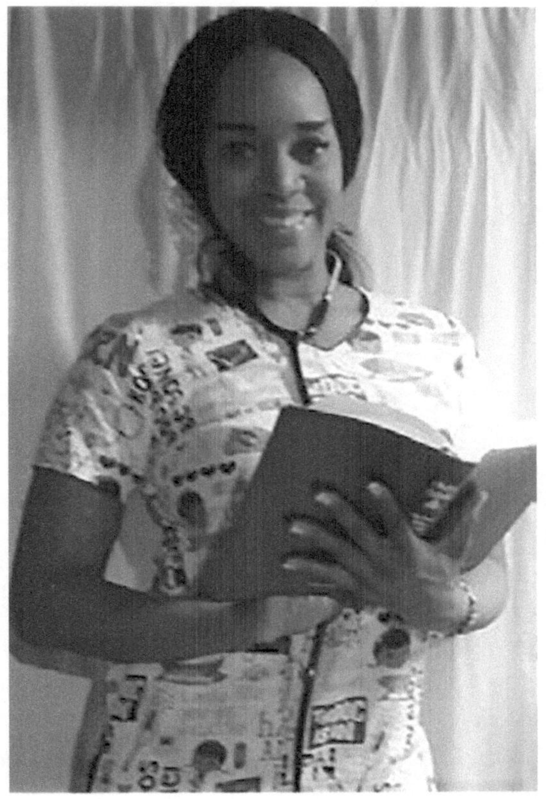

Honor Our Father in Heaven!

Judgment Day is Coming!

Everyone will be Judged, yes we'll all have to give an account on how we spent our lives down here on planet earth, the scrolls don't lie. Get right with God while you still have a chance.

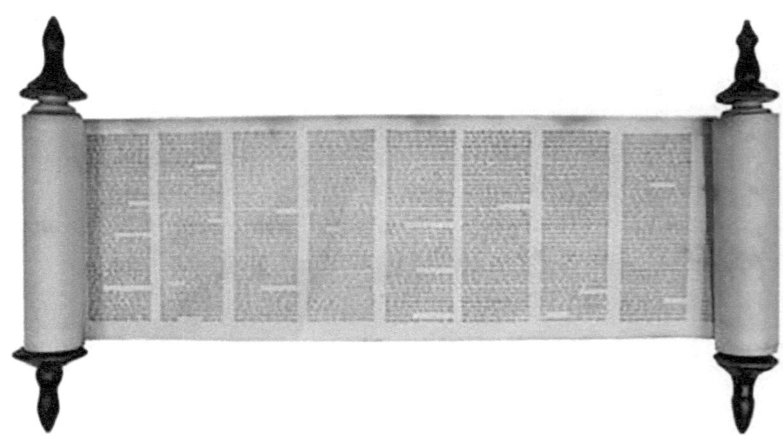

Then I saw a great white throne and him who was seated on it. The earth and the heavens fled from his presence, and there was no place for them. And I saw the dead, great and small, standing before the throne, and books were opened. Another book was opened, which is the book of life. The dead were judged according to what they had done as recorded in the books. The sea gave up the dead that were in it, and death and Hades gave up the dead that were in them, and each person was judged according to what they had done. Then death and Hades were thrown into the lake of fire. The lake of fire is the second death. Anyone whose name was not found written in the book of life was thrown into the lake of fire. **Rev. 20:11-15**

 Miss Asondra StarN'air

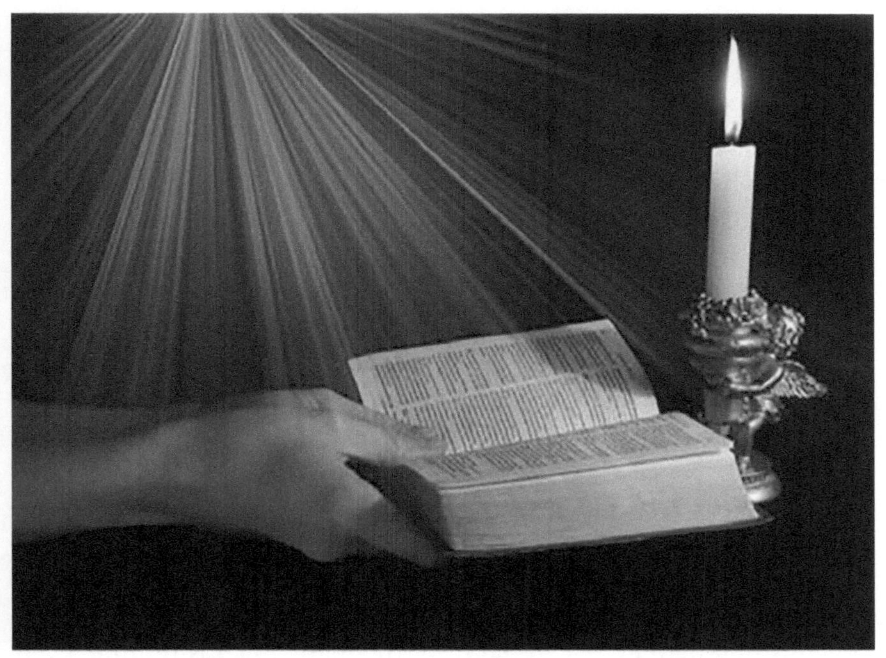

The Bible

Basic things we need to know and do

Instructions we need to follow

Before we make a mess out of our lives and others

Leaving God no choice but to teach us painful lessons, even death if that's what it takes. **Stop Testing God!!!**

Earth is not our final destination, some of us will move on with Christ to eternal life and some will not.

God's Is All Knowing!

Matthew 11:27

All things have been handed over to Me by My Father; and no one knows the Son except the Father; nor does anyone know the Father except the Son, and anyone to whom the Son chooses to reveal Him.

John 10:15

Even as the Father knows me and I know the Father; and I lay down My life for the sheep.

1 Corinthians 2:10-11

For to us God revealed them through the Spirit; for the Spirit searches all things, even the depths of God. For who among men knows the thoughts of a man except the spirit of the man which is in him? Even so the thoughts of God no one knows except the Spirit of God.

Isaiah 40:13-14

Who has directed the Spirit of the LORD, Or as His counselor has informed Him? With whom did He consult and who gave Him understanding? And who taught Him in the path of justice and taught Him knowledge And informed Him of the way of understanding?

Job 21:22

"Can anyone teach God knowledge, In that He judges those on high?

Romans 11:33-34

Oh, the depth of the riches both of the wisdom and knowledge of God! How unsearchable are His judgments and unfathomable His ways! For WHO HAS KNOWN THE MIND OF THE LORD, OR WHO BECAME HIS COUNSELOR?

<u>1 Corinthians 2:16</u>

For WHO HAS KNOWN THE MIND OF THE LORD, THAT HE WILL INSTRUCT HIM? But we have the mind of Christ.

<u>Matthew 10:30</u>

"But the very hairs of your head are all numbered.

<u>Luke 12:7</u>

"Indeed, the very hairs of your head are all numbered. Do not fear; you are more valuable than many sparrows.

<u>Psalm 147:4</u>

He counts the number of the stars; He gives names to all of them.

<u>Isaiah 40:26</u>

Lift up your eyes on high And see who has created these stars, The One who leads forth their host by number, He calls them all by name; Because of the greatness of His might and the strength of His power, Not one of them is missing.

<u>Deuteronomy 29:29</u>

"The secret things belong to the LORD our God, but the things revealed belong to us and to our sons forever, that we may observe all the words of this law.

<u>Job 37:15-16</u>

"Do you know how God establishes them, And makes the lightning of His cloud to shine? "Do you know about the layers of the thick clouds, The wonders of one perfect in knowledge.

Daniel 2:22

"It is He who reveals the profound and hidden things; He knows what is in the darkness, And the light dwells with Him.

Matthew 24:36

"But of that day and hour no one knows, not even the angels of heaven, nor the Son, but the Father alone.

Mark 13:32

"But of that day or hour no one knows, not even the angels in heaven, nor the Son, but the Father alone.

Acts 1:7

He said to them, "It is not for you to know times or epochs which the Father has fixed by His own authority;

2 Corinthians 12:2-4

I know a man in Christ who fourteen years ago--whether in the body I do not know, or out of the body I do not know, God knows--such a man was caught up to the third heaven. And I know how such a man--whether in the body or apart from the body I do not know, God knows-- was caught up into Paradise and heard inexpressible words, which a man is not permitted to speak.

Job 34:21

"For His eyes are upon the ways of a man, And He sees all his steps.

Job 24:23

"He provides them with security, and they are supported; And His eyes are on their ways.

Job 31:4

"Does He not see my ways And number all my steps?

Psalm 33:13-15

The LORD looks from heaven; He sees all the sons of men; From His dwelling place He looks out On all the inhabitants of the earth, He who fashions the hearts of them all, He who understands all their works.

Psalm 139:2-3

You know when I sit down and when I rise up; You understand my thought from afar. You scrutinize my path and my lying down, And are intimately acquainted with all my ways.

Jeremiah 23:24

"Can a man hide himself in hiding places So I do not see him?" declares the LORD "Do I not fill the heavens and the earth?" declares the LORD.

Matthew 6:8

"So do not be like them; for your Father knows what you need before you ask Him.

Matthew 6:31-32

"Do not worry then, saying, 'What will we eat?' or 'What will we drink?' or 'What will we wear for clothing?' "For the Gentiles eagerly seek all these things; for your heavenly Father knows that you need all these things.

Luke 12:29-30

"And do not seek what you will eat and what you will drink, and do not keep worrying. "For all these things the nations of the world eagerly seek; but your Father knows that you need these things.

1 Chronicles 28:9

"As for you, my son Solomon, knows the God of your father, and serve Him with a whole heart and a willing mind; for the LORD searches all hearts, and understands every intent of the thoughts If you seek Him, He will let you find Him; but if you forsake Him, He will reject you forever.

Psalm 44:20-21

If we had forgotten the name of our God Or extended our hands to a strange god, Would not God find this out? For He knows the secrets of the heart.

Psalm 139:1-2

O LORD, You have searched me and known me. You know when I sit down and when I rise up; You understand my thought from afar.

Jeremiah 17:10

"I, the LORD, search the heart, I test the mind, Even to give to each man according to his ways, According to the results of his deeds.

Ezekiel 11:5

Then the Spirit of the LORD fell upon me, and He said to me, "Say, 'Thus says the LORD, "So you think, house of Israel, for I know your thoughts.

 MISS ASONDRA STARN'AIR

Hebrews 4:12-13

For the word of God is living and active and sharper than any two-edged sword, and piercing as far as the division of soul and spirit, of both joints and marrow, and able to judge the thoughts and intentions of the heart. And there is no creature hidden from His sight, but all things are open and laid bare to the eyes of Him with whom we have to do.

Jeremiah 16:17

"For My eyes are on all their ways; they are not hidden from My face, nor is their iniquity concealed from My eyes.

Job 10:14

If I sin, then You would take note of me, And would not acquit me of my guilt.

Psalm 69:5

O God, it is You who knows my folly, And my wrongs are not hidden from You.

Jeremiah 2:22

"Although you wash yourself with lye And use much soap, The stain of your iniquity is before Me," declares the Lord GOD.

Hosea 7:2

And they do not consider in their hearts That I remember all their wickedness Now their deeds are all around them; They are before My face.

Amos 5:12

For I know your transgressions are many and your sins are great, You who distress the righteous and accept bribes And turn aside the poor in the gate.

Isaiah 46:10

Declaring the end from the beginning, And from ancient times things which have not been done, Saying, 'My purpose will be established, And I will accomplish all My good pleasure';

Isaiah 42:9

"Behold, the former things have come to pass, Now I declare new things; Before they spring forth I proclaim them to you."

Isaiah 44:7

'Who is like Me? Let him proclaim and declare it; Yes, let him recount it to Me in order, From the time that I established the ancient nation. And let them declare to them the things that are coming And the events that are going to take place.

Daniel 2:28

"However, there is a God in heaven who reveals mysteries, and He has made known to King Nebuchadnezzar what will take place in the latter days This was your dream and the visions in your mind while on your bed.

Acts 2:23

this Man, delivered over by the predetermined plan and foreknowledge of God, you nailed to a cross by the hands of godless men and put Him to death.

 MISS ASONDRA STARN'AIR

Acts 3:18

"But the things which God announced beforehand by the mouth of all the prophets, that His Christ would suffer, He has thus fulfilled.

Acts 4:27-28

"For truly in this city there were gathered together against Your holy servant Jesus, whom You anointed, both Herod and Pontius Pilate, along with the Gentiles and the peoples of Israel, to do whatever Your hand and Your purpose predestined to occur.

Romans 8:29

For those whom He foreknew, He also predestined to become conformed to the image of His Son, so that He would be the firstborn among many brethren;

Jeremiah 1:5

"Before I formed you in the womb I knew you, And before you were born I consecrated you; I have appointed you a prophet to the nations."

Romans 11:2

God has not rejected His people whom He foreknew Or do you not know what the Scripture says in the passage about Elijah, how he pleads with God against Israel?

1 Peter 1:2

according to the foreknowledge of God the Father, by the sanctifying work of the Spirit, to obey Jesus Christ and be sprinkled with His blood: May grace and peace be yours in the fullest measure.

<u>Psalm 139:4</u>

Even before there is a word on my tongue, Behold, O LORD, You know it all.

<u>Exodus 3:19</u>

"But I know that the king of Egypt will not permit you to go, except under compulsion.

<u>Deuteronomy 31:21</u>

"Then it shall come about, when many evils and troubles have come upon them, that this song will testify before them as a witness (for it shall not be forgotten from the lips of their descendants); for I know their intent which they are developing today, before I have brought them into the land which I swore."

<u>Hebrews 4:13</u>

And there is no creature hidden from His sight, but all things are open and laid bare to the eyes of Him with whom we have to do.

<u>1 Samuel 2:3</u>

"Boast no more so very proudly, Do not let arrogance come out of your mouth; For the LORD is a God of knowledge, And with Him actions are weighed.

<u>Job 34:22-23</u>

"There is no darkness or deep shadow Where the workers of iniquity may hide themselves. "For He does not need to consider a man further, That he should go before God in judgment.

Romans 2:16

On the day when, according to my gospel, God will judge the secrets of men through Christ Jesus.

1 Corinthians 4:5

Therefore do not go on passing judgment before the time, but wait until the Lord comes who will both bring to light the things hidden in the darkness and disclose the motives of men's hearts; and then each man's praise will come to him from God.

2 Timothy 2:19

Nevertheless, the firm foundation of God stands, having this seal, "The Lord knows those who are His," and, "Everyone who names the name of the Lord is to abstain from wickedness."

Numbers 16:5

and he spoke to Korah and all his company, saying, "Tomorrow morning the LORD will show who is His, and who is holy, and will bring him near to Himself; even the one whom He will choose, He will bring near to Himself.

Exodus 33:12

Then Moses said to the LORD, "See, You say to me, 'Bring up this people!' But You Yourself have not let me know whom You will send with me Moreover, You have said, 'I have known you by name, and you have also found favor in My sight.'

Job 23:10

"But He knows the way I take; When He has tried me, I shall come forth as gold.

John 10:14

"I am the good shepherd, and I know My own and My own know Me,

Galatians 4:9

But now that you have come to know God, or rather to be known by God, how is it that you turn back again to the weak and worthless elemental things, to which you desire to be enslaved all over again?

1 John 3:19-20

We will know by this that we are of the truth, and will assure our heart before Him in whatever our heart condemns us; for God is greater than our heart and knows all things.

Revelation 3:8

'I know your deeds Behold, I have put before you an open door which no one can shut, because you have a little power, and have kept My word, and have not denied My name.

Proverbs 15:3

The eyes of the LORD are in every place, Watching the evil and the good.

Psalm 11:4

The LORD is in His holy temple; the LORD'S throne is in heaven; His eyes behold, His eyelids test the sons of men.

Jeremiah 11:20

But, O LORD of hosts, who judges righteously, Who tries the feelings and the heart, Let me see Your vengeance on them, For to You have I committed my cause.

　　　Miss Asondra StarN'air

Jeremiah 20:12

Yet, O LORD of hosts, You who test the righteous, Who see the mind and the heart; Let me see Your vengeance on them; For to You I have set forth my cause.

Proverbs 16:2

All the ways of a man are clean in his own sight, But the LORD weighs the motives.

Proverbs 21:2

Every man's way is right in his own eyes, But the LORD weighs the hearts.

Proverbs 24:12

If you say, "See, we did not know this," Does He not consider it who weighs the hearts? And does He not know it who keeps your soul? And will He not render to man according to his work?

Romans 8:27

and He who searches the hearts knows what the mind of the Spirit is, because He intercedes for the saints according to the will of God.

Matthew 6:4

so that your giving will be in secret; and your Father who sees what is done in secret will reward you.

Genesis 16:13

Then she called the name of the LORD who spoke to her, "You are a God who sees"; for she said, "Have I even remained alive here after seeing Him?"

Exodus 3:7

The LORD said, "I have surely seen the affliction of My people who are in Egypt, and have given heed to their cry because of their taskmasters, for I am aware of their sufferings.

Numbers 14:27

"How long shall I bear with this evil congregation who are grumbling against Me? I have heard the complaints of the sons of Israel, which they are making against Me.

Deuteronomy 2:7

"For the LORD your God has blessed you in all that you have done; He has known your wanderings through this great wilderness These forty years the LORD your God has been with you; you have not lacked a thing.'"

1 Samuel 16:7

But the LORD said to Samuel, "Do not look at his appearance or at the height of his stature, because I have rejected him; for God sees not as man sees, for man looks at the outward appearance, but the LORD looks at the heart."

2 Samuel 7:20

"Again what more can David say to You? For You know Your servant, O Lord GOD!

1 Kings 8:39

then hear in heaven Your dwelling place, and forgive and act and render to each according to all his ways, whose heart You know, for You alone know the hearts of all the sons of men,

2 Kings 19:27

'But I know your sitting down, And you're going out and you're coming in, And your raging against Me.

1 Chronicles 29:17

"Since I know, O my God, that You try the heart and delight in uprightness, I, in the integrity of my heart, have willingly offered all these things; so now with joy I have seen Your people, who are present here, make their offerings willingly to You.

2 Chronicles 16:9

"For the eyes of the LORD move to and fro throughout the earth that He may strongly support those whose heart is completely His. You have acted foolishly in this. Indeed, from now on you will surely have wars."

Nehemiah 9:10

"Then You performed signs and wonders against Pharaoh, Against all his servants and all the people of his land; For You knew that they acted arrogantly toward them, And made a name for Yourself as it is this day.

Job 11:11

"For He knows false men, And He sees iniquity without investigating.

Job 12:13

"With Him are wisdom and might; To Him belong counsel and understanding.

Job 12:22

"He reveals mysteries from the darkness And brings the deep darkness into light.

<u>**Job 22:13-14**</u>

"You say, 'What does God know? Can He judge through the thick darkness? 'Clouds are a hiding place for Him, so that He cannot see; And He walks on the vault of heaven.'

<u>**Job 24:1**</u>

"Why are times not stored up by the Almighty, And why do those who know Him not see His days?

<u>**Job 26:6**</u>

"Naked is Sheol before Him, And Abaddon has no covering.

<u>**Job 28:10**</u>

"He hews out channels through the rocks, And his eye sees anything precious.

<u>**Job 28:24**</u>

"For He looks to the ends of the earth And sees everything under the heavens.

<u>**Job 34:21-22**</u>

"For His eyes are upon the ways of a man, And He sees all his steps. "There is no darkness or deep shadow Where the workers of iniquity may hide themselves.

<u>**Job 34:25**</u>

"Therefore He knows their works, And He overthrows them in the night, And they are crushed.

Job 36:4

"For truly my words are not false; One who is perfect in knowledge is with you.

Job 37:16

"Do you know about the layers of the thick clouds, The wonders of one perfect in knowledge,

Job 42:2

"I know that You can do all things, And that no purpose of Yours can be thwarted.

Psalm 1:6

For the LORD knows the way of the righteous, But the way of the wicked will perish.

Psalm 10:11

He says to himself, "God has forgotten; He has hidden His face; He will never see it."

Psalm 37:18

The LORD knows the days of the blameless, And their inheritance will be forever.

Psalm 38:9

Lord, all my desire is before You; And my sighing is not hidden from You.

Psalm 44:21

Would not God find this out? For He knows the secrets of the heart.

Psalm 66:7

He rules by His might forever; His eyes keep watch on the nations; Let not the rebellious exalt themselves. Selah.

Psalm 69:19

You know my reproach and my shame and my dishonor; All my adversaries are before You.

Psalm 73:11

They say, "How does God know? And is there knowledge with the Most High?"

Psalm 92:5

How great are Your works, O LORD! Your thoughts are very deep.

Psalm 94:9-11

He who planted the ear, does He not hear? He who formed the eye, does He not see? He who chastens the nations, will He not rebuke, Even He who teaches man knowledge? The LORD knows the thoughts of man, That they are a mere breath.

Psalm 103:14

For He Himself knows our frame; He is mindful that we are but dust.

Psalm 104:24

O LORD, how many are Your works! In wisdom You have made

Psalm 119:168

I keep Your precepts and Your testimonies, For all my ways are before You.

 Miss Asondra StarN'air

Psalm 121:3-4

He will not allow your foot to slip; He who keeps you will not slumber.

Behold, He who keeps Israel Will neither slumber nor sleep.

Psalm 136:5

To Him who made the heavens with skill, For His lovingkindness is everlasting;

Psalm 139:1-4

O LORD, You have searched me and known me. You know when I sit down and when I rise up; You understand my thought from afar. You scrutinize my path and my lying down, And are intimately acquainted with all my ways. *read more.*

Psalm 139:6

Such knowledge is too wonderful for me; It is too high, I cannot attain to it.

Psalm 139:12

Even the darkness is not dark to You, And the night is as bright as the day Darkness and light are alike to You.

Psalm 139:14-16

I will give thanks to You, for I am fearfully and wonderfully made; Wonderful are Your works, And my soul knows it very well. My frame was not hidden from You, When I was made in secret, And skillfully wrought in the depths of the earth; Your eyes have seen my unformed substance; And in Your book were all written The days that were ordained for me, When as yet there was not one of them.

<u>Psalm 142:3</u>

When my spirit was overwhelmed within me, You knew my path In the way where I walk They have hidden a trap for me.

<u>Psalm 147:4-5</u>

He counts the number of the stars; He gives names to all of them. Great is our Lord and abundant in strength; His understanding is infinite.

<u>Proverbs 3:19-20</u>

The LORD by wisdom founded the earth, By understanding He established the heavens. By His knowledge the deeps were broken up And the skies drip with dew.

<u>Proverbs 5:21</u>

For the ways of a man are before the eyes of the LORD, And He watches all his paths.

<u>Proverbs 15:11</u>

Sheol and Abaddon lie open before the LORD, How much more the hearts of men!

<u>Proverbs 17:3</u>

The refining pot is for silver and the furnace for gold, But the LORD tests hearts.

<u>Isaiah 28:29</u>

This also comes from the LORD of hosts, Who has made His counsel wonderful and His wisdom great.

Isaiah 29:15-16

Woe to those who deeply hide their plans from the LORD, And whose deeds are done in a dark place, And they say, "Who sees us?" or "Who knows us?" You turn things around! Shall the potter be considered as equal with the clay, That what is made would say to its maker, "He did not make me"; Or what is formed say to him who formed it, "He has no understanding"?

Isaiah 37:28

"But I know your sitting down And you're going out and you're coming in And your raging against Me.

Isaiah 40:27-28

Why do you say, O Jacob, and assert, O Israel, "My way is hidden from the LORD, And the justice due me escapes the notice of my God"? Do you not know? Have you not heard? The Everlasting God, the LORD, the Creator of the ends of the earth Does not become weary or tired His understanding is inscrutable.

Isaiah 41:4

"Who has performed and accomplished it, Calling forth the generations from the beginning? 'I, the LORD, am the first, and with the last I am He.'"

Isaiah 45:4

"For the sake of Jacob My servant, And Israel My chosen one, I have also called you by your name; I have given you a title of honor Though you have not known Me.

Isaiah 48:5-6

Therefore I declared them to you long ago, Before they took place I proclaimed them to you, So that you would not say, 'My idol has done them, And my graven image and my molten image have commanded them.' "You have heard; look at all this. And you, will you not declare it? I proclaim to you new things from this time, Even hidden things which you have not known.

Isaiah 66:18

"For I know their works and their thoughts; the time is coming to gather all nations and tongues. And they shall come and see My glory.

Jeremiah 5:3

O LORD, do not Your eyes look for truth? You have smitten them, But they did not weaken; You have consumed them, But they refused to take correction They have made their faces harder than rock; They have refused to repent.

Jeremiah 10:7

Who would not fear You, O King of the nations? Indeed it is Your due! For among all the wise men of the nations And in all their kingdoms, There is none like You.

Jeremiah 32:19

great in counsel and mighty in deed, whose eyes are open to all the ways of the sons of men, giving to everyone according to his ways and according to the fruit of his deeds;

Jeremiah 51:15

It is He who made the earth by His power, Who established the world by His wisdom, And by His understanding He stretched out the heavens.

Ezekiel 9:9

Then He said to me, "The iniquity of the house of Israel and Judah is very, very great, and the land is filled with blood and the city is full of perversion; for they say, 'The LORD has forsaken the land, and the LORD does not see!'

Daniel 2:20

Daniel said, "Let the name of God be blessed forever and ever, For wisdom and power belong to Him.

God See and Know Everything!

See, I Told "You" God is All knowing!

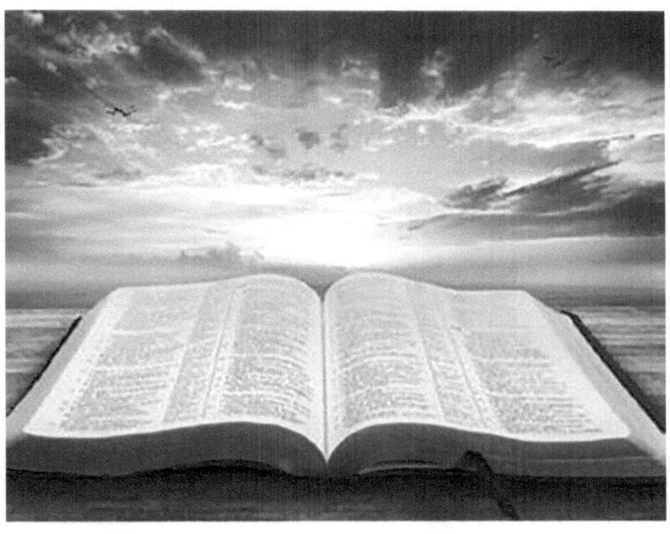

SECTION III

Live Daily

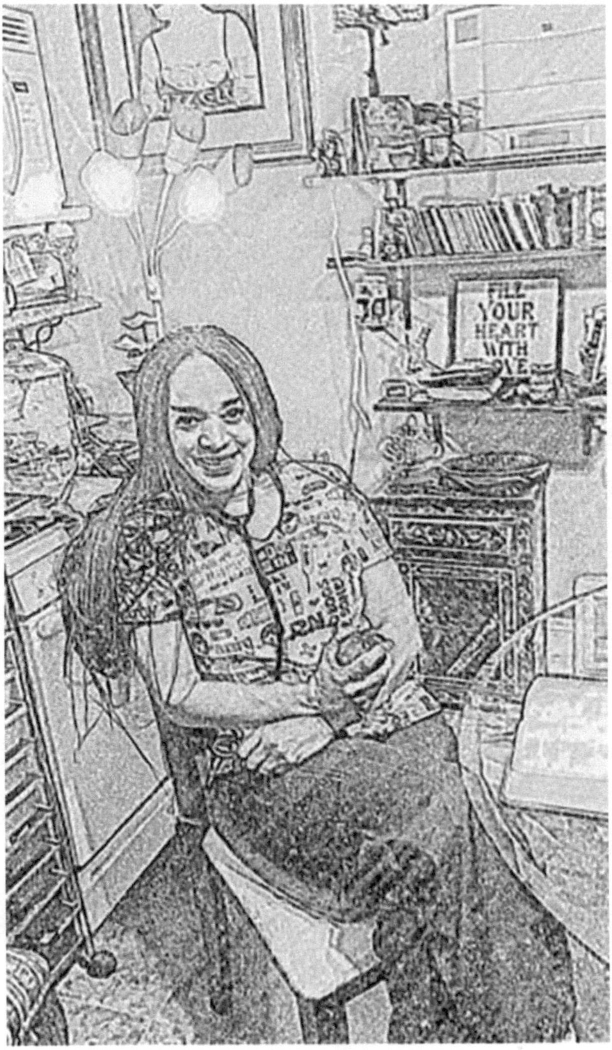

Caregiver's Proverbs

A Proverb A Day, Keeps Negativity Away!

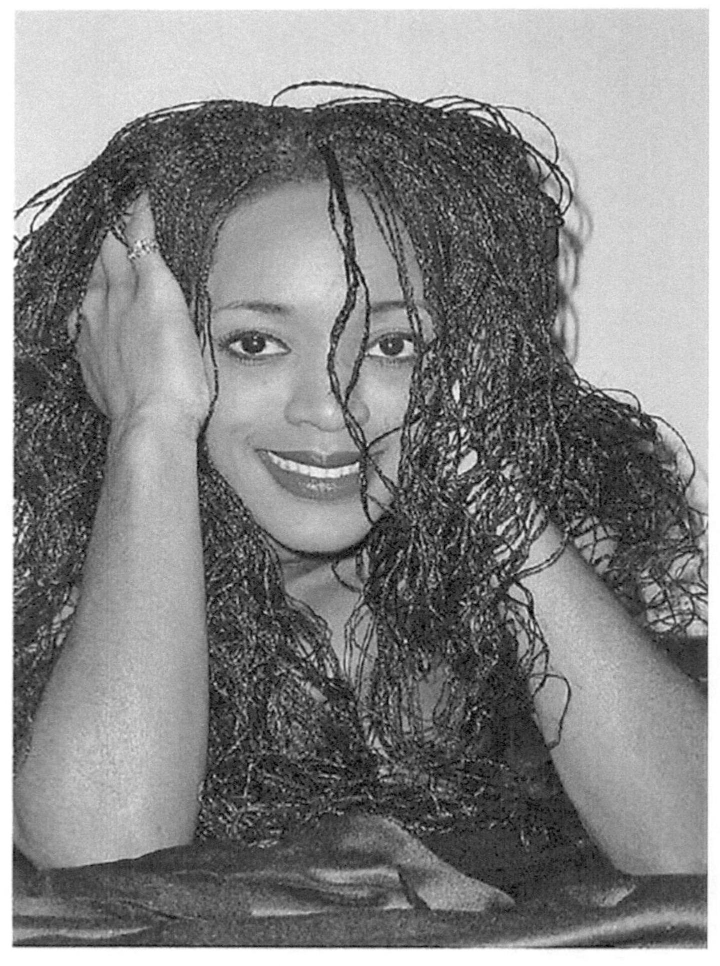

 Miss Asondra StarN'air

31 Caregivers Proverbs

One a Day Vitamins for your Mind, Body and Soul!

A Caregiver's Bible To Excellence!

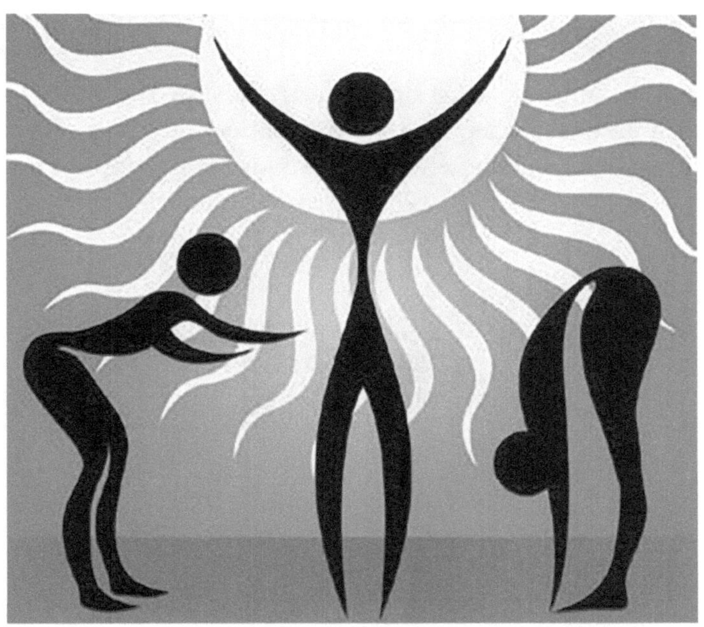

Day 1

Work hard and become a leader, be lazy and never succeed.

If you are going to be a leader, you must be dedicated and committed.

Not lazy, watching others do all the work while you watch or put your feet up.

A wise caregiver is an excellent worker even when the boss is not around.

Smart people continue to educate themselves all the time, some go back to school while others keep getting better and better at what they already love to do. But those who are lazy opens the door to poverty.

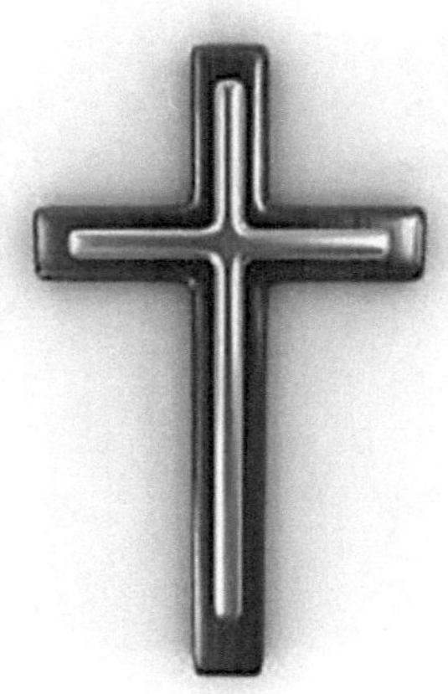

31 Proverbs 12:19

Day 2

Trust stands the test of time; lies are soon exposed!

It's just a matter of time, before an individual true self comes out, many times it shows in the attitudes, work ethics and how we treat other people. Are you really the person you say you are? A lot of people have great resumes, charming personalities, educated with degrees you name it "they've got it all".

But beware, have you ever seen a fake fall? God exposes them one by one, no matter how short or tall.

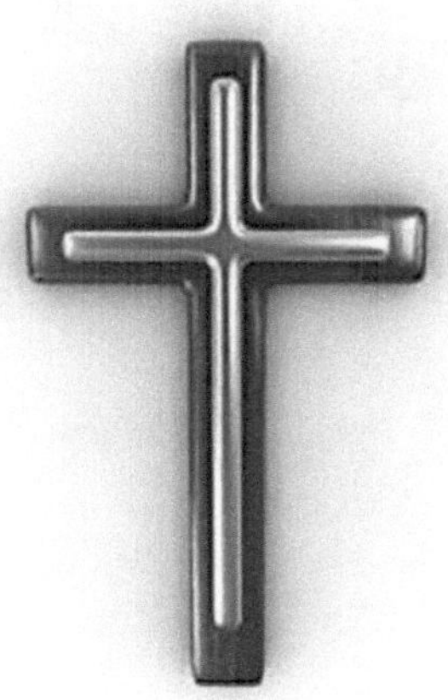

Day 3

Wickedness never brings stability; only the godly have deep roots.

You shall reap what you sow! I don't understand, tell me why can't you love your fellow man? Don't you know if you get stranded, you'll need his helping hand. Stop scheming and being untrue, Go to God for a new heart, that's the first place you start! For he knows what goes on in the light and in the dark! Doctor's order, **"A NEW HEART"**!

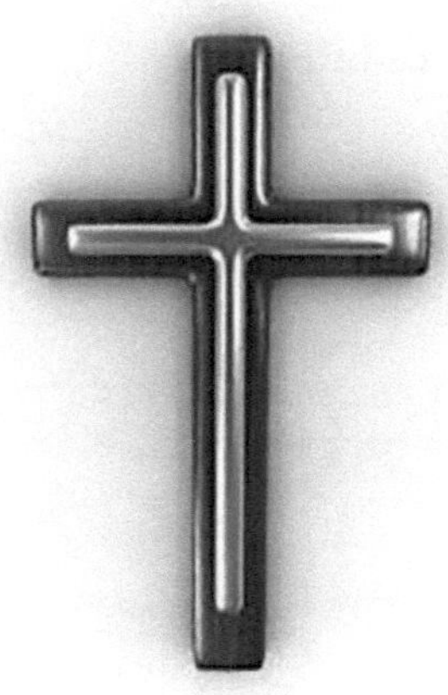

31 **P**roverbs 12:15

Day 4

A fool think he need no advice, but a wise man listens to others.

Constructive criticism from a leader, or true friend can help soar you to the top if you're wise enough to listen.

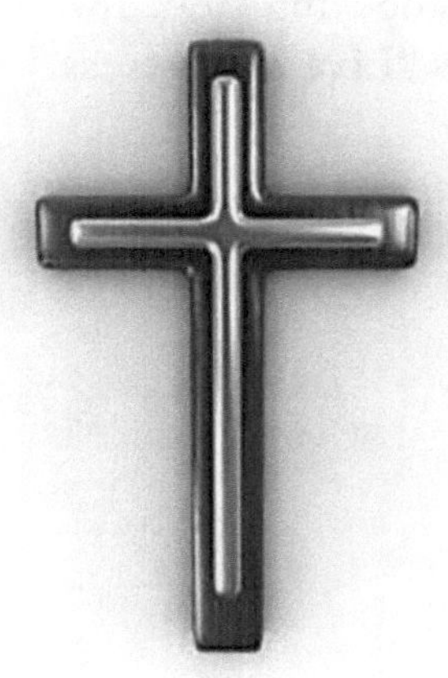

Day 5

Despise God's word and find yourself in trouble, obey it and succeed.

A life without Christ is doom, I see it every afternoon. Too, Fools never play by the rules all they want to do is cruise. People don't you know, living righteous lives and obeying God, always, always, always leads to success. Despise *His ways* **"Live in Distress."**

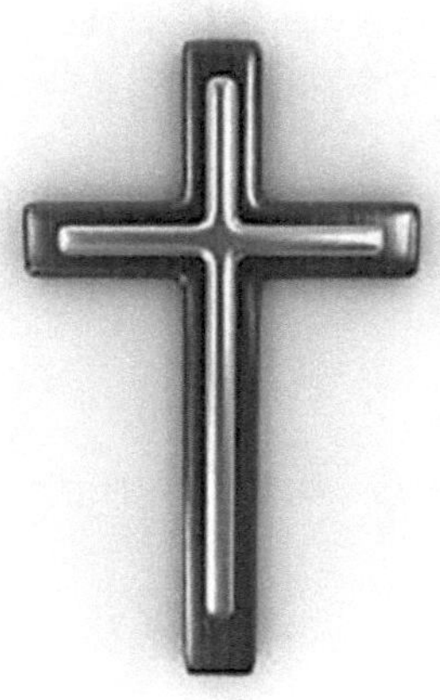

Day 6

An unreliable messenger can cause a lot of trouble, reliable communication permits progress.

Just stay away for gossipers; the truth is not in them. Better yet, if you must know, go find out for yourself. You gather the information.

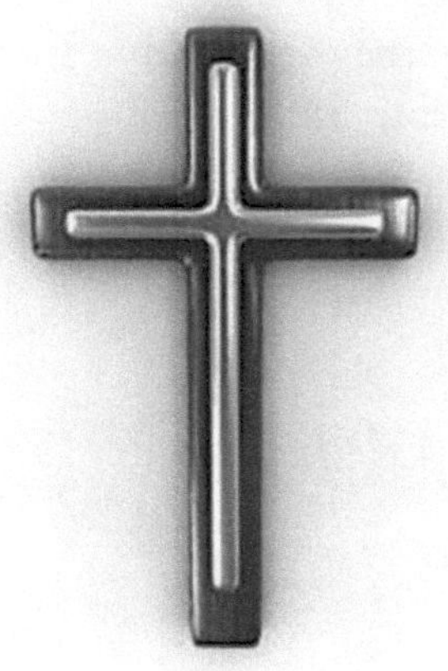

Proverbs 14:7

Day 7

If you are looking for advice, stay away from fools.

Let's take it a step further, don't even eat with them! The Bible says and it is written in 1 Corinthians 5:11 do not associate with anyone who claims to be a brother or a sister but is sexually immoral or greedy, an idolater or slanderer, a drunkard or swindler. You say, what does this have to do with fools? If their into all that, what makes you think they have your back. And too, they've already turned their backs on God it doesn't get more foolish than that!

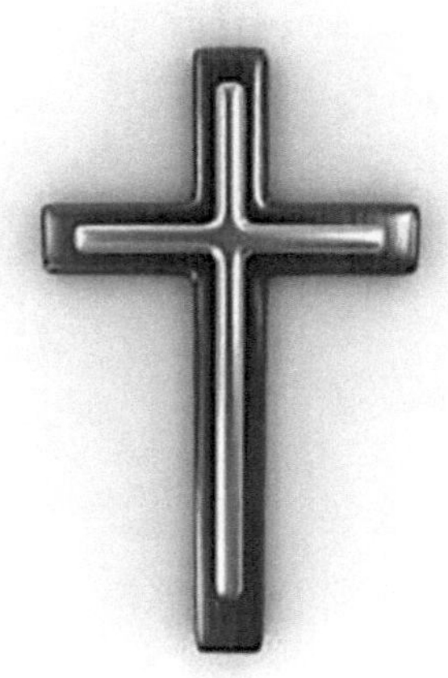

     Miss Asondra StarN'air

31 Proverbs 14:31

Day 8

Anyone who oppresses the poor is insulting God who made them, to help the poor, is to honor God.

This scripture talks about the poor, but if anyone is helpless or sick out there, I do believe God wants us to help take care of them as well, don't you? Of course you do, if you have a **'HEART!'** Well then, today, that's where we'll start. It's simple, To honor God and to show you care, help somebody, be there, don't abandon them or leave them in the dark.

HAVE A HEART!
Don't Have A Heart, Get A Heart,
Can't Get A Heart, Build A Heart!
Studying the **Word of God** is a start!

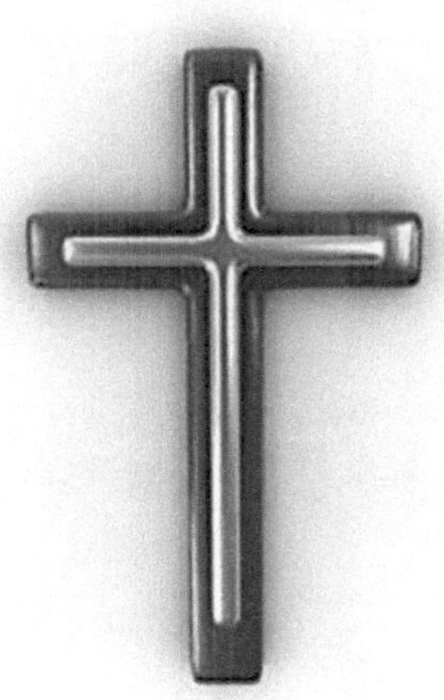

31 Proverbs 15:6

Day 9

There is treasure in being good, but trouble dogs the wicked.

It's dog them all day and night long, you may think you got away with what you did to that other caregiver, talked about that person behind their backs even tried to get them fired, and perhaps you did. But your wicked and evil ways will not go unpunished!

Here's a warning to the evil hearts out there, just when you least expect it, trouble is going to track you down, vengeance is mine says the LORD! Some of you out there might be paying for it right now, no blessings seems to be coming your way, nothing but trouble and heartache, why? I'll tell you why, because ain't nothing good coming out of a person's life who makes trouble for others "Absolutely Nothing"!

Repent, Repent, Repent, In Jesus name, Repent! Take a look in the mirror, and make that change, before it's too late, and one day it will be too late!

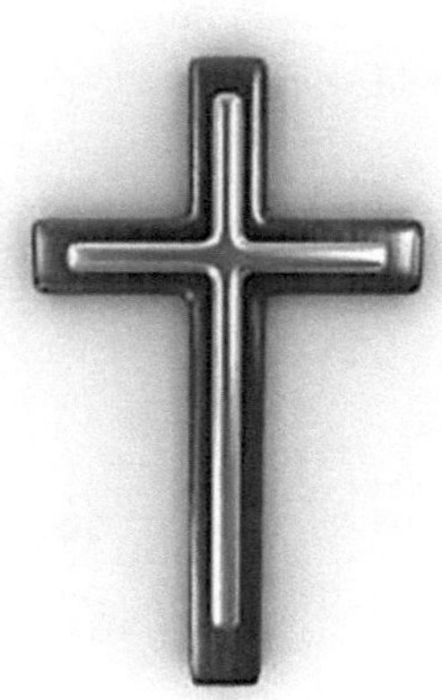

 Miss Asondra StarN'air

31 Proverbs 15:1

Day 10

A gentle answer turns away wrath, but harsh words cause quarrels.

"Listen up" next time there is a misunderstanding, be gentle and kind with one another, just say I'm sorry I miss understood what you were saying, please forgive me. **"And get some rest"** sometimes we're just over worked and perhaps tired too and many times that too can affect our attitudes. "you're not you", you're the worn out you! Here's what to do: clue! **A gentle answer turns away wrath,** have a sense of humor, don't quarrel, work it out, **"Laugh!"**

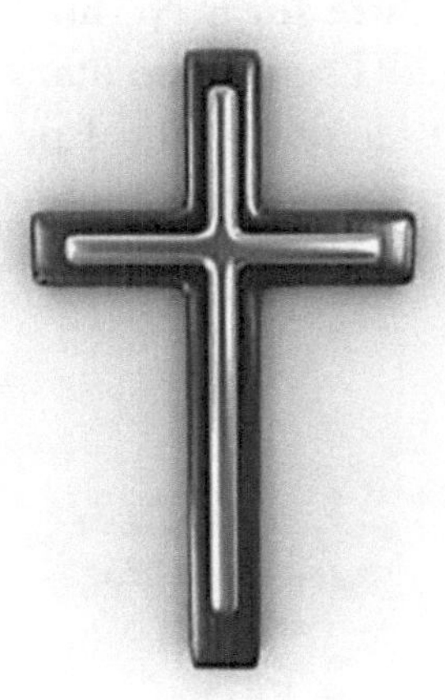

31 Proverbs 15:13

Day 11

A happy face means a glad heart, a sad face means a breaking heart.

So Caregivers, put on a **"Happy Face"** and smile though your heart is aching, smile even though it's breaking, When there are clouds in the sky you'll get by… These are lyrics to an old Charlie Chapin song, but very appropriate here indeed.

In life we are all going to experience what the bible calls "trials and tribulations" but, God's says **"This Too Shall Pass"** or how about this one: **"Weeping May Endure for a Night, But Joy Cometh in the Morning"** how about that! There are so many scripture in the bible to help turn your frown upside down, and I promise you this, that can really, really happen if you keep God around!

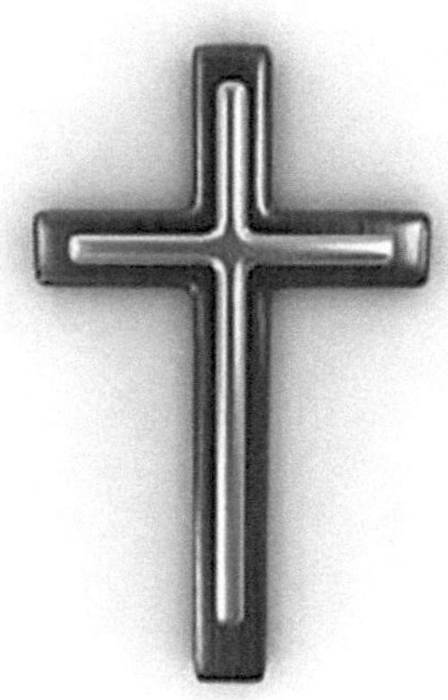

     Miss Asondra StarN'air

31 Proverbs 14:35

Day 12

A king rejoices in servants who know what they are doing; he is angry with those who cause trouble.

Caregivers, stay focus on your task, stay far away from trouble makers, pray for them but, keep it moving, Just say hi and bye!

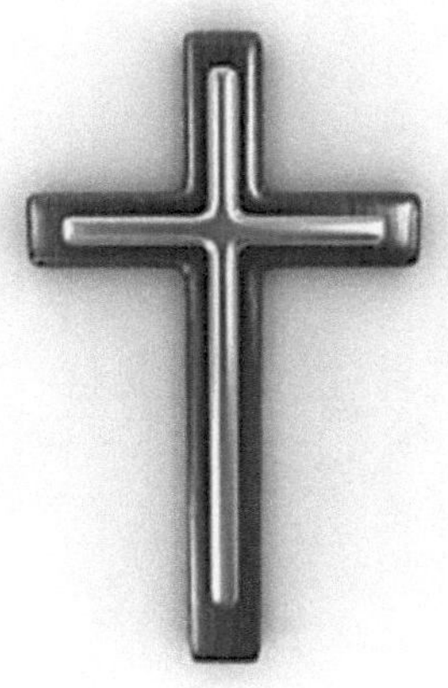

31 Proverbs 16:3

Day 13

Commit your work to the Lord, then it will succeed.

If the Lord's not in it, don't begin it!

Stop chasing the wrong things in life. Seek God's advice. Don't end up like ah candle in the wind never knowing who to cling to" Pray before you proceed. Stay close to **GOD**. He knows the plans he has for you, **READ!**

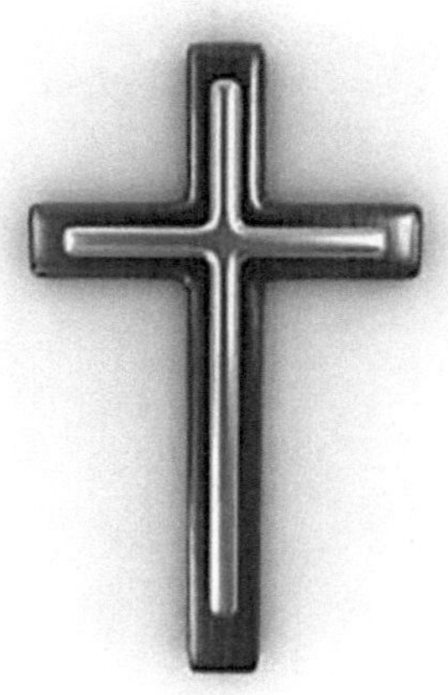

 Miss Asondra StarN'air

31 Proverbs 15:15

Day 14

When a man is gloomy, everything seems to go wrong; when he is cheerful, everything goes right!

How true this is indeed! So what is that telling us caregivers? Don't bring your problems to work, leave them behind or at the door. Better yet, cast your cares on the Lord, ***"Come to me, all you who are weary and burden, and I will give you rest.*** Matthew 11:28.

So, there you have it, Jesus says, come to him, not everybody else, for they can not do what Jesus can do. Remember, He's the savior of the world, Jesus is our healer, our help in times of trouble, and he's also our protector and so much more, when you read the bible you will be aston-ished by all the promises that awaits his people. Besides, Jesus does not want his caregivers filled with gloom, especially since we're told he's coming back soon, Therefore, **Be Strong and Keep on Keeping on!** And If you get tired or thirsty, "gear up"put some **Jesus in your Cup!**

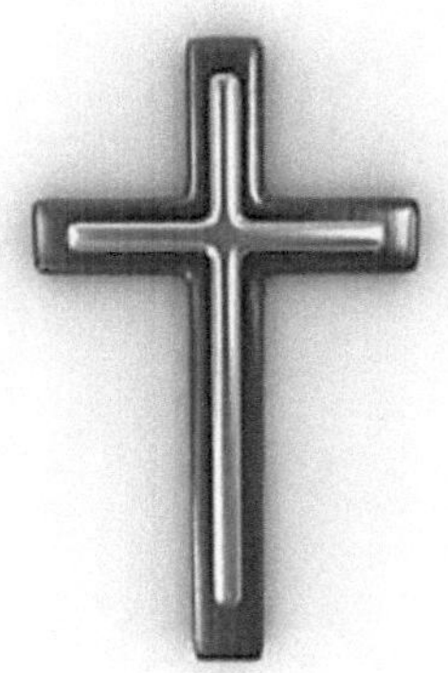

Day 15

A quick tempered man starts fights; a cool tempered man tries to stop them.

The best way to deal with a quick tempered person, is to stay far away from them, because anything can set them off!

Always pray for peace, you never know who you may reach!

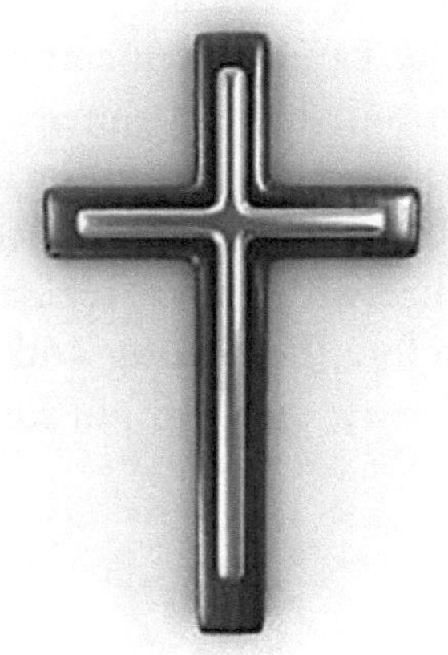

31 **P**roverbs 15:19

Day 16

A **Lazy fellow has trouble all through life; the good man's path is easy!**

Listen up **"Everybody, Everywhere"** If **"You"** don't work, **"You Don't Eat"** and don't study, you won't be approved.

So get off you butt, don't be a fool

No body owes you anything

Anything worth having is worth fighting for

Laziness will not open doors

Skills and Education makes life much easier

Unless you want to be poor

Get up, find a Job, head out the door

Don't go around begging anymore, If **"You"** don't work **"You Don't Eat!"**

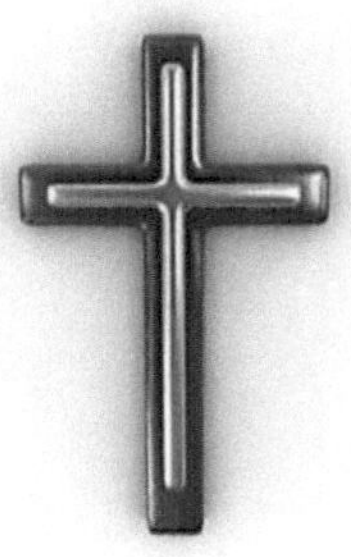

Proverbs 16:24

Day 17

Kind words are like honey- enjoyable and healthful.

Notice this scripture does not say helpful, it says "healthful"

That means we should take a spoonful of kindness everyday to help keep the doctors and Satan away too!

Besides if you don't have anything nice to say do these 3 things:
Zip It! Be Quite! Go Away!

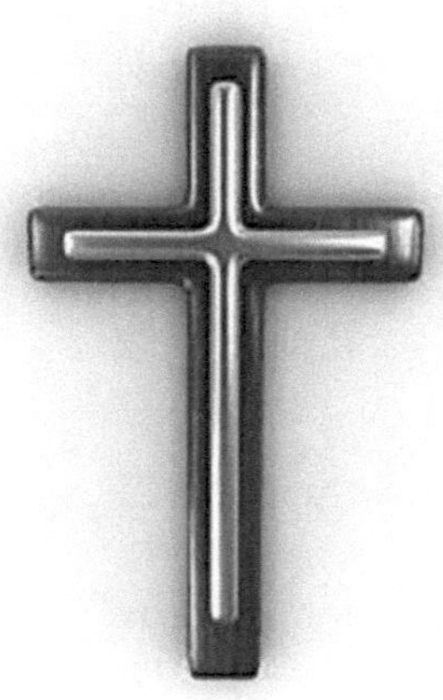

Day 18

Love forgets mistakes; nagging about them parts the best of friends.

No one is perfect, no one and no one is without sin, no one, even those who strive for excellence, like me and you, we still fall short. People make mistakes however we do not need to be reminded of it all the time or be gossiped about behind our backs!

"Just stop it" stop it right now "And get back to work"! Kind words feels good, haven't you heard! When we are not kind to other, we ruin our own reputations.

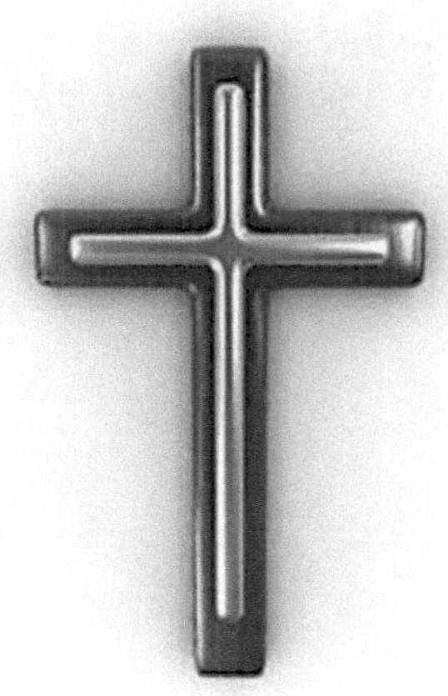

 # Proverbs 17:16

Day 19

It is senseless to pay tuition to educate a rebel who has no heart for truth.

Save your money and time, don't invest in a "Wicked Caregiver"

Trouble follows them everywhere they go. If they ask to have lunch with you, Say **NOOO**, with ah Triple **OOO! NOOO Thank You!**

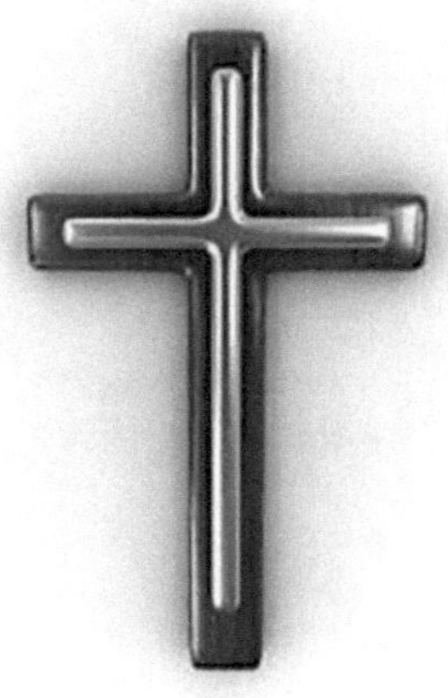

31 Proverbs 17:20

Day 20

A evil man is suspicious of everyone and tumbles into constant trouble.

Have you ever met an employee who has something bad to say about everybody, always suspicious, or ridicules and taunts and mock other co-workers, constantly trying to dig up garbage on someone, just plain old nosy and meddlesome? Well I have and what I have discovered, and soon you will too, their vibe is bad for you. Lord have mercy! Teasing sarcasm, chaff, abortive wickedness at its core.

Pray for them and hope you don't get assigned the same floor!

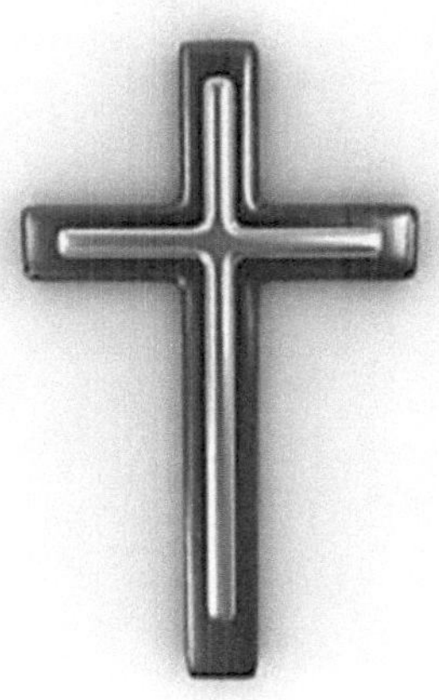

31 Proverbs 17:13

Day 21

If you repay good with evil, evil will never leave your house.

You will always have trouble if you are mean to those who are good to you. Stop taking love and kindness for granted. **"HELLO"** are you listening out there? The world is full of great caregivers, become one!

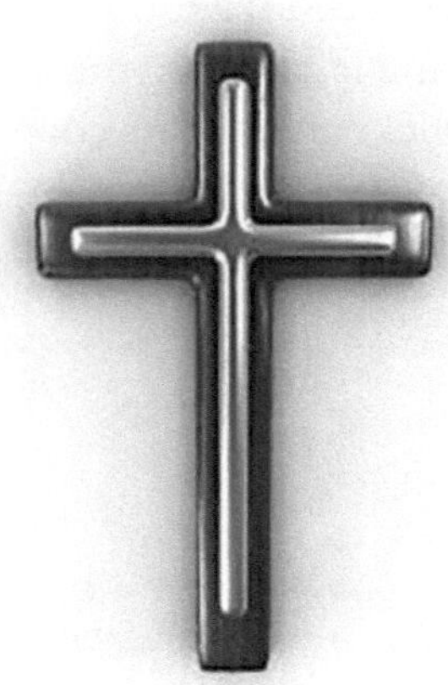

     MISS ASONDRA STARN'AIR

Day 22

The man of few words and settled mind is wise; therefore, even a fool is thought to be wise when he keeps his silent. It pays him to keep his mouth shut.

Too much talking, is just no good anyway. Next thing you know, you are gossiping about others, and that's not good, that's not God!

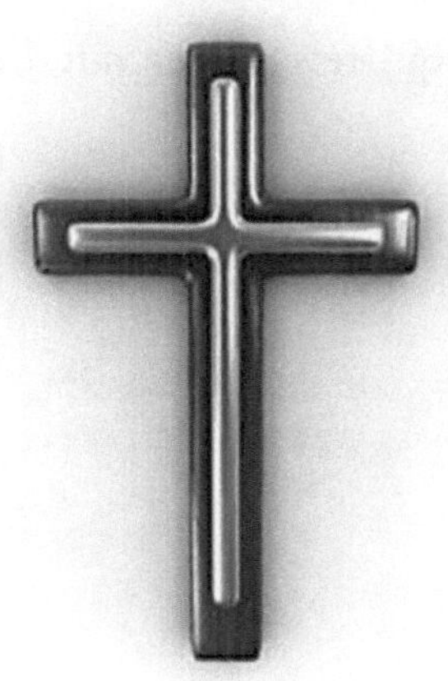

31 Proverbs 17:14

Day 23

It is hard to stop a quarrel once it starts, so don't let it happen.

Caregivers if you have a problem, go to God first, talk to him about it, ask him for advice, or just cast all your cares on him. That's what I do, because if I try to fix it, I'm going to mess it up, and you too. Therefore, stop, walk away, like a kid, go outside and play! Arguing back and forth is not worth all the stress and upset.

Besides quarrels are for squirrels, have a nut, be quite **"Shut Up"**

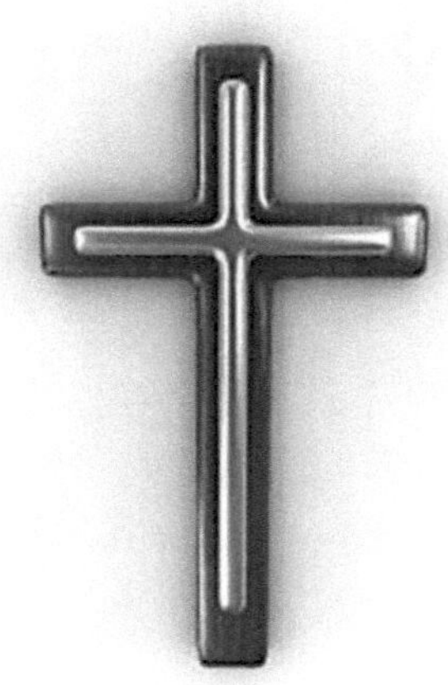

31 Proverbs 16:2

Day 24

People may be pure in their own eyes, but the Lord examines their motives.

Caregivers, I have a question, why did you choose to go into the health-care industry? Be truthful!

____

____

____

It is my hope that you are a caregiver that desires to make a real difference in the world of care-giving. That you want to be used by God to do wonderful things in people's lives. And that you will wholeheartedly serve those in your care well, including the rest of the healthcare team. If this is **"YOU"** then follow your dreams, **God** has planned some good things!!!!!!!

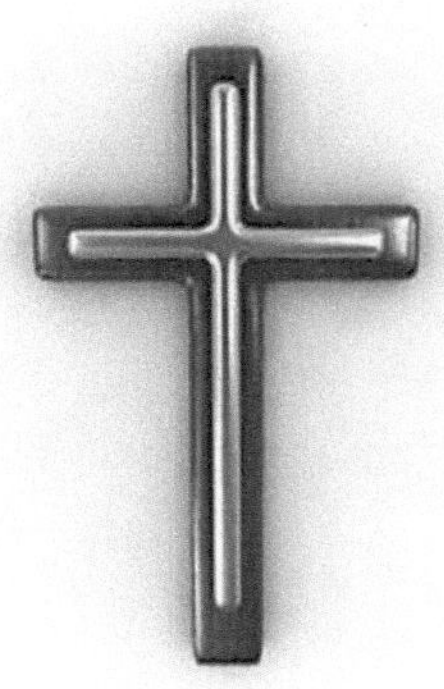

Day 25

We can gather our thoughts but the Lord gives the right answer.

That's right the Lord gives the right answer and his answer is this:

Love No Matter What!

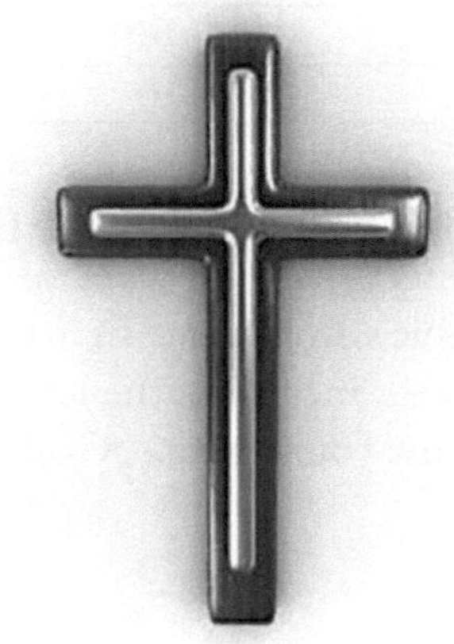

31 Proverbs 15:10

Day 25

Whoever abandons the right path will surely be punished; whoever hates correction will die.

No one's exempt, your Idols included! Hollywood is filled with early deaths and destructions. There's only two paths one that leads to everlasting life and one that makes the devil laugh!

Once **"YOU"** know the truth and turn your back on it, **"YOU"** are playing a dangerous game with **'YOUR'** life. God is no respecter of persons, star or no star!

"Think Twice, Live Right!"

Choose ye this star or no star, sinning against God will not get you far! day whom you will server
Joshua 24:14

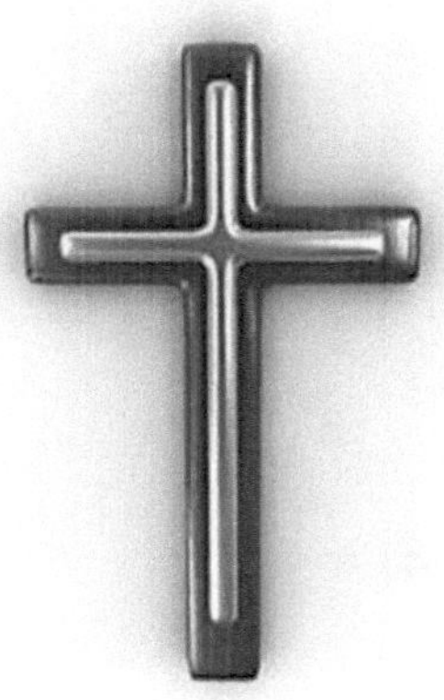

Day 26

A worthless witness cares nothing for the truth-he enjoys his sinning too much.

Today we live in a world where anything goes, people want to be free to do their own thing and can care less about morales or ethics. Many just want to have fun and some want to use their brains, e.g. climb the ladder, get ahead in life but **"Without Christ."**

Isaiah 5:20-21 says, in this dark and evil world we live in today,

Right is Wrong and Wrong is the Right!

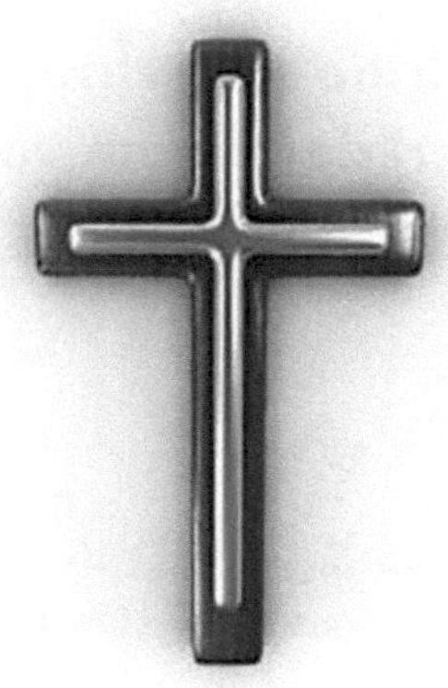

<h1 style="text-align:center">31 Proverbs 20:20</h1>

Day 27

Get all the advice you can and be wise the rest of your life.

Caregivers, humble thyself, don't be a know it all, else you won't grow to reach your full potential. Surround yourself with people who live for the Lord and are going places. Walk away from foolish conversations, don't stay and become two-faced! Learn to respect wisdom, so wisdom can respect you.

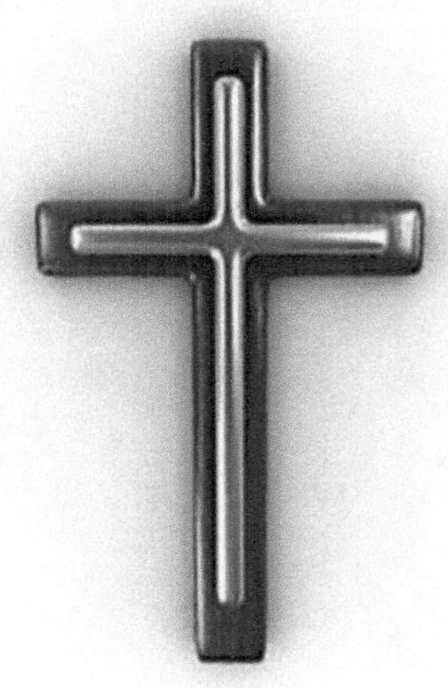

Day 28

The road of the godly leads upward, leaving hell behind.

Come from among them simply means get out of "The World" before we end up in hell!

Caregivers, Jesus is calling, he says, **"Pick up your cross and follow me!"** Matthew 16:24

To be born again is another way we **"Leave Ourselves Behind."**

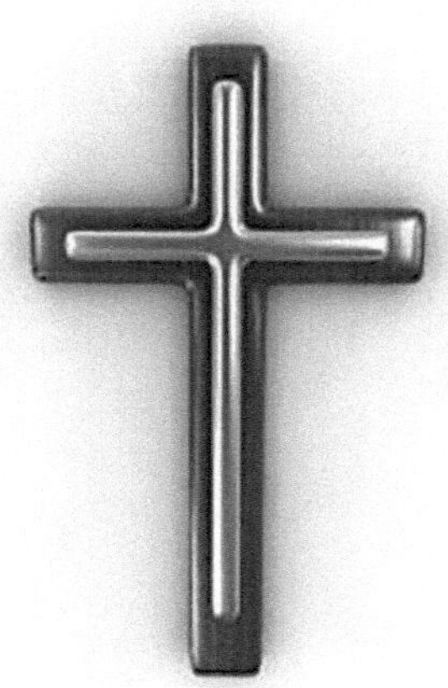

Day 29

When a man is trying to please God, God makes even his worst enemies to be at peace with him.

Just keep on keeping on with God, Stay **Faithful** and **Obedient** and watch **God** have your enemies eating out of the palm of your hands.

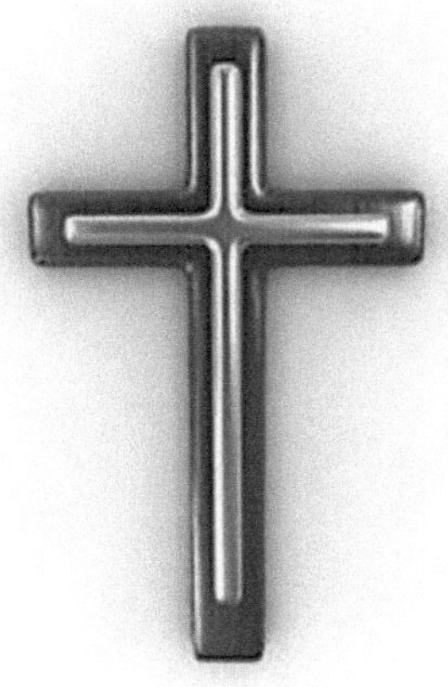

Proverbs 30:5

Day 30

Every word of God is pure; He is a shield to those who put their trust in him.

God rewards the faithful and he will never let us fall; he will help us through it all!

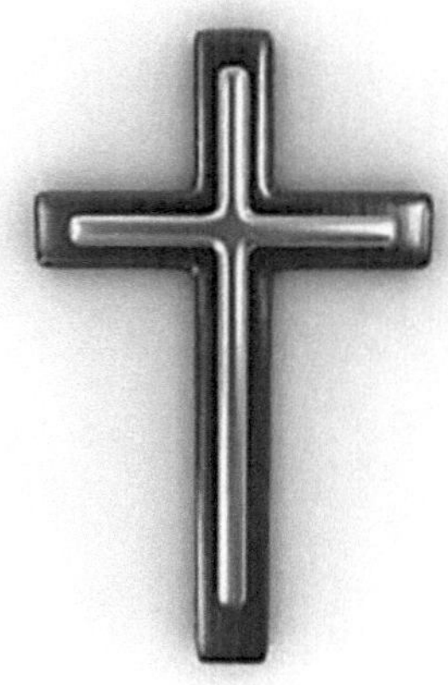

31 Proverbs 16:12

Day 31

It is a horrible thing for a king to do evil, his right to rule depends on his fairness.

Corrupt leaders, will pay a hefty price in the end for hurting God's people!

You know who you are and so does God. **"YOU"** will not go un-punished, Repent!

You may be on top now, but you shall not stay on top! Every wicked ruler drops!

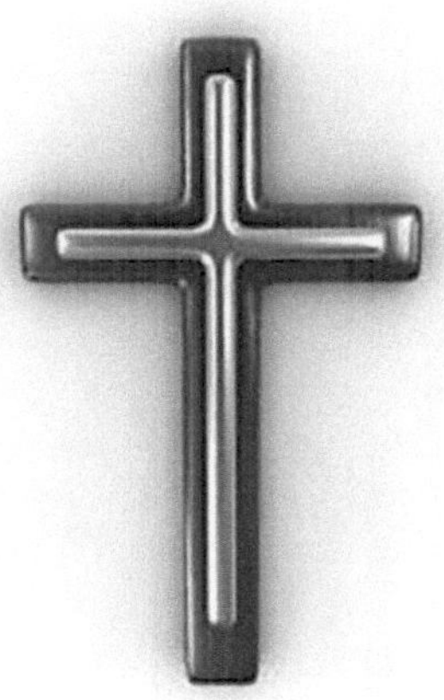

SECTION IV

Caregiver's Tool Boxes

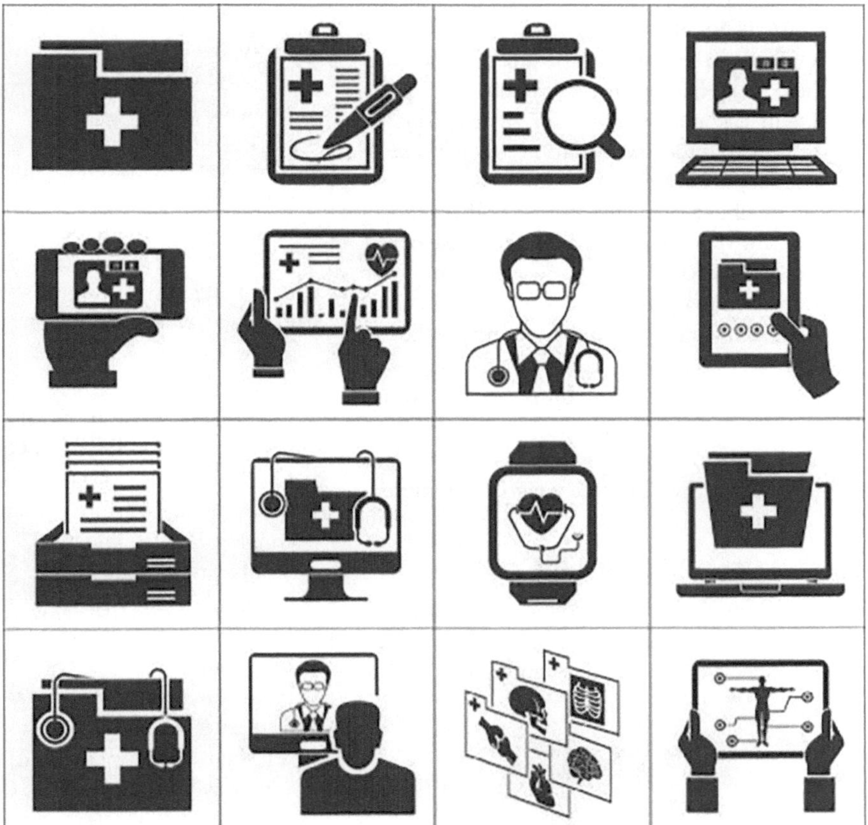

Abuse Pledge for Caregivers

- I will not allow those in my care to hit me.
- I will tell them "It's wrong"!
- I will asks the individual to stop.
- I will not provide personal care until abuse stops, this is for my own protection and theirs.
- I will reassure the person that I am going to take excellent care of their needs and help provide a safe environment for both of us but abuse is not allowed.
- I will take the necessary breaks in between to help bring balance to the situation.
- I will ask management for instructions on how to handle the situation when those in my care are abusive.
- If the abuse does not stop, I will no longer care for that particular person. Abuse of any kind is **WRONG** and must be dealt with by the management team. Caregivers don't come to work to get punched, hit, kicked or spit on.
- My environment has to be a safe place for me to work in at all times.
- I will love and pray for those who hurt other people, but I will not be a victim anymore.

Bottom Line

'Abuse is Abuse' and anyone who does it must be stopped. No one should have to go to work and get abused, especially the caregiver, enough is enough!

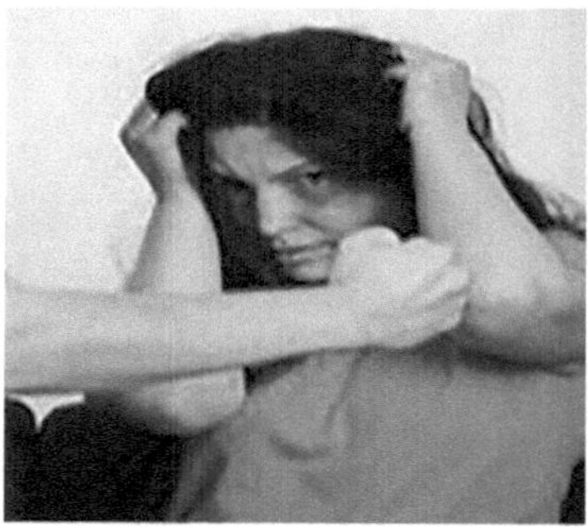

CAREGIVER ABUSE

1. Don't argue with the person.
2. Shift the conversation.
3. Ask, how can I please you?
4. Show me how you want things done
5. Excuse, yourself if it's safe to do so, take a bathroom break and breathe, ask God to help, go back out and start again.
6. Wait, let them talk, you listen. Be humble.
7. Come up with something creative to do with them.
8. If nothing is working, just do your work, give them space and time to cool down.
9. Don't ever take it abuse personal But, **"REPORT IT"**.
10. Ask for help from your company or if you are a family care provider, take a break, use respite care.
11. Document the behaviors times and dates.
12. If the caregiver abuse does not get resolved come off that assignment and contact your ombudsman.

"Caregivers Matter"!

Accepting What Is

Accepting what is, can be the new game changer in just about any person's life, especially for those growing older and older. Growing old does not have to be so rough or depressing.

With the help of family members, friends and caregivers, life can still be full of adventure and joy.

All it takes is a great attitude toward **"Accepting What Is"** and a willingness to be open to try new things.

That's where we come in, lets show them how to have fun again! All we have to do is come up with activities or something that engages their curiosity and gives them a reason to get out of bed every day.

If they are bedbound, yet alert and oriented, you are not off the hook. Get creative, stay creative too, find something you can do together to make the day more enjoyable. look at some images together, watch a movie, play cards, share laughter!

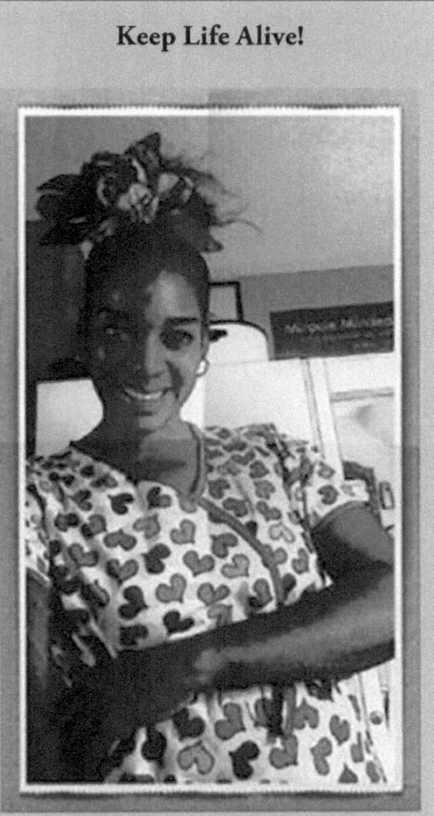

Caregivers it is our responsibility to make sure those in our care especially seniors do not give up hope lets help them keep life alive!

When we do things like this we are gradually aiding them into the mind set of "Accepting What Is" and when this happens, magic happens too.

Suddenly things start to come alive, like stars in the sky, no longer asking God why? Finally they're learned to **"Accept What Is"** Fact of life, **"Everybody Gets Old",** it is written, All go to the same place, all come from dust and to dust all returns. **Ecclesiastes 3:20**

But in the meantime, there is still a lot of living to do. Caregivers we play a vital role in helping them to reach that state of mind. We should never let those in our care, especially seniors give up hope or fall into depression 'Never'.

Get with this, Life isn't over because we're getting older. Oh, no on the contrary, **"Getting Older Is Getting Bolder!"**

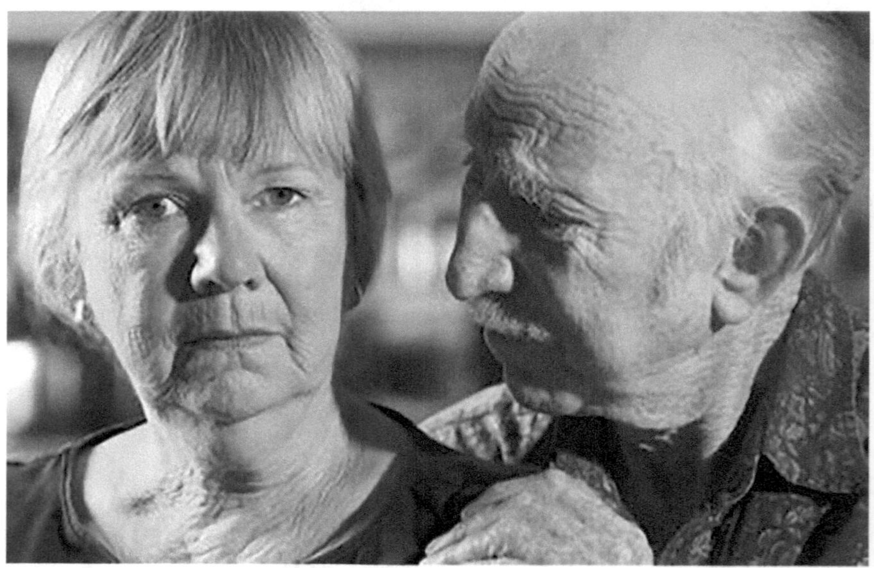

Come On, Let's Go Wheel Chair Bowling!

No matter what age or condition, we owe it to ourselves to live the best life possible. And with God all things are possible!

       MISS ASONDRA STARN'AIR

Acrylic Long Nails

N- Not
A- Allowed
I- In
L- Long-Term Care or Facilities
S- Settings.

Clean hands are the single most important factor in preventing the spread of germs.

Wearing artificial fingernails increases the risk of germs because pathogens now have a place to hide—under the nails.

Professional Caregivers do not wear artificial nails and keep their real nails trimmed low.

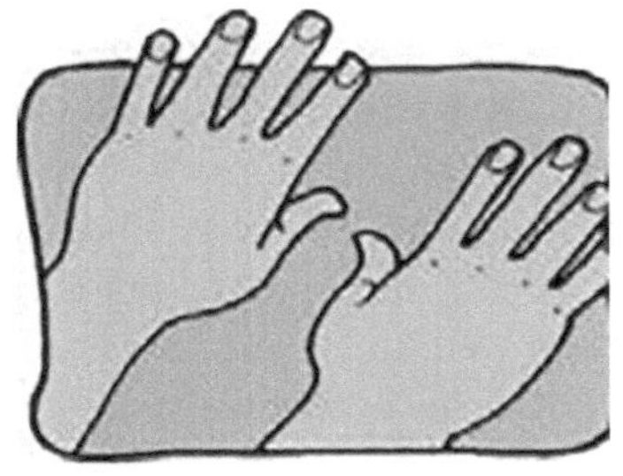

Good Nail Hygiene!

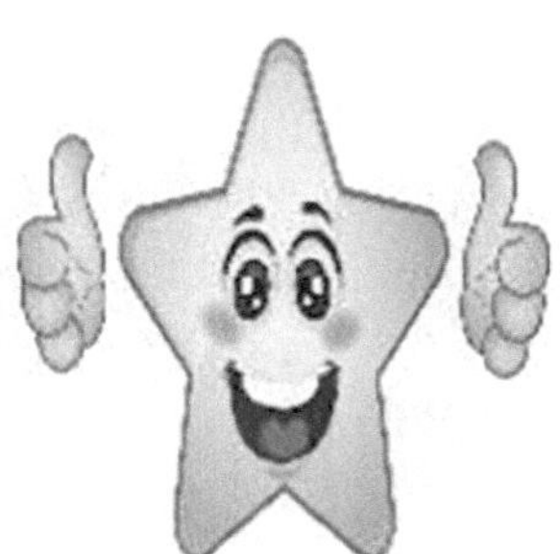

Way To Go!

Activities of Daily Living

Activities of Daily Living also known as ADLs is a term used in healthcare to refer to people's **"Daily Self-Care Activities"**.

The concept of **ADLs** was originally proposed in the 1950 by Dr. Sidney Katz and his team at Benjamin Rose Hospital in Cleveland Ohio and has been added to and refined by a variety of researchers since that time.

Today healthcare professionals often use a person's abilities or inability to perform **ADLs** as a measurement of their functional status particularly in regards to people with disabilities and the elderly. And of course younger children often require help too from adults to perform **ADLs** as well, they have not yet developed the skills necessary to perform them independently.

There are two components of Activities of Daily living (**ADLs**) with that one be-ing the first part then there's Instrumental Activities of Daily Living, (**IADLs**). Usually the Register Nurse (**RN**)or the Occupational Therapist (**OT**) often evaluates **IADLs** when completing patients assessments.

Here is a useful Mnemonic for Caregivers "SHAFT"

Shopping, **H**ousekeeping, **A**ctivities, **F**ood preparation, **T**ransportation/telephone/devices

ADLs Put Simply, "The things we normally do"

ADLs

1. **Bathing/Showering**
2. **Dressing**
3. **Self Feeding**
4. **Personal /Grooming**
5. **Toilet Hygiene, get-ting to and from the bathroom and cleaning oneself.**

Instrumental ADLs

6. **Housework**
7. **Preparing Meals**
8. **Taking Medication as prescribed**
9. **Managing Money/ family**
10. **Shopping for Food/ Clothes**
11. **Use of telephone or other forms of communication**
12. **Transportation**

Note to Caregiver's
Some individuals in your care may not require all twelve. Obtain a care plan for each person in your care.

Activities For Seniors

Research has shown that social interaction offers older adults many benefits. One, it improves their quality of life and Two, it reduces depression and cognitive decline.

"Socialization Matters!"

We as caregiver must encourage those in our care to get up, get dress and participate in activities offered or come up with some of our own to keep our seniors thriving and living the best life possible.

Below I just threw some activities out there, and left you space to add in some of your own. Get a pencil and circle the ones enjoyed the most and try to make them a regular part of your activity plan. If the person is total care,

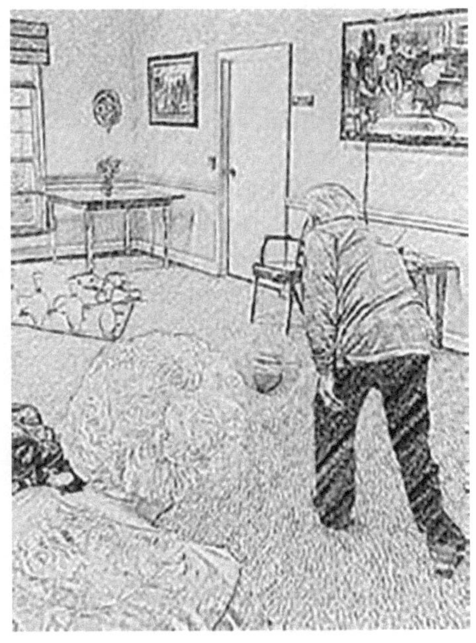

unable to get up and out, no problem, come up with activities that do not require mobility, example, poetry reading, picture books, popcorn and a "movie", together, decide but do something.

Circle Your Favorite Activities

scrap booking dancing photo fun Jewelry making, baking, coloring photography karaoke quilting cooking bingo iPod/computers balloon toss popcorn and a movie oldies but goodies puzzle play birthday parties arts and crafts sing a longs all about the Oscars name that tune jeopardy social dance Ice —cream socials bowling fashion shows board games playing cards current events cross word puzzles guess speakers/singers bible study bingo holiday celebrations fishing television/sports gardening stories poetry exercise painting how to demonstrations glamor day outings tea time indoor tennis or golf balloon tennis shopping Wal-Mart knitting coloring

---

Appearance

The day of your interview it is very important that you are prepared and looking your very, very best.

It's certainly true "First Impressions Means Everything" and I want to make sure Caregiver's are ready and looking fantastic! The way you look matters.

Do not wear Jeans to an interview, period. Orientation, maybe, but not during the interviewing stage.

You want to look fresh, professio nally posed and polished.

Be smart, use the tips in this book, dress for success not for the streets and carry a business bag or tote. Make sure you have writing utensils and a notepad. Employers should not have to find you those important items.

And please, please, please, please ladies, leave the wild colors and extreme hairstyles out. Don't show up to work like that, I know times are changing but still, how we look still matters especially if you want to land a good job. I'm just saying'! Watch what you wear too!

We are **'The New Day Caregivers'** we can't look any kind of way. We have to look like excellence, success! If you don't have the right clothes for the interview just wear a nice pair of scrubs. Employers love that, it shows you are ready to start right away! That's what I wear mostly to healthcare interviews, nice scrubs.

Lastly, smile, **Don't Worry, Be Happy!** You have God and

A Caregiver's Bible To Excellence 'by your side!

Tools You Can Use!

The Way We Look Matters!

Professional Do's and Don'ts

Do's.

- Wear professional shoes
- Black or dark navy bottoms
- Polo or Professional blouse or shirt
- Work wear/ Scrubs that are like new.
- Business Bag or Briefcase
- Notepad and good writing utensils, black ink most preferred.
- Groomed hair/men/hair cut
- Very little make-up, if any.

Don't's

- No Perfume
- Long False Eyelashes
- Fake Nails
- Visible Tattoos, cover them up!
- Hooped Earrings
- Radical hairstyles or colors
- Hats or Scarves
- Tight and Inappropriate clothing or shoes.
- Chew Gum
- Wear Excessive Jewelry
- Smell like Cigarette Smoke
- Don't worry, used these tips, Congratulations,

You Got This!

New Day Caregivers, We Have Arrived!

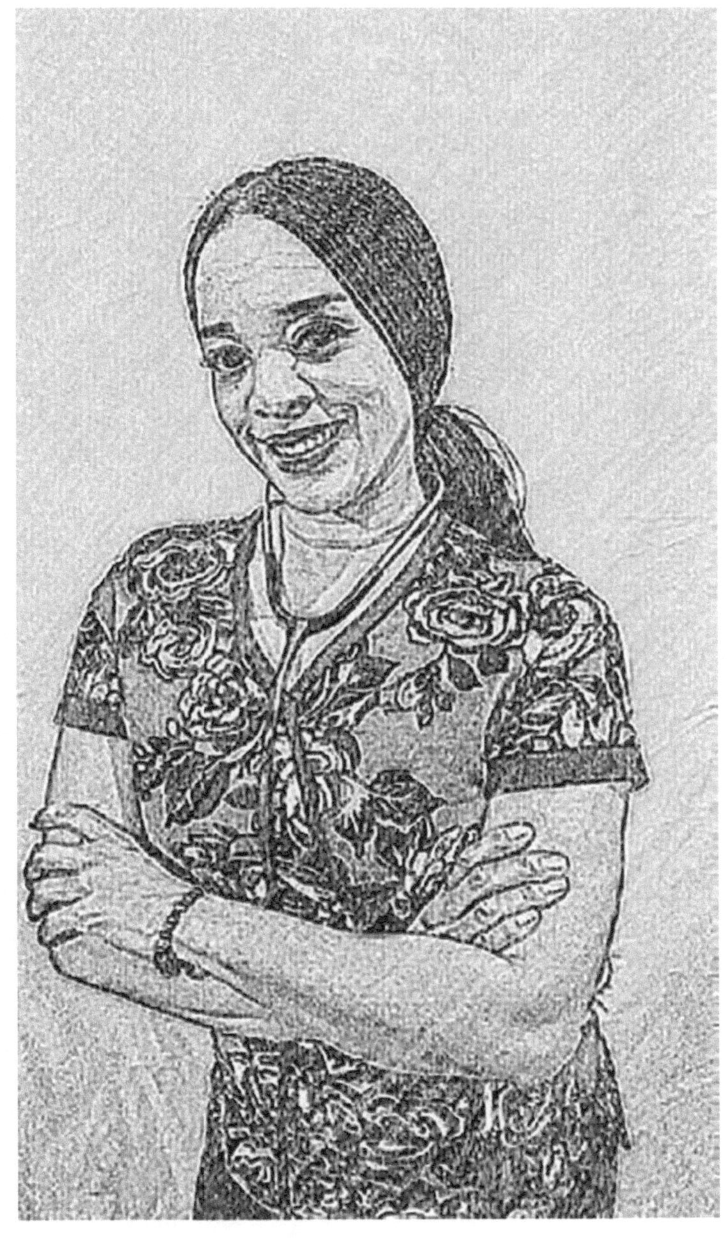

Autism

Autism also known as Autism Spectrum Disorder **(ASD)**

Autism is a serious developmental disorder that impairs the ability to communicate and interact. It involves abnormal development and function of the brain. Furthermore, it can't be cured, but treatment often helps.

ASD is chronic and can last for years or be lifelong. **ASD** requires a medical diagnosis. Signs typically appears during early childhood.

Some of the signs to look for are:

- Language, are there any delays, or spoken words at all.
- Motor Mannerisms, (e.g., hand flapping, twirling objects).
- Eye contact (e.g., looks at you when you are talking, and respond back as if they know what you said or want from them. Or it's little or no eye contact.
- Lack of interest in peer relationships.
- Lack of spontaneous or imaginary play.
- Persistent fixation on parts of objects.

How To Care For Special Needs

AUTISM (ASD)

- Love is the first ingredient.
- Learn all you can about ASD.
- Connect with other caregivers who are experienced/ share and exchange ideas.
- Learn from family members what the individual likes and dislikes. (e.g., hugs, no hugs)
- Create a daily schedule which includes hygiene and personal care.
- Create an open space for relaxation and safety for him or her.
- Reward good behavior!
- Come up with fun activities you both will enjoy!
- If you are the parent/ caregiver, use "Respite Care." Take care of you too, go somewhere and have some fun, you need a life too!
- Always included everyone in on schedules changes and new developments.
- Be flexible, things change! And be patient with all those involved in that persons care. Show lots of love.
- Incorporate, good nutrition and exercise throughout the week make that part of the care plan.

Be prompt, avoid being late, any disruption in routine can set the person off. Lastly,

What's Up Doc?
- **Documentation** is a must!
- **Observation** don't adjust!
- **Communication** you can trust!
That's What's Up!

Autism and Caregivers

In the united States alone according to the Center for Disease Control and Prevention, Autism is on the rise, its doubled since 2004 whereas, 1 in every 125 births to ADS, in 2004 it's 1 in every 68 birth. And still, today scientist are scouring genetic and environmental data to find a cause for the rise in autism, the numbers are still climbing. With that being said, it is very important that 'Caregivers' who work with individuals diagnosed with Autism are thoroughly trained and can meet the needs of the families they serve.

It takes a special kind of Caregiver to help bring out the best in those who are dealing with impairments. **Here's a tip, 'Love's the main ingredient!'** Just do like I do, imagine you're taking care of Jesus!

For more In-depth study visit your local library or Via Internet

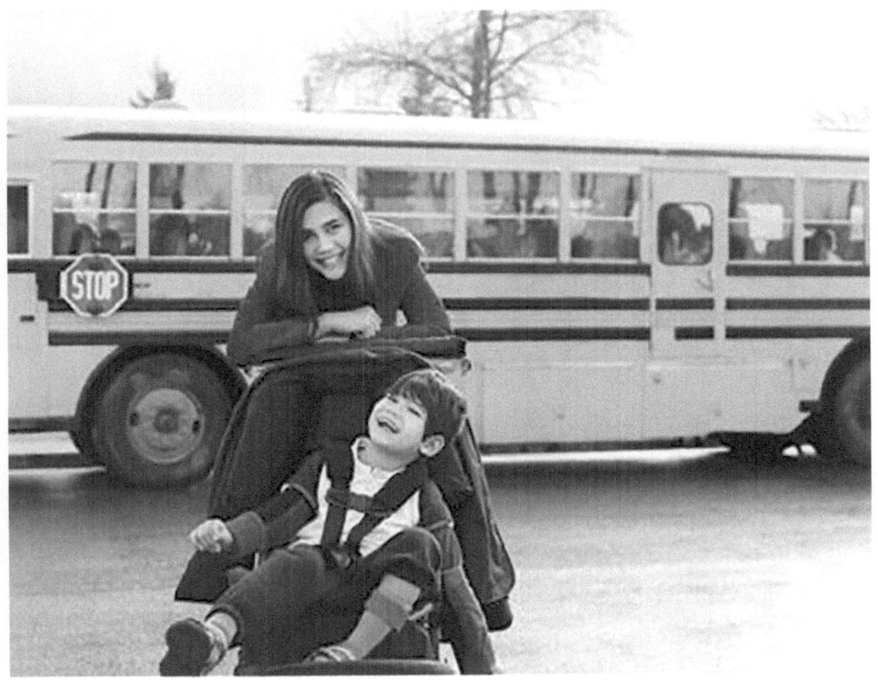

Bad- Weather Driving Conditions

- Make sure your headlights both work and are on.
- Slow down, roads are slippery when wet or snowy.
- Stay two car lengths behind other drivers.
- Make sure you have a good working battery in your car.
- Use caution near intersections. Don't try to beat the light, if it's yellow, just stop and wait for the green light!
- Stay in one lane. Stop switching lanes all the time, switch only when about to exit.
- Keep two hands on the wheel and both eye on the road.
- Get off the Cell Phone!
- Do not Text and Drive. "That Text Can Wait"
- No eating, keep your hands on the wheel, and eyes on the road.
- Stay focus and Alert at all times.
- Turn the Music down or off!
- Make sure you have your seat belts on.
- Leave half an hour to an hour earlier if necessary, so you will have plenty of time to arrive at your destination on time.
- Call your job if you have a car emergency while heading to work.
- Thunder and lightning, if it's unbearable/ pull over and wait in a safe place until it stops. Put your hazard blinking lights on!

Tools You Can Use!

Caregivers Car Supplies

- Food /Non Perishables
- Snacks and bottle water
- First Aid Kit/Flash Light
- Booster Cables
- Ice Scraper and Snow Brush/ Frozen Key Spray
- Fully Charged Cell Phone
- Full or at least a half tank of gas.
- A nice warm blanket
- Sand, salt or cat litter for traction in case you get stuck.
- Shovel
- AAA Membership!
- Keep a Bible and your Caregivers Bible to Excellence handy, reading helps keep you focus and calm while you wait on help to arrive. "God is with you!"
- If you have children, keep an extra bag of healthy snacks, books, blanket, food etc.
- Money and spare change in case you need to put air in your tires.
- Keep a working spare tire in your trunk, if you don't have one, get one.
- No matter what, stay **Calm, Cool** and **Collected**. Getting upset only makes things worse. **Help is on the way!**

Always Check the Weather Report the Night Before.

Back Problems, Is A Problem!

Today more and more caregivers are experiencing back discomfort more than ever before, many are not following the guideline they learned in their lab training classes, and some have no training at all and this is a problem, it's a back problem in the making.

Rule of thumb, my rule of thumb and this is for all those working in facilities nursing home in particular. If that person cannot bare weight, that individual needs a lifting device, e.g. 'Hoyer Lift'. They must be able to at least stand otherwise I don't move them.

Caregivers today, are not only moving individuals who can't bare weight, they are picking them up and transferring them too. Caregivers, "Stop Doing That!" Not only is this not smart, it's risky too and maybe weakening your backs.

It's just a matter of time, years even before you start to feel it's long term affects. Take my advice if you want a good healthy and strong back, stop picking up residence. If they can't be pivoted either, then go and ask the nurse for a **'Reassessment Order'** the nurse has to reevaluate that person health condition and place in the computer the new orders to use lifting devices or place in the care plan the residence is now a two person transfer.

10 BACK PROBLEM SOLUTIONS

1. Do back –strengthening and stretching exercises daily.
2. Stand straight and practice good posture.
3. Avoid heavy lifting.
4. Make every patient a two person transfer, that means working all your rooms with another team member.
5. If you are overweight, do my caregiver's boot –camp, drop those pounds, it will put less strain on your back.
6. Soak in the tub after a full day of work, relax for an hour and read your bible or just talk with God, tell him about your day.
7. Reduce work schedule, over-time, puts a lot of stress and strain on your body.
8. Make sure your rest and sleep on a good firm mattress!
9. Use proper body mechanics at all time.
10. If the problem persist, time to go see the doctor.

For those working in home care, don't do it either, don't lift a person who can't pivot or bare weight, or your back will eventually start to ache! Last time, 'Everybody, Everywhere, Caregivers all over the world, Family care providers too, I'm also saying this to you: **Do Not Lift Those Who Can Not Bare Their Own Weight! Don't Do It!** You will regret it later, you all have been warned! Advice for caregivers working in home care, contact your agency and ask them for advice, what to do, because once your back is out, so are you.

Now you can't work or perform the job you once loved to do. Never leave it up to the employers or others to determine if you need help or not, we are all supposed to be a team. Don't pay any attention to those who brag and say, "I can do it by myself, it doesn't bother my back, (not yet, not yet). Just wait one day they will eat those words. **Back Problems Is A Problem!**

Millions of caregivers are at risk for some kind of chronic pain, back problems being high on the list, other areas are shoulder and knee pain from trying to help others, stop it, if you are hurt, you can't help others.

Caregivers, listen to me, our bodies are not our own, it was bought with a price, we must keep our bodies in shape as a spiritual discipline so that we can be used by God greatly!

We have a long journey ahead of us! Jesus's got big plans for us, so we must be physically ready and able to act when called upon. We are God's caregivers for life, we must protect our vessel!

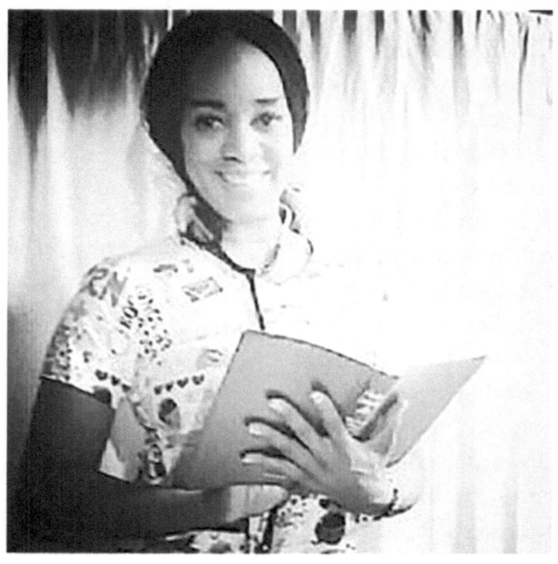

 MISS ASONDRA StarN'air

Beauty Tips For Caregivers

Appearance says a lot about us!

It is very important that "Caregivers" realize the importance of good appearance, individuals in our care, appreciates it more than they can say, people like seeing care-givers look fresh and vibrant, pretty or if you are a guy, well groomed too.

Caregiver who take pride in how they look tend to be the ones who are more professional, at least that's what I've noticed.

Therefore, caregivers look the part, I tell you, there is absolutely nothing wrong with loving what you do and looking good too! But remember, dress for success, how we look says a lot about us.

If you want to be taken seriously dressed appropriately.

Looking Good, is Good!

Beauty Tips For Caregivers!

- Wear nice and neat work apparel that match well together.
- Wear a 'SMILE', and ladies add a flower in your hair, why not? I do!
- Wear professional work shoes
- Keep your hair well groomed.
- Remove fake nails, don't wear loud colors, unpolished is best.
- Wear conservative makeup/ or none at all but, moisturize your wonderful face.
- Carry professional work bags.
- Wash Up! Body Clean, Teeth Clean, Smell Clean!
- Wear love in your heart!
- Wear Jesus 24/7 it does wonders for the mind, body and soul!

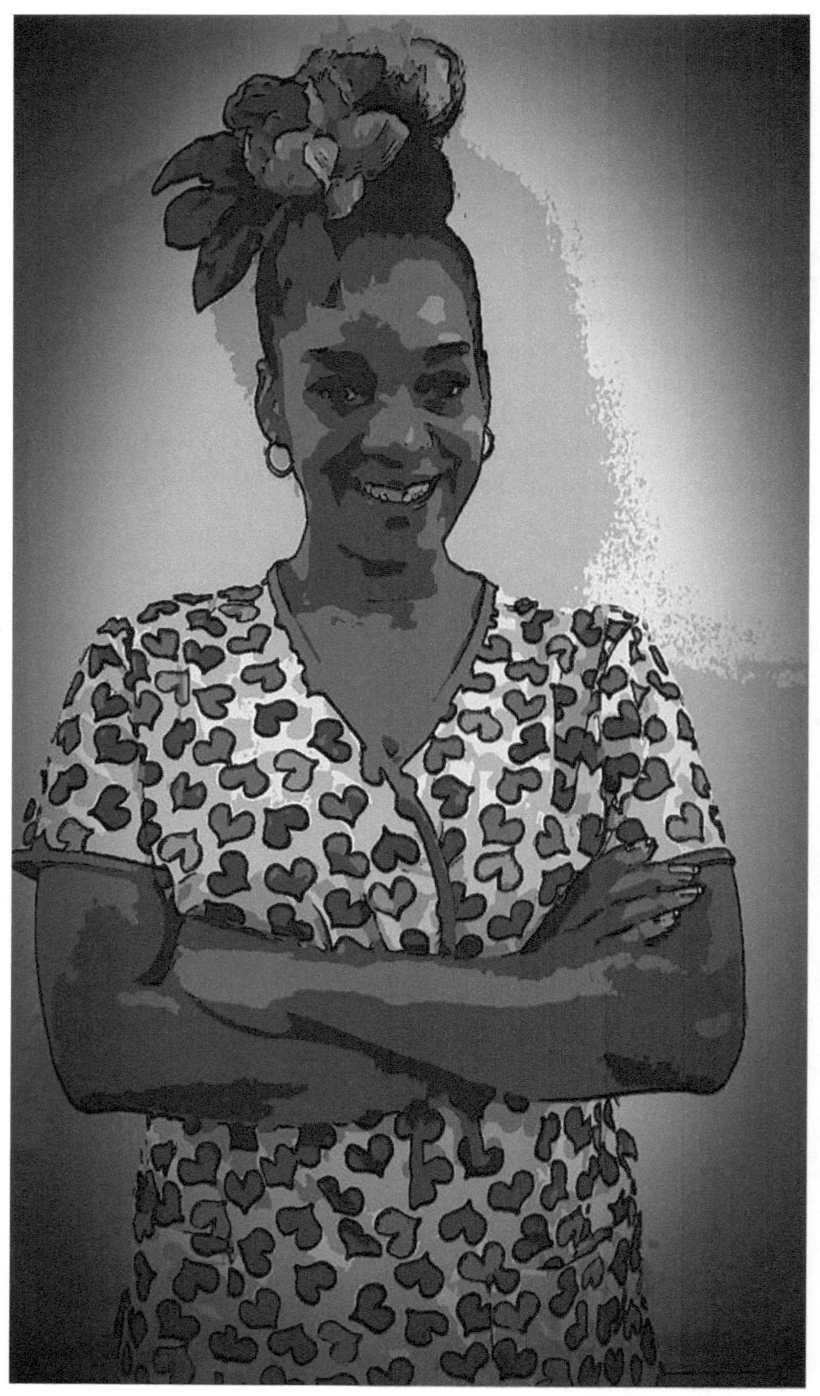

 Miss Asondra StarN'air

Bereavement, Grief and Loss

Losing a love one is hard, it seems no one can fully understand your loss, your pain, not even you. No amount of comforting will do. When that persons gone, part of you is gone too, I've been there. Losing my dad was the hardest thing I ever had to endure. But we must go on "We Must!"

After a serious loss we want something to ease the pain, but we must be careful not to harm ourselves in the process; we must be strong and choose healthy and Godly ways to cope.

Cry, and keep crying if you have to but, at some point stop and realize that life goes on... We all have to leave this place too one day, so we have to learn to embrace life and death as it comes.

The best place to turn to when this happens is to Jesus, He will get you through it all, He will heal you completely if you let him, but the more you resist his loving and comforting arms the more you stay stuck in that grief, we don't want that. God wants you healed, up and going again.

If there is anybody else out there experiencing a loss of any kind, a job loss, death of a marriage, a dear friend or have loss a pet, whatever your losses are God can help and He wants to. He's known for healing the broken-hearted, and binding up all kinds of wounds. In fact, the bible says

COME TO ME ALL YOU WHO ARE WEARY AND BURDENED AND I WILL GIVE YOU REST
Matthew 11:28

- Turn to God!
- Read scriptures on healing.
- Keep embracing your faith.
- Do uplifting activities.
- Be with family members and close friends.
- Turn to your pastor /church family
- Prayer works so keep praying for your healing, everyday pray!

Stay Close to God!

- Keep a healthy lifestyle.
- Don't over eat, incorporate exercise during this time it will take the edge off the physical symptoms of grief giving you better control over your body and emotions.
- Give yourself all the time you need to grieve. Cry it's okay.
- Men, it's okay too for you to cry. **'Real Men Do Cry'**, Jesus wept. John 11:35
- Get away for a while if you can, if not find a special place in your home to be in spirit with that person you loss. It's perfectly fine to still talk to the deceased, and celebrate the good times shared, go for it, whatever helps.

Everyday Losses

- Accept the things you can't change.
- Trust God to work things out in your favor.
- Wait on God because He has the perfect person for you.
- God gives, God takes away, trust him, listen, do what he say!
- When God closes one door, He always opens another, you're on your way!

Some Loses Are Good For Us!
"In God We Trust!"

He is closer to the broken hearted, and saves those who are crushed in spirit. *Psalms 34:18.*

So if there's anybody out there, that has had a lost, or hurting in any way, call on the name of Jesus. Let him care for you, after all, He is the **"Ultimate Caregiver"** Yes indeed, He is **'The Greatest Caregiver Of All!'** He will heal you, put you back together again. Make you whole and give you knew life with purpose if you let Him. Just know that, healing takes time so be patient, keep reading his word and allow the master to do his thing.

Again, don't rush the healing by settling for quick fixes such as alcohol, substance abuse, overindulgence on foods or sinful pleasures. Jesus cares about what happens to you, don't do that! Just try to take things one day at a time and you'll be fine.

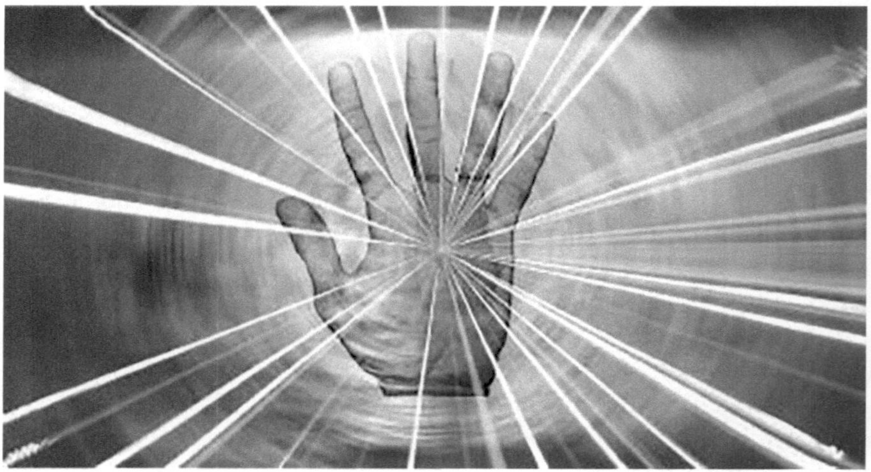

Have mercy on me, Lord for I am faint; heal me, LORD, for my bones are in agony. My soul is in deep anguish. How long, LORD, how long? Turn, LORD and deliver me; save me because of your unfailing love. **Psalms 6:2-4**

 MISS ASONDRA StarN'air

Breast Cancer Awareness

As Caregivers, we spend so much of our times helping and caring for others and many times forget about ourselves, our health is just as important as anyone else.

According to The National Breast Cancer Foundation 1 in 8 women will be diagnosed with breast cancer in their lifetime.

What is **"Breast Cancer"**? It is a disease in which malignant cancer cells form in the tissue of the breast. But, when it is detected early and is in what's called the Localized Stage, the 5 year relative survival rate is 100%.

Don't Put It Off, "Get Tested"

Breast Cancer are diagnosed through several testing methods

- **Test**
- **Mammograms**
- **Ultrasound**
- **MRI**
- **Biopsy**

Let's all get tested. Call today for an appointment, early detections saves lives, yours and mine.

Here are some other things ladies we can do, we can create our own early detections plan. Yes we can, we can start by staying informed, charting our own monthly breast exams and paying special attention to our bodies and overall wellness. Ladies, 'Yes We Can'! And also, we can donate, give back, and become sponsors too. Oh, there's just so many wonderful loving things we can do!

God Bless You!

For More Information Go to National Breast Cancer Foundation.org

Calm Cool and Collected

Maintain Professionalism

Sometimes **"Accidents"** happens and when it does, it is very important **Caregivers Master** what I call **"The 3C's of Emergencies"**

Stay **Calm** take a deep breath, so you can think straight, and take better care of the situation.

Stay **COOL** Remind yourself you are a Professional Caregiver, ask God to order your steps. Tell you how to handle the situation and he will.

Stay **Collected** decide right away if you need to call 911, if not, looks at the situation, map out in your mind what to do and **Do it!** If you need to contact your supervisor **Follow Protocol!**

You're a skilled professional caregiver now, so act like one. Just stay Calm, Cool and Collected!

Caregiver Bullies

There are rising problems of bullying in the workplace, both from other caregivers and seniors. You may not want to talk about it, but it must be addressed.

I have experienced them both, mainly from other caregivers but also from some seniors in my care.

Yet nothing is being done about it. I have lost or resigned from too many jobs to count, leaving me depressed and wondering how I was going to make it. No one should ever, ever have to live like that. For most of my care-giving career at facilities I have been persecuted and bullied on the job. One day I hope to help changes the laws, my life mission is to help put a stop to bulling worldwide.

What it is, is, hurt people, hurting people. And they keep getting away with it too. Because a lot of employers are not doing anything about it. They want to keep it hush, hush, some even try to accuse the victim, and say things like, maybe it's something you are doing? Or per-haps the way you speak to others maybe it's your tone etcetera. They come up with all kinds of things to make you think somehow it's your fault. It's not, employers are not the top, God is! He knows and sees everything.

A Change Is About To Come!

Today it's one of my missions in life to publicly speak out against work place bullies and help support those who have been affected by it. My plan is to use some of the proceeds from this book to get that campaign up and running soon. Bullies must be stopped! Something has to be done worldwide. Bullying is a serious

HOW TO PROTECT YOURSELF

- Cry out to the Lord!
- Tell somebody, don't keep quite!
- Document, each time it happens.
- If you have to, stop and go to the police department.
- Report the company who ignores the problem; make them accountable.
- Write a letter to your local TV station.
- Nip it in the bud, quickly, before the intimidator gets out of control.
- Find witnesses if you can.
- Contact an attorney or legal aide.
- Try to find a friend who will help keep an eye on you.
- Come off of cases that intimate and mistreats you.
- Know that, God is with you, he will open another door. You've tried and tried, but enough is enough! Leave, do not be trampled on anymore.

Children: Tell your mom and dad when it first starts to happen. Or you go straight to the principal's office and tell someone. Tell everyone who will listen, what's happening and find out the bully's first and last name.

Lastly, don't leave the school building afraid. Stay there until your parents come.

problem, and not only in the workplace. It's also happening in our schools too. Today our children are being attacked or made to fear others, or else. In my case, it was my job. For our kids, it's their safety and self-esteem that's being attacked. Bullying is wrong and those who do it must be stopped. It's a wicked form of evil and dark intimidation set out to frighten and destroy other people's lives. The Bible calls it a form of murder. **1 John 3:15** says, *"Everyone who hates his brother is a murderer, and you know that no murderer has eternal life abiding in him."*

We —as sisters and brothers in Christ must look out for those being bullied by other by reporting it when we see it happening. And people we must disassociate ourselves with these kind of people or we too will have to answer to God.

If You See Something, Say Something!
"Speak Out", 'Be A Friend"
"Fight for the Rights of Others"
"Bullying Has To End. Let Love and Peace Begin!

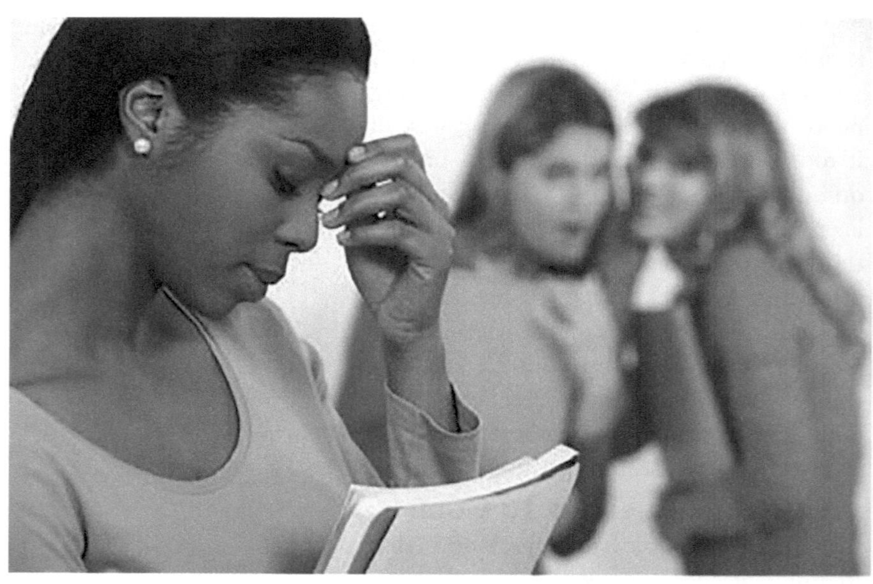

 Miss Asondra StarN'air

COPD

COPD or Chronic Obstruction Pulmonary Disease it is a progressive disease that makes it hard to breath. Because it is progressive that means the disease gets worst over time.

Cigarette smoking is the leading cause of COPD yet many will not stop smoking.

Most people who have COPD smoke or use to smoke.

Long term exposure and other lung irritants such as air pollution, chemical fumes, or dust may also contribute to COPD.

Therefore, I encourage everyone including caregivers if you smoke, **"Quit"**! Life or Death is now in your hands. Is smoking worth it? **"Absolutely Not"**!

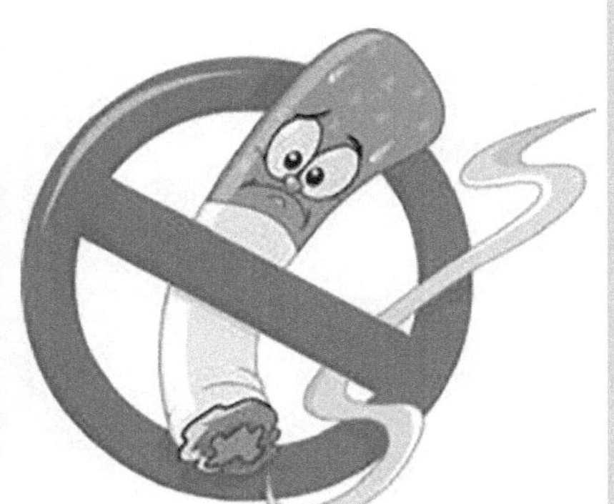

Caregivers In The Know

Quit Smoking Today!

Here are some smoking tips for caregivers who do not smoke:

- Ask smoker to provide a non-smoking room /area for you.
- Work smoke -free cases only!
- But if you need that case, find out all the tricks and tips to help that individual quit. Remember, second hand smoke is just as deadly.
- Make sure you know how to care for individual with COPD and how to use an oxygen tanks, as a Caregiver it is YOUR JOB to be in the know!
- Carry a pulse oximeter and be ready to do CPR, this book and other resources are all at your fingertips. Call 911, CPR coaches are standing by, they'll help walk you through the process if you forget.

Be a healthcare professional, grow, do not sit and smoke with the person in your care, if you smoke, get the help you need too, to quit. Our job as Caregivers is to help promote good health and wellness first and foremost. Don't be a stumbling block! Help them and yourself to want to quit.

"Smoking Kills"
Stop and Live!

CPR

What is CPR? The word **CPR** stands for **C**ardio-**P**ulmonary **R**esuscitation.

That is Cardio, which refer to the "Heart" whose main function is to pump blood around the body.

When someone is unconscious and not breathing, they are not getting oxygen and if they don't get **Oxygen – Rich Blood** flowing back into their bodies, they will die. We don't want that, that's why we do **CPR** to help save individuals lives. All Caregiver should be certified in **CPR** including those caring for loved ones.

When should we do **CPR**?

We should do **CPR** when a person is not responsive or not breathing.

It is important to ask the victim "Are you Ok" first and if you get no response have someone call 911, **YOU**, yes, **YOU** Start **CPR** immediately"!

Come on, You Can Do It!

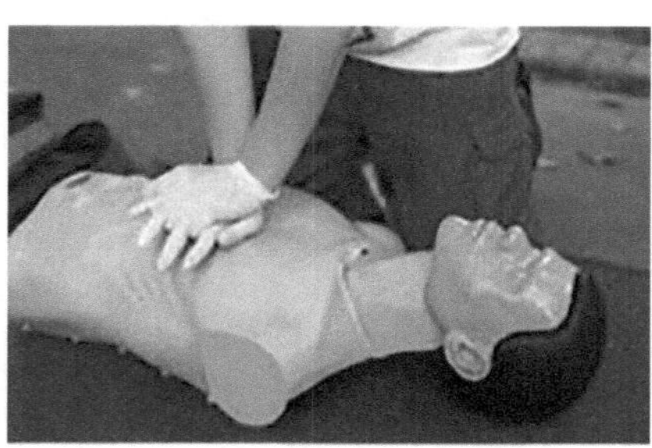

You Can Do It! CPR

First: Check the scene
Check the victim
Call for help

Second: If the person is not responding put your phone or cell phone on speaker mode. **LISTEN** to dispatcher, Start **CPR.**

If you do not have a phone, here's what you do.

1. Pump the chest 30 times by placing the heel of one hand in the center of the chest and place your other hand on top of it. Press chest down at least 2 inches, at a rate of 100 to 120 per minutes.
2. Open the air way by tilting the head back, lift the chin up.
3. Breath air in to the victim, all you do is pinch their nose so air doesn't escape, place your mouth over theirs and blow out breaths (life) back into their bodies otherwise they will die. Look for the chest to rise.
4. If the chest doesn't rise, open airway again and re-peat all **CPR** steps until help arrives. We are caregivers we **MUST** help save lives.
5. Just remember to stay

Calm, Cool and Collected
You Got This!!!!

You Can Do It!

CPR for Infants and Children

If you are alone with the unconscious infant give 2 minutes of **CPR** before calling 911.

Time is of the essence when dealing with **CPR** especially for infants, permanent brain damage or death can occur within minutes if a baby's blood flow stops. So no time to be scared to do **CPR**, you MUST do **CPR**! Many times the need for **CPR** happens after drowning, suffocation, Chocking, and in children it may be due to some other injuries.

CPR involves Rescue Breathing, which provides oxygen to the lungs and Chest compressions, that helps keep the blood flowing.

Anyone working with children should be certified; anyone who is a parent too, should be certified. And anyone who is neither should be certified!

CPR Saves Lives! And too, people we never know in life what we may be faced with, mightiest well be prepared to help infants, the **Zero** become a real live **Hero** a real superwoman or superman!

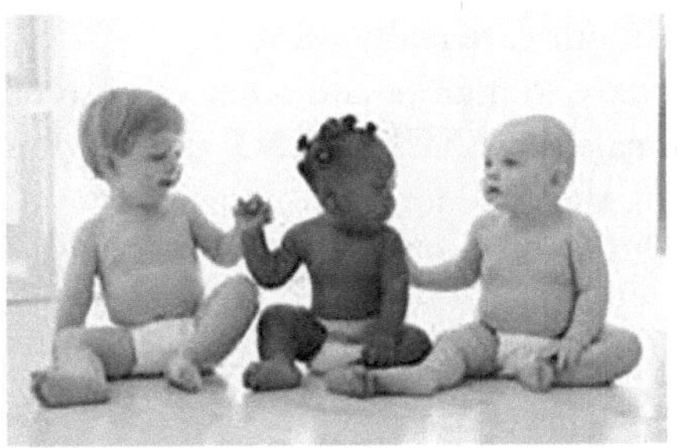

You can do it **CPR**

First   Check the scene
          Check the victim
          Call for help

Second If the child is not responding Put phone on speaker mode **LISTEN** to disputer, Start **CPR**

If you do not have a phone, here's what you do.

1. Shout and tap the child feet or if the child does not respond, isn't breathing or is breathing but not normal. position the baby on its back and start **CPR**
2. Give 30 gentle chest compressions at a rate of 100 to -120 per minutes. Use two fingers, your index and middle fingers place those fingers directly in the center of the child's chest just below the nipples. Now press down about one – third the depth of the chest, which is about 1 and a half inches.
3. Open the air way by tilting the head back, lift the chin up gently do not tilt the child head back too far.
4. If the chest doesn't rise, open airway again and repeat all **CPR** steps until help arrives. We are caregivers we **MUST** help save lives.
5. Just remember to stay:

Calm, Cool and Collected
"You Got This!"

You Can Do It!

Don't Cross the Line
It's a Thin Line Between Professionalism and Friendship!

What's crossing the line? "Glad you want to know" it means we are starting to behave in ways that are not socially acceptable. For the caregiver it means, we are not behaving like professionals. We are starting to mix things up a bit shall we say, for example, becoming to personally involved with the client.

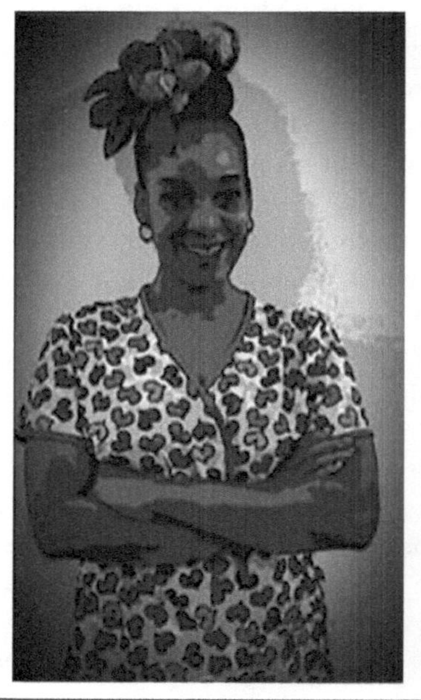

Kissing and hugging on the way out the door, that's not professional. Here's what is: "with a smile" say, 'it was a plea-sure taking care of you today, do you need anything else before I leave, if not. Have a great evening, I'll see you tomorrow now that's a professional caregiver! The latter is crossing the line in my opinion. We should not be kissing our clients, ok, maybe after many, many years of service, but certainly not within weeks or months into the **WORKING** relationship. Again, I say it's unprofessional! But some may disagree that's okay too.

Let, truth be told, we all want to be liked, but your work ethics is what's most important here. Our Attitudes, hospitality, how well we give service, are we on time? Do we know want we're doing? Are we skilled, Competent? These kinds of Qualities are what individuals in our care really want.

Caregivers, listen to me, we do not have to manipulate other ways to be liked or become favorites. Stay Professionals, **Be EXCELLENT** at what you came there to do, and they'll keep calling the back for you!
One more time, Don't Cross The Line!

Be Professional, Yet Kind!

Debt Free Caregivers

Today there are so many caregivers working past exhaustion trying to get out of debt. I too use to be one of them, but not anymore. Now I live within my means and found new ways of doing things.

Caregivers did you know that when you are in debt you are also in "Slavery", yes "YOU" are a slave now. Now you have no choice, you have to work, work, work and keep on working until you are used up or dead.

Sorry, but there is no other way to wake some of you up.

Did you know that working a lot of over time causes stress and that stress kills? Well it does, stress is sneaky. Stress is known as 'The Silent Killer' you want to know why? Because it shows very little symptoms until it's too late.

So Caregivers, You cannot continue on this way, you just can't! Too much overtime is not your friend, there are other ways to get out of debt that won't cost you your health, or your life. "Choose Christ!" That's the first thing you do if you want financial freedom, "Choose Christ!"

Now, after that, caregivers you must acknowledge that you are in financial trouble and that you need

DEBT FREE CAREGIVERS

StarN'air saving tips for Caregivers

- **Make changes inside your home, down grade services.**
- **Telephone, Cable, Cell**
- **Homeowners, turn down your hot water tank /saving of 20 to 30 dollars per month. Want to save even more, put your hot water tank on vacation in the summer time.**
- **Do all your own personal grooming, no more solons**
- **Cut up all your Credit cards except one, for emergencies**
- **Contact A Debt Consolidator**
- **Choose free entertainment**
- **Have your wine at home, drink ginger ale at social events.**
- **Reduce grocery bill by 30% or more if you use coupons.**
- **Eat at home, I cook all my gourmet meals! I even set a beautiful table.**
- **Purchase newly use car, never pay sticker price.**
- **Shop at trendy thrift stores**

Ask for a modification on your mortgage, I did and got 375.00 reduced. Just call your mortgage company and apply.

- **sisters, save lots of money, wear braids for 6 months and learn to do your own lashes. I do my own.**

Lastly, anyone sixteen or older and in good health living with you must work or they don't eat! That's a scripture, look it up!

help. Next, ask God to help you get out of debt that's what I did many years ago, He still manages me and all my business affairs; let him do that with you too.

Keep in mind, not all debt is bad, I still owe on a mortgage most people do, and of course many have Car Notes, Student Loans, and **"Now"** "Mandatory Healthcare" just those alone can be financial burdens, so we don't want to keep adding to that, No! We cannot afford to keep spending like "Movie Stars" we're not. It even catches up with them at some point, I'm sure you've read or heard about celebrities whose gone bankrupt.

In your Tool box on the right I have shared with you what I did to get out of debt and hope you will take heed to all I have provided for you.

Pretty soon you will be on your way to debt free living and let me tell you, it won't be easy but it will be worth it in the end. It's going to take a lot of discipline over fleshly desires, determination and patience. Caregiver's You can do it! Start right **NOW!** Take back control over you finances and begin to live a more balanced life, free of financial stress and worries, don't put it off or delay, hurry!

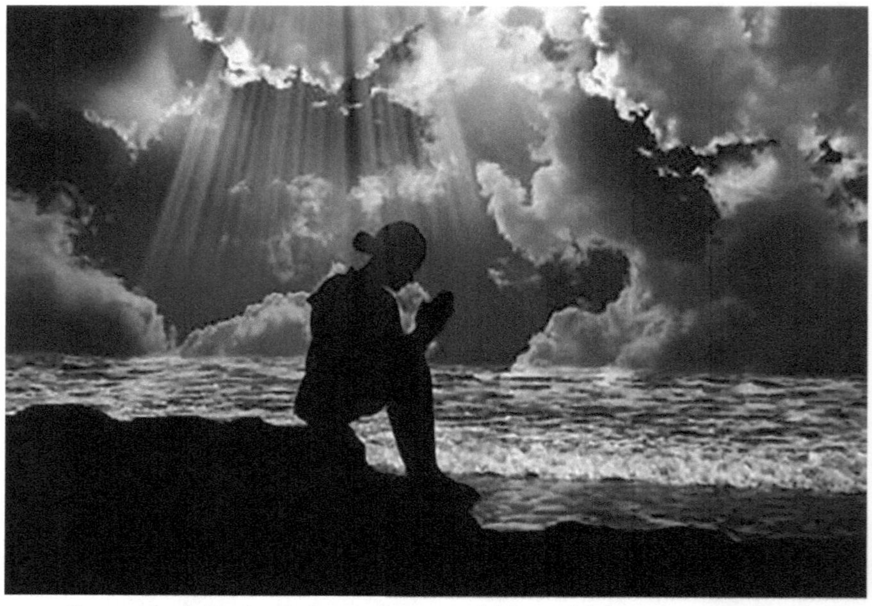

Pray and ask God to help get you out of debt and keep you out of debt!

     Miss Asondra StarN'air

Dementia

Dementia is a general term for loss of memory and other abilities severe enough to interfere with Activities of Daily Living **(ADL's)** it is caused by physical changes in the brain.

Alzheimer's disease is the most common type of dementia, accounts for 60 to 80 percent of cases.

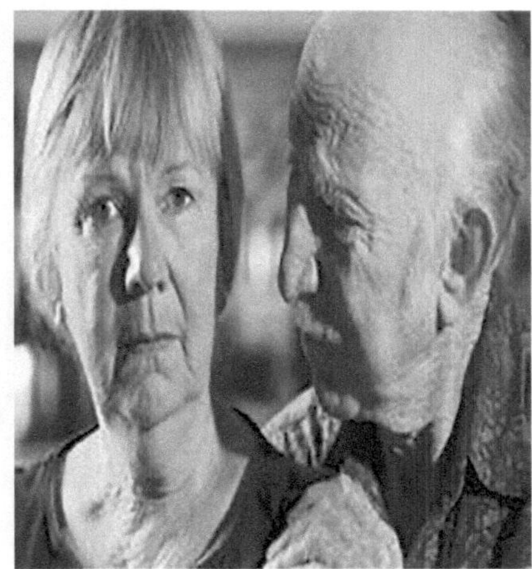

Alzheimer's Disease

The 7 Stages

Stage 1: No impairment.
Person functions normally, undetected by the medical professional.

Stage 2: Very Mild Cognitive Decline
It could be related to normal aging or early signs of Alzheimer's.
The individual may be having memory lapses, forgetting familiar words, location of everyday objects still undetected by doctors, family, friends or co-workers.

Stage 3: Mild Cognitive Decline.
Early stages of the disease can now be diagnosed in some, but not all, who have these symptoms.
Now everyone is starting to notice something is wrong. Unable to complete task in social or work setting. Losing and misplacing valuable objects. Increase trouble with planning or organizing.

Stage 4: Moderate Cognitive Decline.
Now clearly detectable. Mild or early stages of Alzheimer's impaired ability to perform counting exercises/problems paying bills/ personal history. They also can become moody and withdrawn.

Stage 5: Moderately Severe Cognitive Decline memory and thinking are quite noticeable now. Help is needed with Activities Of Daily Living however, still require no assistance with eating or toileting. Some confusion about where they are or what day it is etc. Can't be left alone anymore.

Stage 6: Severe Cognitive Decline: need full time help with just about everything. Trouble controlling bladder or bowels. need ADL's Incontinent care, major personality and behavioral changes, tend to wander or become lost. Changes in sleep patterns or remembering loved ones names.

Stage 7: Very Severe Cognitive Decline.
At this stage the individual is unable to respond to their environment total care is now required. Does not recognize or remember loved ones and friends.
This is the last and final stage of Alzheimer's disease.
For more in depth studies go to Wikipedia. org /search under Alzheimer's Disease or go to your local library.

Dementia

More about dementia and things you need to know, there are more than 3 million cases per year and growing.

Dementia can't be cured but treatment may help.

Dementia is chronic can last for years or be lifelong.

Dementia requires a medical diagnosis, lab test or imaging often required.

It is very important those caring for Dementia/Alzheimer patients be thoroughly trained, in fact it should be 100% mandatory.

Dementia caregiving is a world of its own, normal rules don't apply.

Therefore we need all the training and support we can get, Caregivers **WE** will be the ones to motivate and keep them safe. Family Caregivers and Professional Caregivers alike, must master working with memory care individuals if you are going to be effective.

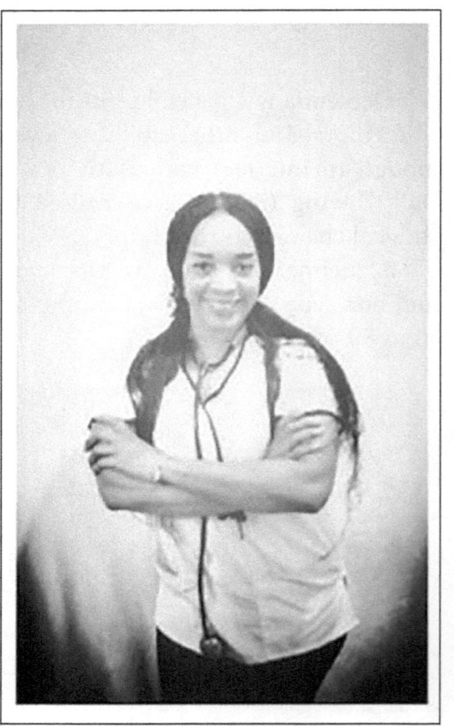

We must stay informed, competent, and professional at all times.

Welcome to the world of Caregiving, we are not the caregiver's of our parents' generation. Today we are truly "Healthcare Professionals".

Stay Educated!

Diabetes Mellitus

Commonly called Diabetes, people with this disease either cannot produce enough insulin or cannot effectively use the insulin they do have to produce or control their blood sugar (glucose) level.

Yet it's still on the rise here in the United States. Everyone should be aware of this potentially fatal disease according to 2014 statistic report CDC 29.1 million people here in the united states alone has diabetes and 27.8% which is about 8.1 million people have it and don't know they have it. There are two types of diabetes:

Type 1 and Type 2

Type 1: also called **Juvenile Diabetes** or insulin dependent the pancreas produces little or no insulin. It's a chronic condition/ongoing, cannot be cured, but treatment and special diet along with exercise makes this disease manageable can last for years or lifelong.

Type 2: also called, **Adult Onset Diabetes,** it's very common, more than 3 million people are diagnosed with type 2 diabetes. It is characterized by high blood sugar, insulin resistance and relative lack of insulin. This type is treatable by a medical professional, however, chronic and can also last for years or be lifelong.

DM GUIDE FOR CAREGIVERS

Signs and Symptoms

- Hunger
- Fatigue
- Blurry vision
- Extreme thirst
- Frequent urination
- Unexplained weight loss
- Soars that don't heal
- Frequent infections

Caregivers Care Plan

- Encourage dental checks.
- Never put lotion between the toes.
- All meals served as scheduled do not skip meals.
- Encourage shoes or slippers when up on the floor.
- Encourage physical daily activities and exercise.
- Wash feet and thoroughly dry between the toes
- Do not cut toe nails.
- Report any lesions found on body to nurse or supervisor.

Give insulin if directed by nurse and certified to do so.

Lastly, when checking blood sugar apply lancet to the chosen finger, never the pad. Rotate finger to avoid callus formation.

Diabetes

Caregivers, Rock On. **"Stay In The Know'** that's right, know the blood sugar levels, what's normal what's not. Normally, blood sugar level should fall between 70-110. It's too high when it's above 120, this is called **"Hyperglycemia"**. When blood sugar is too low (below 70) it is called **"Hypoglycemia"**.

Signs and Symptoms

Hyperglycemia
- Feels weak
- Drowsy, sleepy
- Pain in abdomen
- Nausea, vomiting
- Dehydration, dry mouth and skin
- Spuporous, not alert
- Skin flushed, red and warm
- Slow and lethargic movements
- Rapid respirations

Hypoglycemia
- Nausea,
- Headache
- Fast pulse
- Feel hungry
- Blurred vision
- Unsteadiness
- Tingling in the hands, feet or face
- Feels too hot or cold
- Tremors, shakiness
- Feels dizzy, light headedness, heart pounding
- Excessive sweating, slurred speech

Documentation

CareGivers, can't stress enough how important that we document. Documentation is a vital part of our professional job as caregivers. Not only does it provide clear and important information to the healthcare team, it protects us, you and me "The Caregiver".

When documenting, only document Factual and Actual Information, "nothing more, nothing less"

No Opinions or Assumptions. Write neat and use black ink if possible, in fact "Every Professional Caregiver "should keep a note pad and a black ink pen with them at all times.

And if you make a mistake, never scribble out, just initial and draw a straight line through it, and keep documenting.

Follow your Companies "Protocol" and summit documents in their allotted time.

Tools You Can Use!

DOCUMENTATION

Document The Following

- Time
- Date
- First name
- Last name
- Correct Spelling
- Your Full Name
- Your Title
- Location of Incident/or
- Brief Description
- Actual and Factual Info..
- Manager or Supervisor or person you contacted, First and Last Name.

Be ready to provide a 24 hour number you can be reached at, a working cell phone number is acceptable.

- Names and Contact information of witnesses if applicable.
- Give Information if 911 was called
- Where did they take them and did you follow?
- Private Caregivers, so what, document!
- Document what you were told to do and by who?

Lastly, print your full name, sign and date.

__________ Thank You!

Elderly Abuse

What is Elder Abuse? According to Administration on Aging, (AoA) "In general, elder abuse is a term referring to any knowing, intentional, or negligent act by a caregiver or any other person that causes harm or a serious risk of harm to a vulnerable adult.

Unfortunately each year hundreds of thousands of Senior Citizens are abused. They are the ones who are older, frail and vulnerable and cannot help themselves, these seniors depend on others to help meet their most basic needs. The bible says once and adult twice a child. And with all due respect, we owe it to our seniors to look out for them and provide the best care possible.

As professional caregivers it is our job to make sure these individual are taken care of properly and kept safe. If you suspect that there may be some signs of abuse **REPORT IT RIGHT AWAY!**

Just so you know, abusers of older adults is usually someone they know, family members, friend or "trusted other."

WARNING SIGNS

- Unexplained bruises or marks.
- Broken bones
- Burns
- Neglect, no food in house.
- Significant weight loss.
- Bed Soars, unattended medical needs.
- Poor hygiene and appearance.
- Sudden change in financial situation.
- Missing medication
- Verbal and Emotional Abuse.
- Threats and belittling.
- Strain or tense relationships.
- Frequent arguments between "The Caregiver/Other and the elderly person, may also be signs.

That's why it is very, very important "Caregivers" that we be very professional and not cross the line. We are there to provide a service. We are not there to try to become their best friends, by doing this, we may be opening up a can of worms if you know what I mean, what if they get mad at you? Or vise-versa, therefore, do not try to build private relationships. Stay very professional and you'll have nothing to worry about!

Caregivers, please don't let it be you. God See's Everything! And too, every move you make, God is watching you. He is watching all of us!

Nothing in all creation is hidden from God's sight. Everything is naked and exposed before his eyes, and he is the one to whom we are accountable.

"Caregivers" we have a loving job to do, God trust us to deliver Tender Loving Care (TLC) to those who can't take care of themselves anymore, that's what we're here for **"RIGHT"**! Caregivers let's say it together **"RIGHT"**!

Each one of us have a responsibility to keep vulnerable elders safe from harm and abuse. If you suspect abuse call 1800-667-1116 Administration On Aging. Let's do our part to keep them safe!
Thank You!

Emergencies

Knowing how to act in an emergency can save a life. First and foremost stay **Calm, Cool and Collected**. Otherwise you can make matter worst. Do your basic lifesaving steps, **CHECK** the person, **CALL** for help, **CARE** until help arrives. If you don't remember the detailed steps to **CPR** go back to your tool box or call 911 they can walk your through it. **Emergencies are just that,** "Emergencies" as caregivers we must always be prepared to act. But don't forget to get permission, just say this, are they ok? Can I help you. Afterwards, contact your case manager, or office staff and they will quickly contact the family. Follow office policies and procedures, incident reports etc.

At some point in life, emergencies are bound to happen, when it does caregiver, we must be prepared to act.

> ### Quick, Call 911
>
> - Chest pain.
> - Unconsciousness
> - Possible spinal or neck injury
> - Uncontrolled bleeding
> - Disorientation
> - Sudden server pain
> - No Breath or Pulse
> - Shortness of Breath (SOB)
> - Medication Overdose
> - Server Injury
> - Suicide Threats and Attempts
> - Life treating episodes /fighting, physical incidents
> - Falls, unable to get back up or move.
> - When you just don't know what to do? **Quick call 911**
>
> **Doing Nothing Is Not An Option!**

Again, stay **Calm, Cool and Collected**
You can handle it!

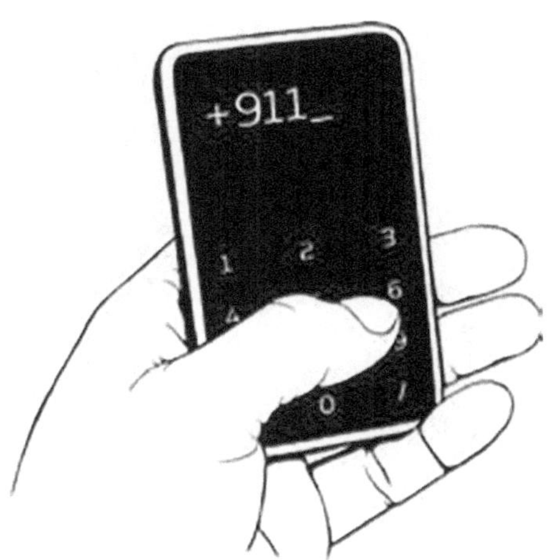

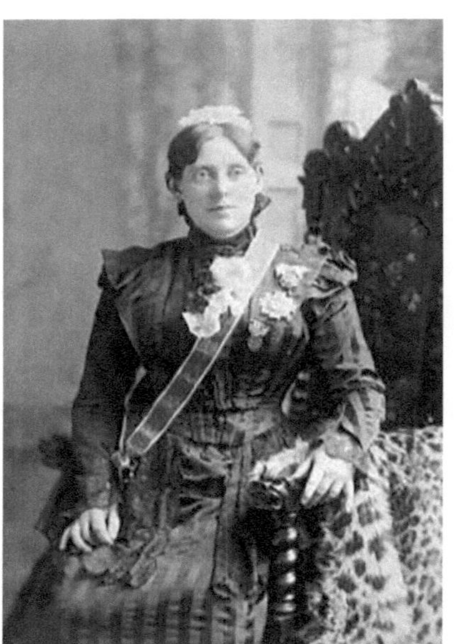

Florence Nightingale
(1820-1910)

LADY WITH THE LAMP

Florence Nightingale, also known as the 'Lady with the Lamp' was a care -giver like us, she went on to become a philosopher of modern nursing and a social reformer.

Florence, was from a wealthy family and believed she had been called by God, to go out and serve, help those in need. Although her family was against this, she said no to them and yes to God. She answered the call.

It is very important that those caring for the sick, or disabled really have a heart for the job, and feel it's a calling and could not imagine doing anything else.

Florence Nightingale was not a RN or LPN, as we know it today, but went on to greatly influence the nursing industry worldwide. She was a hands on Caregiver, "A Real Caregiver!" touched by God. She made a huge impact on the world and so can we!

Make Your Mark, Be All 'HEART'

Florence Nightingale speaks, **"Listen":** *I attribute my success to this: "I never gave or took an excuse. I am of certain convinced that the greatest heroes are those who do their duty in the daily grind of domestic affairs whilst the world whirls as a maddening dreidel."*

"To be a fellow workers with God is the highest aspiration of which we can conceive man capable".

 MISS ASONDRA STARN'AIR

Florence Nightingale Work Bag

Look, if you are serious about your career as a "Caregiver Professional" then you need to invest in your own supplies.

Let me introduce to you our "Florence Nightingale Bag" (**FNG Bag**) This bag is a reminder that as professional caregivers we must come to work equipped and ready to act. Yes become real live Florence Nightingale's, yes, caregivers, both women and men that deliver, get the job done; within our scope of course! If you want to be the best **"Invest"** Purchase your own supplies.

Florence Nightingale was unstoppable she never let anything get in the way of success. Ms. Nightingale, 'The Lady with the Lamp, used her own money to get what she needed, she did not wait or take no for an answer, nor should we. If what you desire is going to help people thrive and survive then go for it! Caregivers, let's be the Florence Nightingale of our time, **"Let's Shine"**!

Now it's time for **US** to show the world what we can do. Florence Nightingale, **WE SOLUTE YOU!**

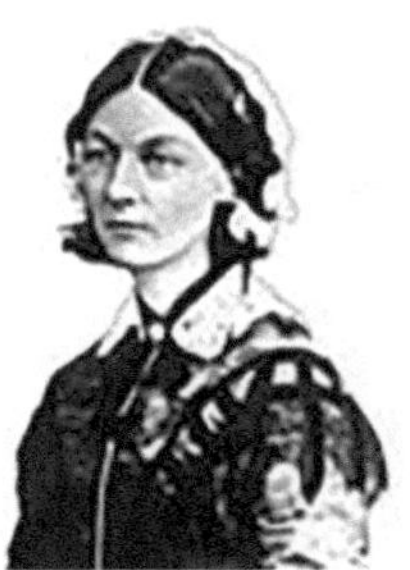

FLORENCE NIGHTINGALE FNG Bag!

1. Flash light
2. Mini first aid kit
3. Gait Belt
4. Gloves and a few towels
5. Stethoscope
6. Digital Thermometer
7. Plastic Waste Bags
8. Scissors/Tweezers
9. Note pad, & writing utensils.
10. The Book, (Holy Bible)
11. This Book (ACB to Excellence!)
12. Professional Business Phone
13. Reading Glasses
14. CPR Barriers, and Mask Kit.
15. Hand Sanitizers and Soap

On The Side Personal Bag

Your own food
Snacks & Beverages
Spending Money
Change of Shoes
Extra uniform/dinner Clothes
"Freshen Uppers"
"Hello New Day Caregivers"
Welcome To your New

Fng Bag!

Foot Care for Caregivers

Being on your feet all day can be harmful to your feet. When your feet hurt, you hurt!

Caregivers we need to be mindful of good foot care and make it a priority as part of a daily routine to take better care of our feet.

By addressing the problem early we can decrease the chances of a more serious condition that sometime require injections or surgery.

Caring for the feet is relatively simple, it starts with wearing the right shoe and foot care on a regular bases.

Tools You Can Use!

TLC FOOT CARE

1. Don't wear cheap shoes.
2. Avoid wearing flat shoes.
3. Wear special work shoes designed for comfort and arch elevation.
4. Sit while you chart, if possible.
5. Sit on your breaks, take a load off
6. Pray over your feet ask God to heal them.
7. Soak and pamper your feet at least three times a week.
8. Relax on your off days, Keep your feet elevated, feet up, read your bibles. have a cup of tea!
9. Wiggle your toes and feet daily for stretching and circulation.
10. Keep toenail cut low.
11. Do foot massages regularly.
12. See a Podiatrist, to find out the underlying problems if these tips are not helping.

In your tool box over to right, I have provided you with some tips on how to tender love and care for your feet, something we don't do enough of, until we are in pain, or hurting and forced to see a doctor.

We don't have to let it get that far, if we began now, early, our feet can do what Jesus did, walked! Jesus Walked and So Must We!

God Bless You!

Growing Older

The challenge of growing older can be cumbersome on both par-ties the one who needs care and the caregiver. It doesn't matter if you are caring for a family member or a formal caregiver working for an agency.

It's going to take a lot of empathy, understanding and patients to help that other individual get comfortable with having to have someone care for them because they are growing older.

Caregivers keep in mind too, and it's not personal but many times some older adults will act out and refuse the personal care. When this happens back off and try again later. They'll come around soon. It is not easy being a senior, some really do have a difficult time adjusting.

However, this is where we come in at, we don't take the rejection or unfriendliness personal, we simply ask ourselves how would we feel if we could no longer do the things we use to love to do, or be able to jump in our vehicles and go and come as we please? With that being said, we must shake it all off and find a way to make their day!

CAREGIVER TIPS

- Growing Older
- Medication
- UTI
- Incontinent issue/constipation
- Aches &Pain
- Medical Conditions/
- Diagnoses/memory care
- Environmental changes
- Loneliness
- Boredom
- Physical Inactivity
- Fatigue, Restlessness
- Worry, financial pressure
- Life and everyday stuff!
- New housing and community
- Death of spouse or love one
- Personality Conflict

Could Be Supremacy Behaviors, like **POP!**
- **P**rejudice
- **O**bnoxious
- **P**ride

If this is happening report it, or it will never stop!

All I can say is be creative, Ask God to help you and He will, He help me in all my difficult times. Here's the thing, Getting older for many is no fun, if they lash out at you, don't run, **"STAY!"** We are "Caregivers", let's help them find their way!

Lastly, keep in mind that some of the behavior issues may not be related to just growing older, there could be a real medical issue such as beginning stages of some kind of dementia such as Alzheimer disease, it can also be a UTI, anything so, we can't assume at all. But **"Growing Older"** is a topic in this book and something that needs a second look. Let's just be mindful and pay close attention to everything during this time in their lives. Report any lingering behavior to your supervisor and if it's a family member, speak with their doctor, we can't take any chances of thinking their behavior is something it's not. Because again, Some behaviors can be a medical cry out for help. Caregivers just stay put, and be patient, kind, loving and alert. Keep a close eye on them unfortunately, we cannot turn back the hands of time but, we can make sure they are free, safe and fine.

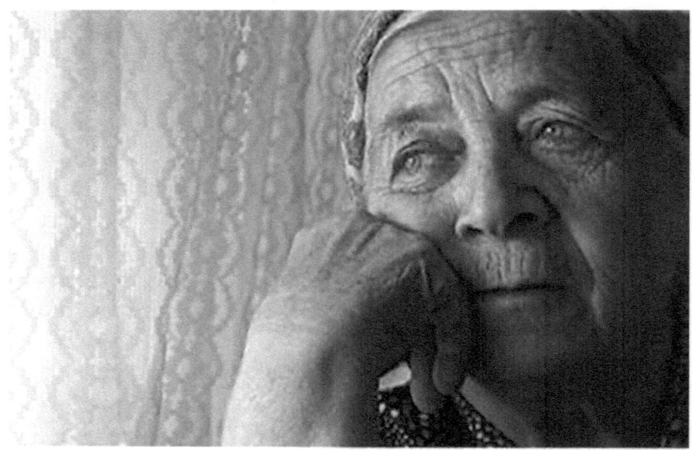

Caregivers, *"You shall rise up before the gray headed and honor the aged and you shall revere your God, I am the LORD."* **Leviticus19:32**

 Miss Asondra StarN'air

Hospital

Hospital are the last place anyone wants to go to, let alone be in. As a caregivers it is our job and responsibility to not only provide quality care, but provide hospitality as well.

We do this when we, do more than what is expected of us, that's right, we do this when we go the extra mile to make sure all the patients' needs are met within our power.

The power I am referring to is the power of LOVE. That's what God needs from his caregivers, He doesn't want us to just go in an collect a paycheck. He wants us to really, really love what we do. In the hospitals these people are sick, they need you.

Caregiver let's not be caregivers for ourselves anymore, let's be caregivers for Christ! We are not working for man, we are working for our father in heaven. So when you arrive at work, or wherever you go everyone should be able to see there is something different about you. That God has sent another person with A lamp, some-one who really wants to be there and really cares. O' how I hope and pray today that, that person is you. If it is, know this, God is there beside you, he is with you. Go, be the next Florence Nightingale, female or male, there is nothing, great caregivers, can't achieve or do.

God is with **"You!"**

Housekeeping Rules

Whether you work in a facility or in homecare, caregivers it is very imperative that we remember some housekeeping rules when serving individuals in our care. Why? Because the way that person wants things done still matters, that's why. We are not to go in and take over. Although the individual may not be feeling well, if they are still able to talk and make decisions for themselves, well then, they still have a say in everything including the kind of care they receive, and again, how they want things done.

Many of them may be sick or elderly but that does not give us the right to take over. We still must respect their home or place of residency we cannot go in and take over. It's one things to be excellent at what you do, but when you start doing what you want to do because you are good, then **'Huston We Have a Problem"**

I don't care how good or excellent you are, caregiver we still must be humble and remain teachable, furthermore, we must not forget that the person in our care is our boss when we're with them.

That's right, you heard me, they are our bosses too, what they say and want matters and must be respected.

Of course, if what they want is going to do more harm than good, try to explain that, or let the office know so they can talk to that person or the family. Meanwhile, show some **RESPECT.**

HOUSE KEEPING RULES

1. Do not move their things around or rearrange items unless they ask you to.
2. If it's a safety issue tell them why you think it needs to be moved, however, they have the final say safety issues, **"Inform The Office".**
3. Do not leave work for other caregivers. Put away your own dishes and don't do the laundry unless you can finish the entire task.

"YOUR SHIFT, YOUR CHORES"

4. If you notice a housekeeping problem, solve it, don't just push it off on another caregiver, be a leader, be great at what you do, take the initiative and see the problem through. Call the office if you need advice or coaching.
5. Always, always respect the customers wishes.

Stay Professional, Be a Team Players too!

In A Nutshell!

Caregivers, do your due diligence and your absolute best when serving those in your care. Make sure you put into practice hospitality awareness. And too, recognize,

They are the customer, We are the providers.
Caregiving is an art, lots of work and all heart!

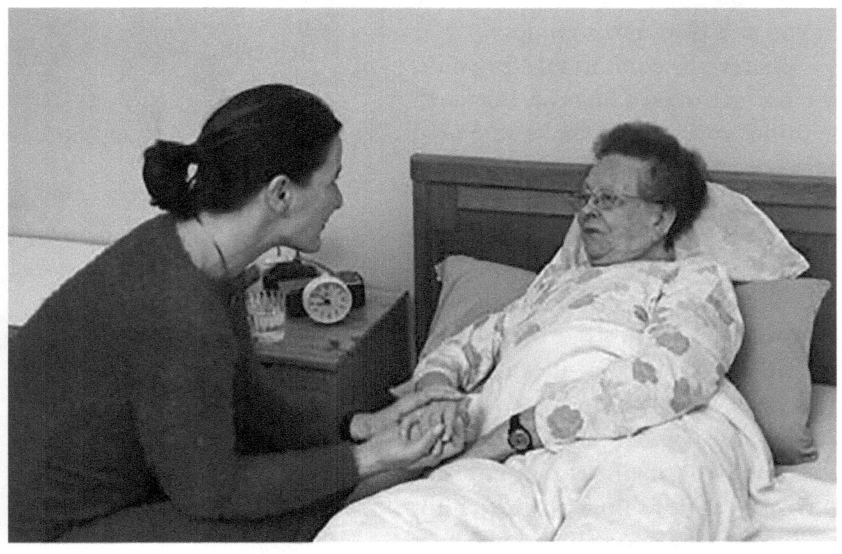

Good Morning, Mrs. Robinson, my name is Sarah Parker, I will be your caregiver today. What would you like to do first?

Now that's what I'm talking about
"Caregiving At Its Finest!"

How to Study the Bible

Basic Instructions Before Leaving Earth There are many different ways one can approach bible reading. Some like to study in groups where everyone is reading the same thing and then have discussions afterward.

But I think, if this is your first time reading through the bible, it should be just you and God, not a group.

Whatever is comfortable for you is the most important I suppose. But here's the thing, you want to make sure God and you are bonding intimately, just you and him, what He says to you, He may not say to the group.

Groups are great after you have studied the first year with God. Because now you are ready to share testimonies, revelations, ask questions and fellowship with other Christian and not feel lost or intimidated by "Christian Intellects", those who know it all, yet may not have a personal relationship with God at all.

By studying God's word the first year by yourself, just you and God, you'll be able to weed out "Counterfeits" see, everyone in bible study groups are not necessarily there for real christian living, some have hidden agendas.

Again, get to know God for yourself first and foremost then join study groups. Because fellowshipping is a good thing and encouraged.

Tools You Can Use!

TURN THE TV OFF AND TURN GOD ON

- God will meet you where you are at. So find a book in the bible that speaks to your current situation.
- Start a prayer life, everyday start praying to God. You are his now!
- Find a special place in your home to begin your journey with God.
- **"Bible Study"**, give yourself at least a year to get rooted.
- Don't worry about full understanding, that will come as you continue to live for Christ.
- Ask God to penetrate your mind body and soul to want to change and follow Christ.
- Commit to the same time and days to study your bible without any distractions.
- Let your family know on this day at this time, you will not be available.
- Pray, tell God how much you need him and how you are lost without him.

Listen for God, *He* will speak to you, God may want you to read from the **New Testament** first, or the **Old Testament**. The Holy Spirit will guide you.

- Lastly, Don't get in front of God, surrender to God and allow him to slowly mold you into what *He* wants you to be.

How To Make An Occupied Bed

1. Tell the person what you about to do.
2. Gather all the linens and laundry bag.
3. Roll the bedbound person over to center of bed.
4. Loosen the bottom soiled linen behind bedbound person back.
5. Roll soiled bed linen toward center of bedbound person and tuck under the person back as far as possible.
6. Begin placing clean fitted sheet and tuck under bedbound person without touching the soiled linen.
7. Go over to the other side roll individual over slightly onto the clean side now, pull old soiled linen sheets from under bedbound person back and place soiled linen in laundry bag.
8. Pull clean linen threw and tuck in sheet, make sure wrinkle free, no creases, sheet needs to be tucked in tightly and smooth.
9. Change both pillow cases.
10. Get rid of the old flat top sheet and replace with a clean one, then place a clean blanket over the bed-bound person.

"That's It, You Got It!"

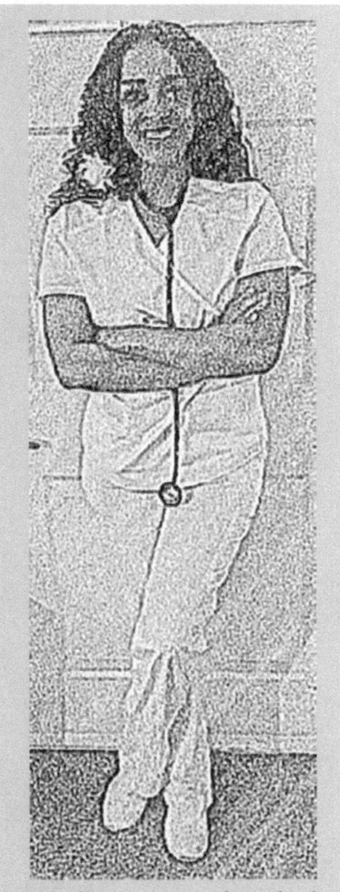

Don't forget to re-adjust bed positioning and place call light button within persons reach.
Thank You!

Miss Asondra StarN'air

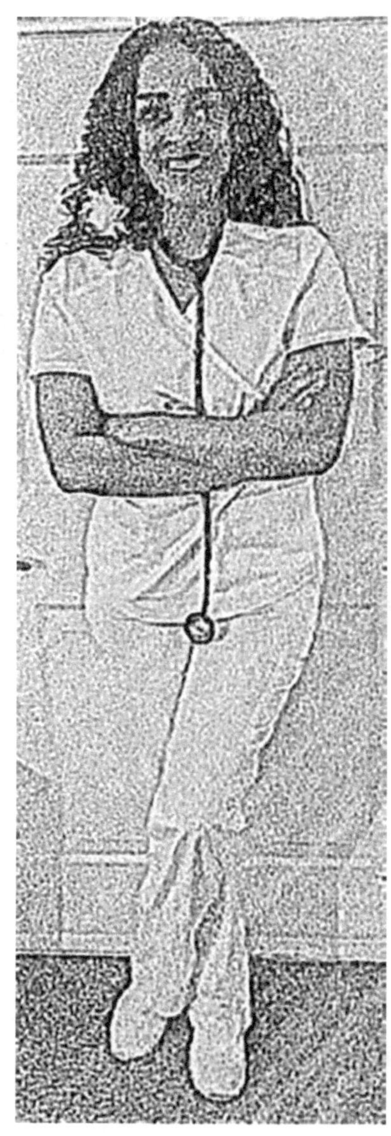

My oh, my, caregivers we've covered a lot haven't we? Yes we have.
Take a break then, let's keep going, let's keep growing.....

How To Prepare Thicken Liquid

People who have difficulty swallowing thin liquids often must drink thicken liquids. Drinking thicken liquids can help prevent chocking and stop fluids from entering the lungs. There are 3 common consistency, **Nectar,** (pourable) like cream soup, next there's **Honey**, pours like honey too and finally **Pudding** which does not pour, as a rule of thumb these are the 3 ways caregivers thicken liquids.

To thicken a 4oz serving of liquid drink or soup add:

- **Nectar :** 1 ½ teaspoon s thickener
- **Honey :** 1 ½ tablespoons thickener
- **Pudding :** 2 table spoons thickener

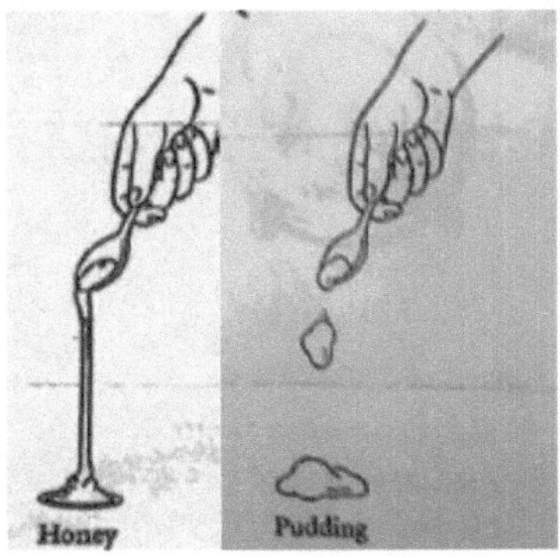

SWALLOWING DIFFICULTIES

Possible Solutions

Drooling : Cue to close lips.
Food falling out of mouth: Give small bites, place food on strong side of mouth.
Spitting : May dislike taste, offer alternative food items.
Pocketing /storing food in mouth : Alternate liquids and solids during meal time and, clean mouth after every meal. **Increase chewing time**: Offer small bites, offer liquids often.
Coughing before, during or after the swallowing: Stop feeding and notify the charge nurse.
Wet, gurgly voice after meal: Notify the charge nurse.

Possible Causes

Drooling : Poor sensation, weak lips seal, excessive saliva.
Food falling out of mouth : Poor lip closure.
Spitting : Dislike the texture and taste.
Pocketing in mouth and cheeks: Reduced cheek or lip strength, weak tongue movement, or decrease sensation.
Coughing Episodes : Aspiration, reduced control of bolus, ineffective airway closure, residue in throat or vocal folds.
Wet, gurgly voice: Residue in throat or vocal fold.

How to use a Hoyer Lift

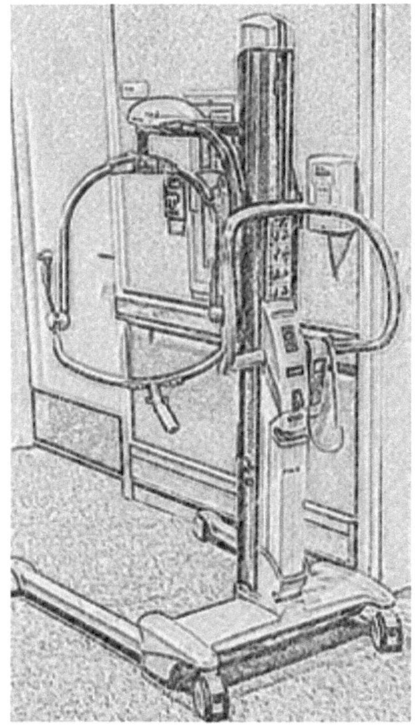

HOYER LIFTS REQUIRE TWO PEOPLE AT ALL TIMES TO OPERATE!

- Following the instruction manual or training given by instructor.
- Make sure person is feeling very secure and safe before lifting.
- Do not attempt to hoyer lift without a second person if working in facilities.
- Private care, makes up their own rules. Make sure you know what you are doing, if not, don't do it!
- Disinfect equipment daily.
- Make sure the battery is always fully charged.
- Store in a safe place when finished.
- Laundry hoyer sling to ensure cleanliness once a week or when necessary.

Using a hoyer lift is the most safe and pratical way to transport individuals who can no longer support themselves or bear weight. It helps to keep everyone safe from injury, caregivers should not try to lift or physically transfer anyone who can not bear their own weight, period. Doing this can have consequences later on. Please be advised.

How To Take Temperature

There are 3 ways to take temperature.
Rectally-Orally-Axillary
For babies and children under five, rectal temperature is the most accurate.

For older children and adults Oral is best.

As an alternative for people of any age, axillary (arm pit) is another way but not as reliable as the other two options.

Use a mutiuse or oral digital thermometer. Some digital thermometer are design to be used either rectally, orally or under the armpit while others are designed for mouth only.

Glass thermometer are considered unsafe now because they contain mercury, which is poisonous to the touch.

After each use, clean and place back inside of case. Return it back to your **FNG Bag** or First-Aid Kit, **"Don't Forget!"**

Tools You Can Use!

How To Take Temperature

1. Wash Your Hands!
2. Use a clean thermometer.
3. Rinse it in cold water first before using.
4. When finish rinse again and clean with rubbing alcohol.
5. Do not eat or drink any-thing for at least 5 minutes before taking temperature
6. Keep mouth close during this time.

If you are using a vital cart at a hospital or facility, discard disposable tube slot and wash your hands again before going to your next room.

Document your reading, if it's too low or high contact the doc-tor or the case manager on duty.

Humility

2 Chronicles 7:14 NIV)

If my people, who are called by my name, will humble themselves and pray and seek my face and turn from their wicked ways, then I will hear from heaven, then I will forgive their sin and heal their land.

So I created this acronym just for you, I believe this will help you realize that you need a savior, yes, **YOU** and all of us need Jesus Christ to run things now.

We can no longer run our own lives anymore if we want our lives to blossom in every area then realize this, you must give you up for Jesus like he gave himself up for you. Whether it cost you something or not, and it will, but in the end it will be worth it.

Allow him to be the role model, the commander and chief of every area of your life from now on.

> **Humility**
>
> **H**umble yourself
>
> **U**nderstand
>
> **M**an /woman
>
> **I**s
>
> **L**ower
>
> **I**n
>
> **T**he trinity so
>
> **Y**ield

Humble yourself, understand man/woman is lower in the trinity so yield! The bible says we ought not think of ourselves more highly than we ought too.

Isaiah 64:6 puts it in our face like this, *All of us have become like one who is unclean, and all our righteous acts are like filthy rags; we all shrivel up like a leaf, and like the wind our sins sweep us away.*

Humility says to me these words "I'm a sinner Lord, and I know that I am not worthy, but please Father God allow me to change. Let me work at becoming all you want me to be. Remove all uncleanliness out of my life, teach me to live right. Make me Holy". **You're next, what do you say to our Lord and Savior?**

Humble Thyself!

How to Wash Your Hands

1. Make sure you have a clean towel or paper towels in advance.
2. Turn on the water, make sure it's warm.
3. Wet your hands well.
4. Lather your hands with soap
5. Wash under warm water.
6. Keep washing, scrub both sides, don't forget to scrub between the fingers, wash your wrist too, combined all of this for about 20 seconds or more. (Sing the hand washing song, or make up one).
7. Now rinse your hands, don't touch the sink.
8. Dry your hands with a towel, make sure that you dry between the fingers, dry your wrist too.
9. Use paper towel to turn water off.
10. Apply moisturizing cream or lotion.

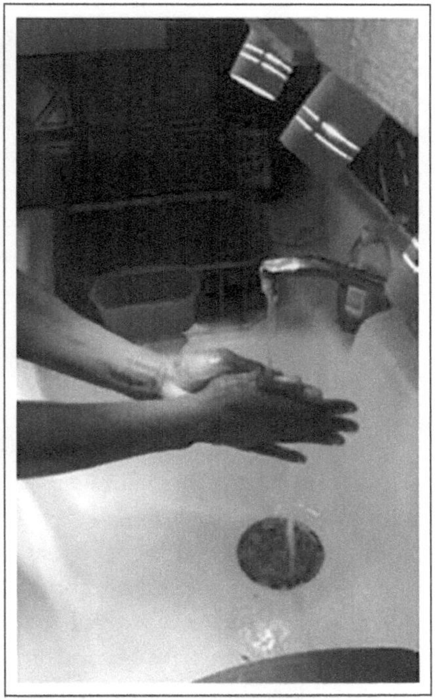

"Good to GO"
Great Job!

Is Your Smartphone Really Smart?

Is Your Smart Phone Really Smart? No it is not, if it has you making foolish decisions like, text messaging or talking on the phone when you are supposed to be working. Cell phones have become the biggest pest since mosquito. It's taken on a life of its own. People are becoming so addicted to their phones. It's seems we just can't live without this pesky device.

I say, and some may or may not agree, but I think employers ought to have **"Zero Tolerance"** for personal cell phone use in the work place, especially in the healthcare industry. To take it a step further, new laws need to be enacted making it harder for employees to operate phones while at work. And here's why I say this, **"Smart Phone"** are becoming problem phones. Healthcare workers, nurses included are putting their private calls before care. What about work, the patient, the customer, come on, is that really fair? No it is not! **When on the job, do your job!** Stop talking and texting or showing off pictures on your smart phones. Let's not leave those in need of help or care, **'ALONE'** while you sit and chill with your phone!

Everybody, Listen Up!

We all know by now that it's not cool or safe to text and drive, so we don't do it. **'It Can Wait!'**
But work world, so can our phones, **'It Can Wait Too!'** We have a job to do!

Smart Phone Apps that helps!!!

- CPR
- First Aid
- Note pads
- Calories Tracker
- The Holy Bible
- Scripture of the day
- Nutrition/food pyramid
- Navigator
- Dictionary
- Phone book
- Dementia/Alzheimer's
- Medical Dictionary
- *A Caregiver's Bible to Excellence!* e-book

Wow!
Now that's a Smart Phone!

The Messiah Speaks to His Caregivers

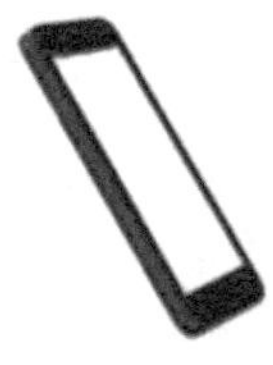

Listen, Listen, Listen!

Caregiver, regarding phones at work, we don't have times to mess around with them, God is depending on us; we have much work to do. Now Jesus wants to talk to you, **Shurr... be quite, listen:**

When I was hungry and you gave Me something to eat; I was thirsty and you gave me something to drink; I was naked and you clothed Me; I was sick and you took care of Me; I was in prison and you visited Me. "Then the righteous will an-swer Him 'Lord, when did we see You hungry and feed You or thirsty and give You something to drink? When did we see you a stranger and take You in, or without clothes and clothe You? When did we see You sick or in prison and visit You? "And the King will answer them 'I assure you; Whatever you did for one of the least of these brothers of Mine, you did for Me." (Matt. 25:35–40)

See, now this call is over, put up your phones and get back to work! Caregivers, need I say more?

Use Your Smart Phones, Godly!

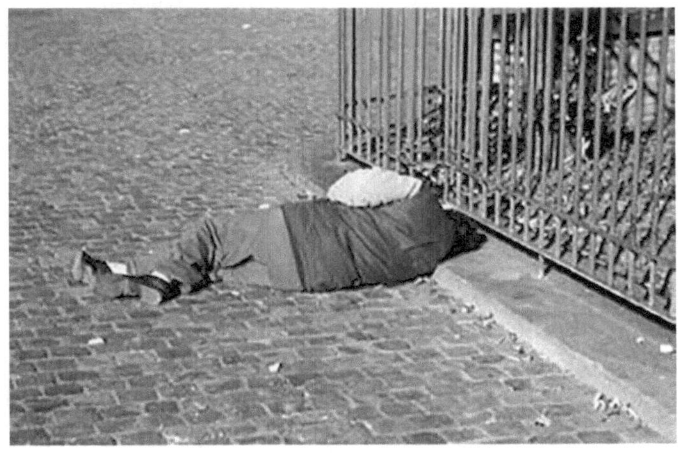

Normal Vital Signs

Blood Pressure:

Adults: defined with 2 measurements on 2 different dates at least 2 weeks apart
- Normal BP <120/<80 mmHg
- PreHTN: 120-139/80-89 mmHg
- HTN Stage I: 140-159/90-99 mmHg
- HTN Stage II: ≥160/≥100 mmHg

Children:
- Birth (12 Hr, <1000g): 39-59/16-36 mmHg
- Birth (12 hr, 3 kg): 50-70/25-45 mmHg
- Neonate (96hr): 60-90/20-60 mmHg
- Infant (6 mo): 87-105/53-66 mmHg
- Toddler (2 yr): 95-105/53-66 mmHg
- School Age (7yr): 97-112/57-71 mmHg
- Adolescent (15yr): 112-128/66-80 mmHg

Heart Rate:

Adults:
- Female: 55-95 bpm
- Male: 50-90 bpm

Children:
- Neonate: 100-180 bpm awake / 80-160 bpm asleep
- Infant (6mo): 100-160 bpm awake / 75-160 bpm asleep
- Toddler: 80-110 bpm awake / 60-90 bpm asleep
- Preschooler: 70-110 bpm awake / 60-90 bpm asleep
- School-aged child: 65-110 bpm awake / 60-90 bpm asleep
- Adolescent: 60-90 bpm awake / 50-90 bpm asleep

Respiration Rate:

Adults:
12-18 breaths per minute

Children:
- Infants: 30-60 breaths per minute
- Toddlers: 24-40
- Preschoolers: 22-34
- School-aged children: 18-30
- Adolescents: 12-16

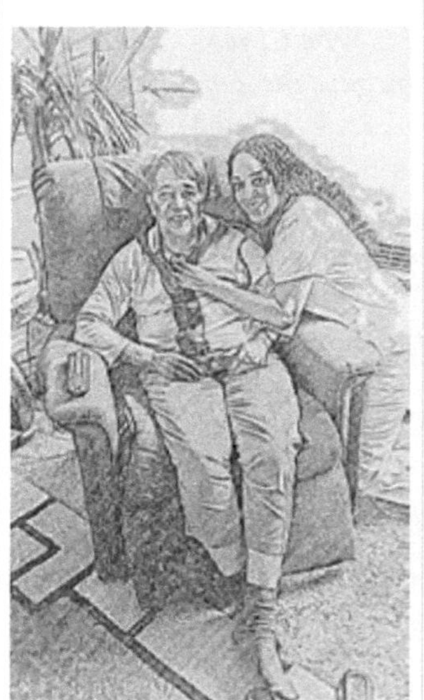

MISS ASONDRA STARN'AIR

Vitals Signs

The chart of resting heart rates below are there for you to check and see where you measure, as well as the heart rates of different ages of people with different levels of activity. If it's poor, see a doctor.

MEN						
AGE	18 -25	26 -35	36 -45	46 - 55	56 -65	65+
ATHLETE	49-55	49-54	50-56	50-57	51-56	50-55
EXCEL'T	56-61	55-61	57-62	58-63	57-61	56-61
GOOD	62-65	62-65	63-66	64-67	62-67	62-65
ABOVE AV	66-69	66-70	67-70	68-71	68-71	66-69
AVERAGE	70-73	71-74	71-75	72-76	72-75	70-73
BELOW AV	74-81	75-81	76-82	77-83	76-81	74-79
POOR	82+	82+	83+	84+	82+	80+

WOMEN						
AGE	18 -25	26 -35	36 -45	46 - 55	56 -65	65+
ATHLETE	54-60	54-59	54-59	54-60	54-59	54-59
EXCEL'T	61-65	60-64	60-64	61-65	60-64	60-64
GOOD	66-69	65-68	65-69	66-69	65-68	65-68
ABOVE AV	70-73	69-72	70-73	70-73	69-73	69-72
AVERAGE	74-78	73-76	74-78	74-77	74-77	73-76
BELOW AV	79-84	77-82	79-84	78-83	78-83	77-84
POOR	86+	83+	86+	84+	84+	84+

Parkinson's Disease

"Floats like a butterfly, sting like a bee, his eyes can't hit what the eyes can't see". Those were the famous words and charm of the late, great **Mohammed Ali.** He was a world renowned boxers and so much more. Yes, He was one of the greatest boxers of all times, he died of 'Parkinson Disease'.

What is Parkinson's Disease?

It is a disorder of the central nervous system that affects movement, often including tremors. More than 200,000 cases per year have been diagnosed according to research.

Those living with this disease can still fight to live the best life possible, Ali did, this boxer never gave up, he fought right up until the very end. And so can others, caregivers, stay on top of your game, work with those who have this degenerating disease, but also encourage them tofight, not to give up on life. Find a way to let those with Parkinson know that as long as they have breath and can breathe they can still enjoy theireveryday life.

Caregiver's Information Center

It Ain't Over Until It's Over!

Daily Care for those with Parkinson Desease.

- Read up on the disease, it's progressive so know the stages, signs & symptoms
- Adapt the environment/home
- Simplify ADL routines keep them easy and consistent.
- Keep Pathways Open

Remove floor rugs or tack them down.

Use red of blue paint or tape to color water facets red or blue to designated which one is hot or cold.

- Encourage activities, and never let them give up on life.

Remind them that when life knocks us down. like the great boxer Muhammad Ali, we keep getting back up, again and again.... Parkinson is not the end.

Remind them of the late great Mohammad Ali, encourage them to put their gloves on, keep their head up and fight, that right! "Float like a butterfly, sting like a bee" that disease can't hit, what the eyes cannot see.

The same goes for **"Everybody, Everywhere"**, especially struggling care-givers, no matter what life throws at you, put your gloves on and fight, don't give up, be the champion, God knows you can be! "Float Like A butterfly, Sting Like a Bee". Say to this world **"You Are Not Going To Rule Over Me"!**

   Miss Asondra StarN'air

We Will Never Forget You!

Mohammad Ali!
January 17, 1942 - June 3. 2016
We Will Never Forget You!
The Greatest Boxer of All Time!

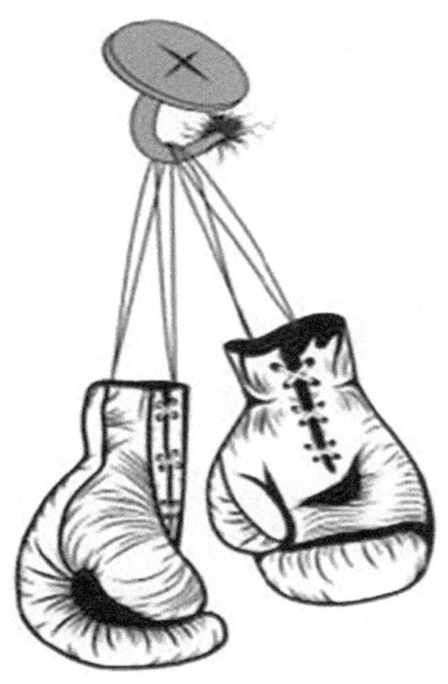

RIP

Parkinson's Disease

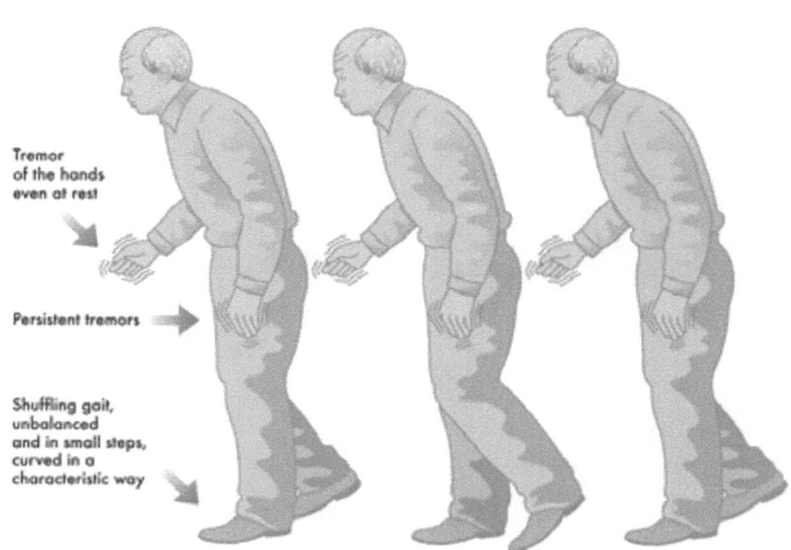

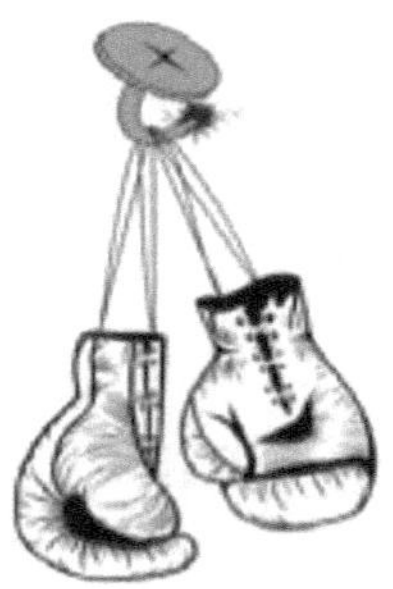

'Fight The Good Fight Of "Faith!"

MISS ASONDRA STARN'AIR

Pill Box

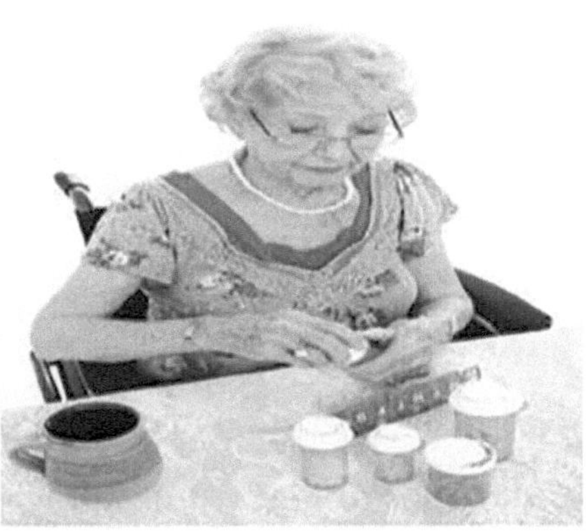

Caregivers **"Stop"** we do not pass meds unless we are certified to do so. Now that you are aware, do not allow the client or family members to talk you into filling pill boxes. Don't do it! Because it can get you in a whole lot of serious trouble if something goes wrong. That person could die, from your mistake, you can end up in a court room, and you don't what that, do you? I don't think so!

Well then 'Caregivers" stay in your lane! You must be an **RN, LPN** or have a med pass license to fill pill boxes, or be a family member, and "you are not!" Rule of thumb, **'WRONG'**, always gets caught!

It's the client or family members that are responsible for this task. However, if that person is alone and have no family, just us, we are caregivers, we can help, and we must, we can assist them by making sure they are filling their pill boxes correctly. Over to the right, I have given you tools you can use to help you stay professional and out of trouble. **'Caregivers'** we don't fill pill boxes but we do fill hearts when we help!

The Client:

Put pills in the pill box.
Instructing them is ok.
Let them take their time.
Look out for mistakes.

Both should read the labels.
Opening the tops are Ok.
X-ray the pill box!
Meaning, make sure your client filled his or her pill box correctly!

More Tips

- The Medicated Person reads the drug label.
- The Caregiver reads the drug label too but, only the **'Medicated Person'** or family members, fills the pill box! **Not us.**

Quick Tip: TIT

They Read What to Do!
Read What to Do!
They Fill the 'Pill Box'!

Not Me!

Pulse Reading

Did you know that measuring the heart rate helps determine the fitness level of an individual? Well it does! For example, when you hear a quicken or fast pulse that is an indicator that the heart is working overtime. That may be okay if you are working out but if you are just sitting and relaxing it's not okay. Something may be wrong and needs to be checked out.

Checking your pause regularly is a simple way to get health information and help prevent heart attacks in older adults.

Heart Rate Ranges

Highs and Lows
Birth 1 years old: 100 and 160
Toddlers 1-3 years: 90 and 150
Preschoolers 3-6 years: 80 and 140
School Age 6 to 15 years: 70 and 100
Adults 18 and older: 60 and 100 depending on persons physical condition and age.

HOW TO TAKE PULSE
2 Quick and Easy Ways

Taking Pulse is Simple and Easy Here's What You Do:

1. Place 2 two fingers on the person's wrist between the bone and the tendon over the radial artery, that's located on the thumb side of the wrist.
2. When you feel the pulse, start counting for 15 second.
3. Now, multiply that number by 4 this will calculate your beats per minute.

The 2nd Quick and Easy Way: count for 30 seconds and multiply by 2, that gives you your number too!

That's It!
record time and date.
You're Done!

Taking Pulse is Soooo Easy!!!

Practice on yourself, what's your fitness level?

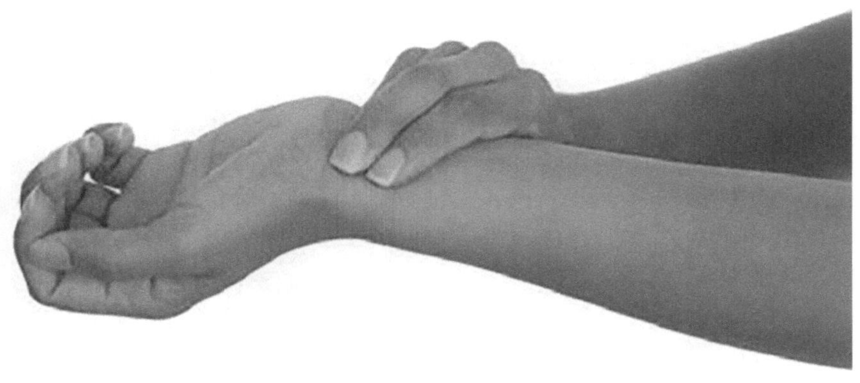

Count 15 Seconds, Next, Times It By 4
1.2.3.4.5.6.7.8.9.10.11.12.13.14.15
Who Can Ask for Anything More!
Now Record Your Score.

Range of Motion

Range of motion is how far the patient's joints can be moved in different directions. Exercises helps the individual move all the joints through their full **Range of Motion.**

Caregivers, there are three types of **ROM** exercises.

1. **Passives:** No effort from patient.
2. **Active:** No assistance needed.
3. **Active Assist:** Assistance needed.

Passive Range of Motion(PROM) is when someone else has to help them do it, example, they may not be able to lift their legs so we help lift it for them until they get stronger and able to do it themselves. that's passive range of motion.

Caregivers Information Center

PASSIVE RANGE OF MOTION

- Do the exercises every day, or as often as prescribed.
- You may do them in any order.
- You may also spread them out over the course of the day.
- Slow and gentle movements.
- Avoid fast or jerky motions
- Always support the area near the joints.
- Extend, move joints as far as it will go.
- If there is any pain or discomfort, **STOP!** Contact your case manager before proceeding.
- Do the exercises on both sides.
- Play soft music, make it relaxing.
- Allow breaks in between the session and offer a cool drink of water.
- Document your sessions date, time. and how many sets completed.
- Try to establish a weekly routine for best results.
- Return **ROM** material/ equipment back to the same location for future use.
- Allow patient to rest after session if desired.

Caregivers "ROM" Poster

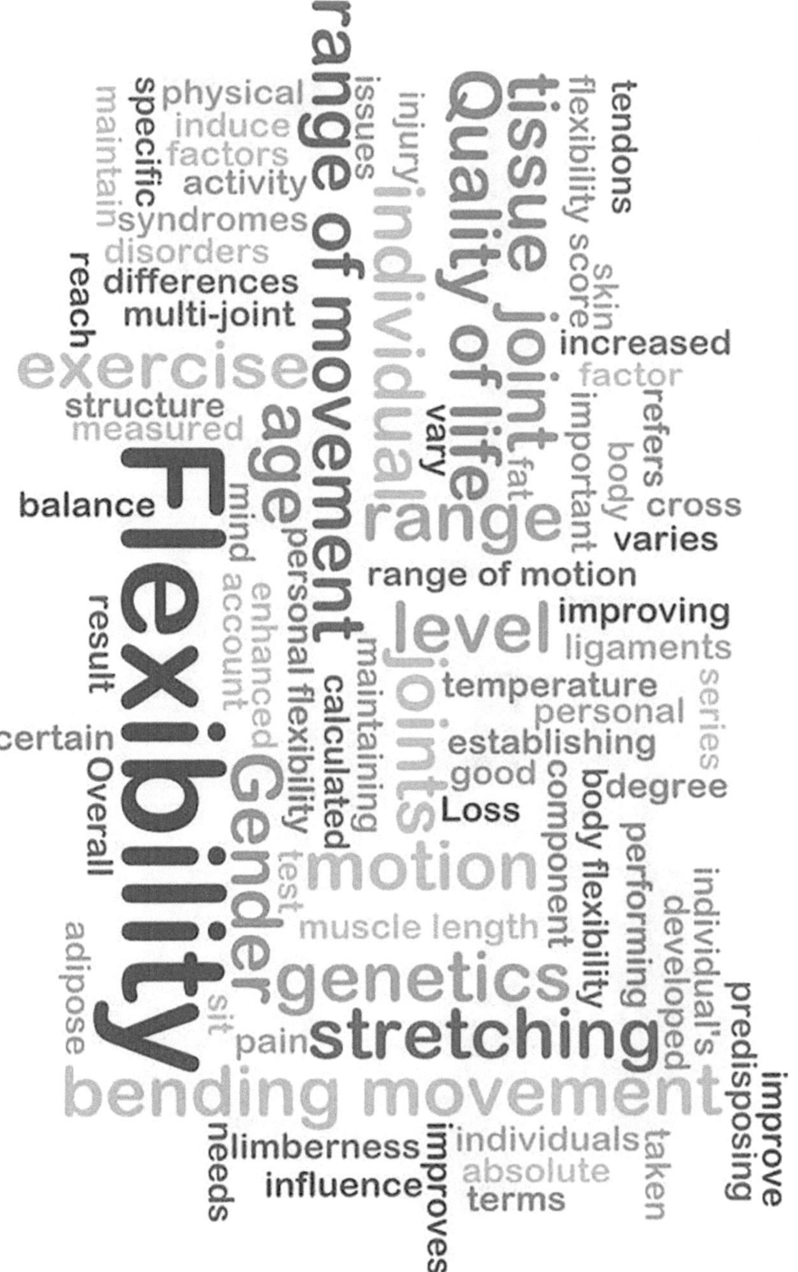

Get Ready!

Remember

Education

Always

Delivers Success

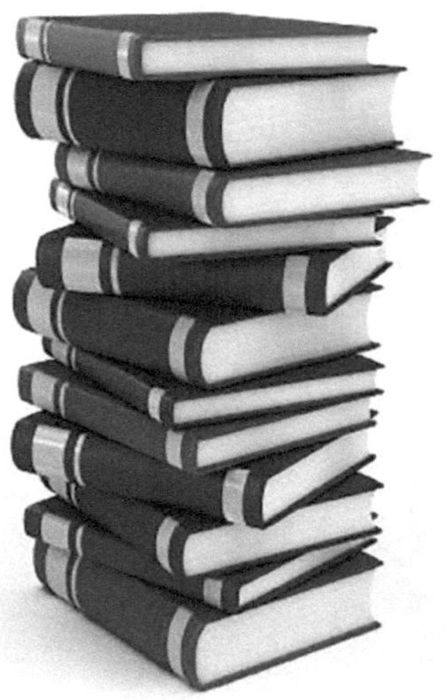

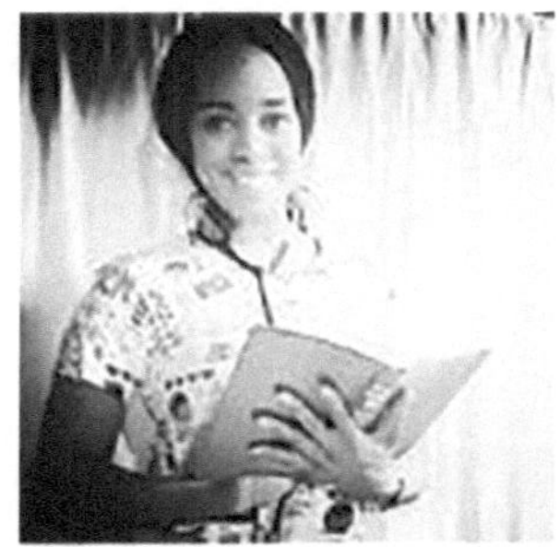

So, READ!

1. Read Daily
2. Welcome, 'Tea Time' reading
3. Make your time reading enjoyable.
4. Choose your material carefully
5. Own your own bibles
6. Take classes
7. Go back to school, it's never too late.
8. Read on your lunch breaks instead of gossiping.
9. Read to those in your care
10. Go to the library more often,
11. Sit, **Read and Relax!**
12. Learn also to read between the lines, if you know what I mean.
13. Read the fine print, before you sign.
14. Read to grow, to know, to show you are competent!
15. Read about things you don't know, that's how we get intelligent and grow.
16. Keep a book with you at all times.
17. Read what saith the **LORD!**
18. Read **'A Caregiver's Bible to Excellence'** often.
19. Read for others!
20. Read my lips, **"I Love You!"**

Standard Precaution

Standard precautions are for everyone. It's not just for healthcare workers. It's good practice for children and adults. Everyone around the world should be washing their hands several times a day. Practicing good hand hygiene is very important. It helps reduce the spread of germs that can cause us to get sick; and the sooner we start, the better.

Clean hands save lives—yours and mine!

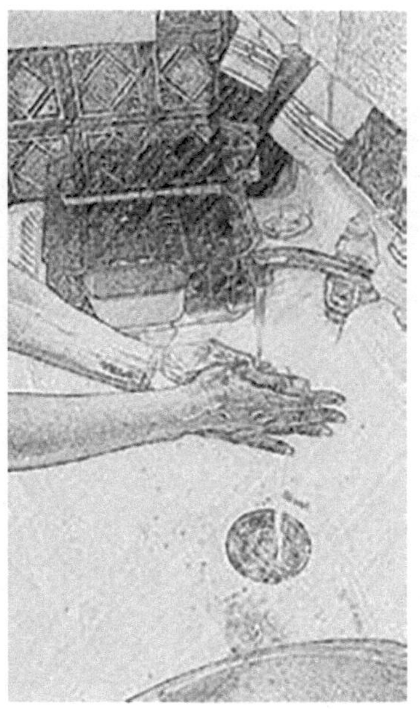

Wash those germs right out of your hands and send them on their way.

1. After arriving and leaving.
2. After sneezing or coughing.
3. Before making or eating food.
4. After playing with animals.
5. Before and after toileting.
6. After being outdoors, gardening, etc.
7. Before changing contact lenses.
8. Before and after patient care.
9. After shopping.
10. During and after social and entertainment events.
11. After intimacy.
12. Before and after personal grooming.
13. Before and after using office and computer/machinery.
14. Before and after child care.
15. After public exposure to elevator buttons and doors knobs.
16. Wash your hands more than once during public events, parks, concerts, rallies, sport events, baby showers, board games, cards, movie theaters, garage sales, parties, and celebrations— any time there is public inter-action. Wash your hand several times throughout the day.

Wipe and Clean Your Smart Phones Too!
"Cleanliness, Looks Good On YOU!"

Wash Your Hands Everyday!

Standard Precaution & Fingernails

Standard Precautions are a set of infection control practices used to prevent the spread of diseases. We should always follow standard precaution of course, but, it doesn't stop with our hands, we also need to keep our nails free of dirt and germs too. Health care professionals, especially nurses and caregivers, our nails are supposed to be kept low and unpolished at all times. They should look like the picture sample below. Pause a minute and look at your own hands and nails, are they clean and are your nails unpolished and cut low? If your answer is yes good, but if it's yes and no, hands clean, but, long fake nails then something's wrong. You're not practicing Standard Precaution. 'YOU" are out of compliance, correct this, your hands and nails should look like that picture below **'Clean, Tidy and Ready to Go!** Those long or acrylic nails you're wearing right now, sister, **Not Cool, Not Professional at all.**

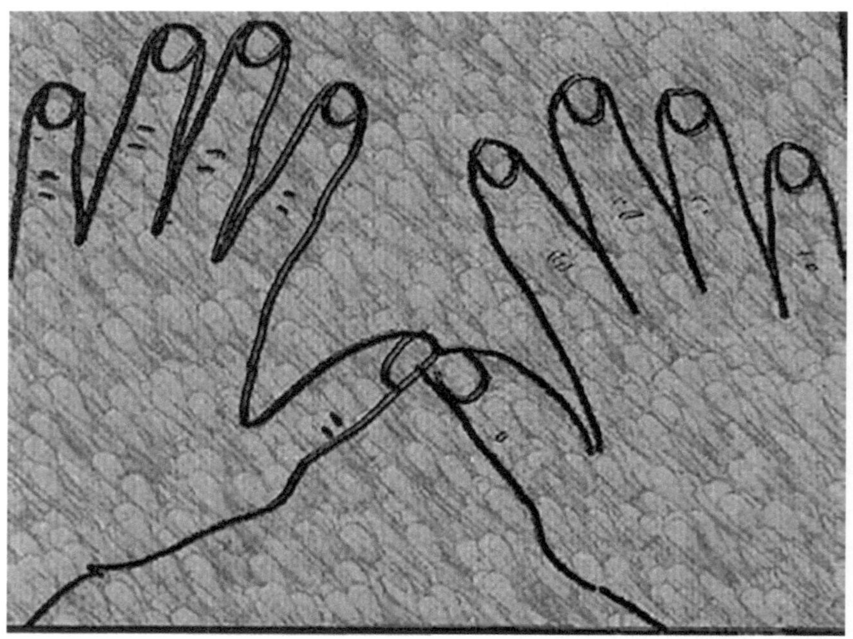

Get With The Program
Groomed Clean Hands, Short and Unpolished Nails Matters!

 Miss Asondra StarN'air

Stages of Dying

The stages, popularly known by the acronym **DABDA**, include:

1. **Denial** – The first reaction is denial. In this stage individuals believe the diagnosis is somehow mistaken, and cling to a false, preferable reality.
2. **Anger** – When the individual recognizes that denial cannot continue, they become frustrated, especially at proximate individuals. Certain psychological responses of a person undergoing this phase would be: "Why me? It's not fair!"; "How can this happen to me?"; "Who is to blame?" "Why would this happen?".
3. **Bargaining** – The third stage involves the hope that the individual can avoid a cause of grief. Usually, the negotiation for an extended life is made in exchange for a reformed lifestyle. People facing less serious trauma can bargain or seek compromise.
4. **Depression** – "I'm so sad, why bother with anything?"; "I'm going to die soon, so what's the point?"; "I miss my loved one, why go on?"

   During the fourth stage, the individual despairs at the recognition of their mortality. In this state, the individual may become silent, refuse visitors and spend much of the time mournful and sullen.

5. **Acceptance** – "It's going to be okay."; "I can't fight it, I may as well prepare for it."

   In this last stage, individuals embrace mortality or inevitable future, or that of a loved one, or other tragic event. People dying may precede the survivors in this state, which typically comes with a calm, retrospective view for the individual, and a stable condition of emotions.

Stroke

Stroke, also known as **Cerebrovascular Accident (CVA)** and **Cerebrovascular Insult (CVI)** or brain attack, is when blood flow to the brain results in sudden death.

My research from the Stroke Association says there is a quick and easy way to help identify the signs of a stroke. So that, 'Caregivers' will be able to spot it FAST, "Take a Look"

F—Face on one side droops and is numb. Ask the individual to smile.

A—Arm weakness. Is one arm weak or numb? Have the person raise both arms. Does one arm drift?

S—Speech difficulty. Speech is slurred or unable to speak. Can you understand what they said? Ask them to repeat a simple sentence like "Hello. How are you?" Can they? If not, pick up the phone.

T—**Time to call 911** If the person shows any of these symptoms, they may be having a stroke.

FAST! Go Call 911

A Caregiver's Guide

How To Dress and Undress A Stroke Patient

Follow These Tips

- Caregivers pick out clothes that are going to be easy to put on first.
- Make sure you have plenty of time to dress the person. No rushing.
- Dress the arm or leg of the weak side first. Have the patient sit down, if they can. Allow them to use the strong arm to dress the weak side first.
- If you have to dress them, tell them what you will be doing so they are comfortable receiving assistance.
- When it's time to undress, un-dress the strong side of the arm or leg first.

**A New Way To Remember
First Weak, Last Strong
When I do that, I can't go Wrong!**

Taking Blood Pressure

As Professional Caregivers, Family Caregiver and Caregivers in general, everyone whose responsible for the care of others whether you're Husband and Wife, First time moms etc. Should know how to take blood pressure both, manually and electronically.

1. Make sure caregivers your device is not defective, no small hole or cracks in any part of the device.
2. The device must be in good shape and make sure you have the right size fit for each person. Otherwise your reading will be off.
3. Make sure the individual is comfortable and relaxed.
4. Have the person sit with their arms slightly bent on the same level of their heart and resting comfortably on a table or if there is no table, any flat surface will do.
5. Place the inflatable blood pressure cuff securely on the upper arm, doesn't matter which arm unless one's injured or soar, if that is the case use the strong side upper arm.
6. Place the cuff approximately one inch above the bend of the elbow. It is best that the cuff touches the skin for a more accurate reading; may have to roll up sleeve.
7. Close the pressure valve on the rubber inflating bulb and pump the bulb rapidly to inflate the cuff. Take note: flat the cuff so that the dial reads about 30 mm Hg higher than the individuals at rest systolic pressure. Tip, If at rest pressure is unknown, inflate to 210 mm Hg or until the pause at the wrist disappears.
8. If using a Stethoscope, place the earpiece in your ear and the bell of the stethoscope over the artery, which is just below the cuff.
9. Now slowly release the pressure by twisting or pressing open the pressure valve, located on the bulb. The patient pressure should decrease about 2 to 3 mm Hg per second. Listen through the stethoscope and note on the dial when you first start to hear a pausing or tapping sound. This is the top number called **Systollic Blood Pressure**. Record that number, exp. 120 is

where you first heard that pausing or tapping, you saw it on the dial as 120. Again, that's your top number. Write it down!

10. Continue letting the air out slowly, now the pausing and tapping sounds will start to become dulled and eventually stop. That bottom number is called **Diastolic Blood Pressure** now record that one as your bottom number. Exp. It stopped completely at 70 on the dial.

11. Release the remaining air to relieve the pressure from the arm.

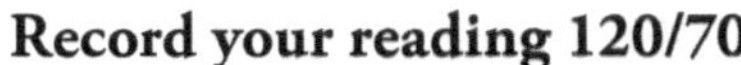

Record your reading 120/70

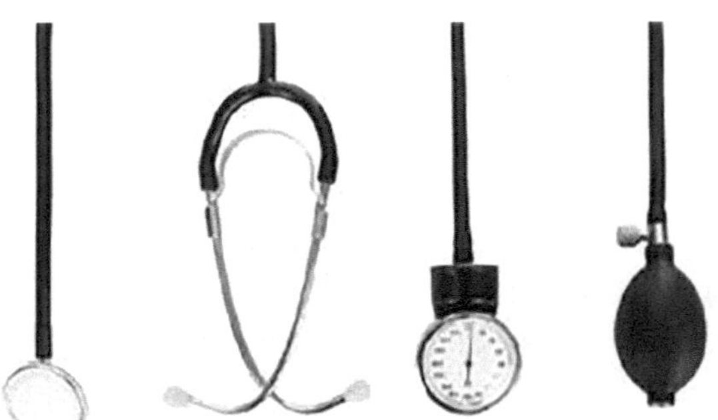

New Day Caregivers

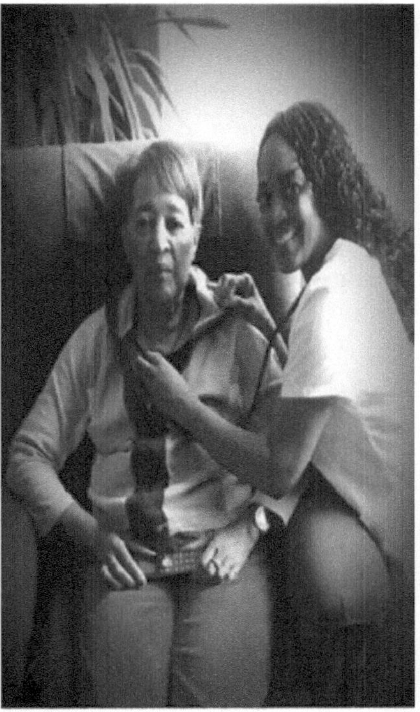

Did you know that monitoring blood pressure levels is import-ant because if the blood pressure is high, it is putting extra strain on the arteries also on the heart; which can cause heart attacks and strokes. So if you run into a 'high reading' stop and report it immediately or call 911.

BP

Caregiver Tips

- Take BP 30 minutes before meals and exercise.
- Allow individual to rest, relax 15 minutes before hand.
- Do not offer coffee, tea or anything with caffeine before taking BP.
- Take BP first thing in the morning because:

    1. Stress levels are lower
    2. Biological rhythms naturally cause pressure to be high in afternoons and evenings.

- Take BP several times while lying, sitting and standing.

Why? Because reading often skyrocket as you change positions. Which means it may not be high blood pressure after all instead weak adrenal glands.

Make sure the person is relaxed and elbows are at the same level of the heart, then start.

- Have BP taken three times with one minute rest in between each one.

Record, time and date and keep a log book handy.

Alert!
Dangerously Low or High BP
Call case manager or 911
Immediately
Taking Blood Pressure Matters!

Ten First Aide Tips For CareGivers

1. Grab your **FNG Bag** (Florence Nightingale Bag) all your tools from the list should be in there, right? If the injured person has a first-aid kit and other supplies you need, use theirs first.
2. Contact your supervisor if it's out of your scope or call 911, better safe than sorry!
3. Remember the **3C's** and stay **C**alm, **C**ool and **C**ollected!!!
4. First always ask for permission to help a person, e.g "are you okay? Is it alright if I help you?" If they are unconscious, Start CPR, **Check, Call, Care!**
5. Follow Universal and Standard Precautions, wash your hands first, put on gloves, and pull out your Personal Protective Equipment **(PPE)**.
6. Keep the injured person safe and calm and do not move them, unless it becomes absolutely necessary to move the injured person from the scene, e.g. a fire! Why? Because there may be some internal bleeding or broken or damage limbs that we can't see, it could be anything. Just keep them breathing and safe, wait for **(EMT)** Emergency Medical Technicians Paramedics to arrive.
7. If it's just ah first aid situation, and you can handle it, explain what you are going to do first.
8. After you are finish, wash your hands again and monitor the person. Ask that person, say are you okay now? If they say no, call for help.
9. Take Vitals, **(VS)** Temperature, Pulse, Respiration **(TPR)**
10. Document, and follow companies protocols. Private Caregivers contact family member in charge. **"Caregivers We Rock!"**

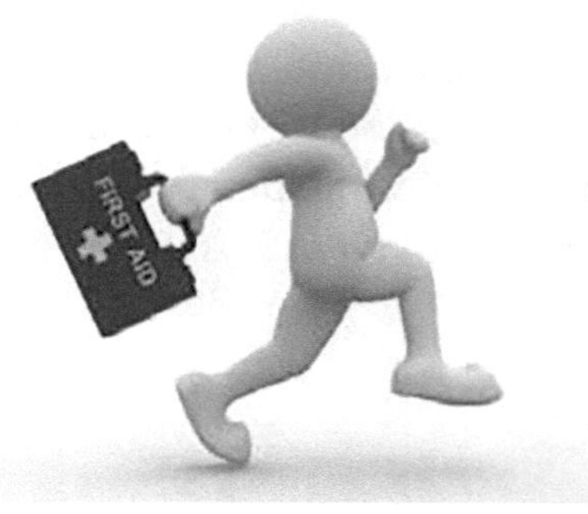

 Miss Asondra StarN'air

The Dangers of Overload

Today working two and three jobs have become a normal for many and the stress that comes with it has become a way of life.

Healthcare workers are choosing work, work, work, over health, and quality care. Customers are not getting what they are paying for and are becoming unhappy and frustrated. They will blame the employers in the end, see nobody wins. **Fatigues takes toll on patient care!**

Furthermore, when caregivers don't take the time out to rest they are setting themselves up too for health problems.

Some of the dangers of overload for the caregivers are: heart disease, digestive problems, depression, skin conditions, black circles under the eyes, weight gain, low energy levels and some can become horrible co-workers too. Yes, they can be-come lazy anger worker that sabotage and hurt other employees. I know this to be true because, they came after me. The lack of sleep can bring out a beast!

So, come on yawl, with all I just mentioned, sickness, circle under the eyes, weight gain and so on.. think for a minute, is it really worth it in the end? Of course not! It's time to reclaim excellence, that won't happen if you don't slow down and rest, sleep and take better care of yourself.

AVOID OVERLOAD

- Get a calendar, place all you work schedule on it and other priorities so you can see with your own eyes how book up you are.
- Look for flexibility, on your schedule, if there is none, red flag, this looks like overload to me.
- Check for family and fun time, if there is no room for that, your priorities off.
- Try to lighten your load up a bit, by asking others to help out at home, instead of always cooking, go out to eat, or order in Chinese, relax, do nothing for a change. Relax and spend some quality time with God.
- Live within your means so you don't need to work overtime or work two jobs.

Ask Jesus to help you bring balance to your life, so you can rest and enjoy life.

- Exercise daily, and spend time with God, let him plan your week, not you.
- When asked can you work over-time? This time say **NO!** Have no fear, God will provide all the things you truly need and right now it's rest and good health.

Caregivers, don't play games with your life. Over time can turn into hospital time, high blood pressure time, no time to eat nutritious food time, instability time, speed up aging time, and the awful list goes on... you've been warned!

Rest, Get Plenty of SLEEP!

Even God, Himself, rested on the seventh day, come on, what do you say? Are you ready to make that change? If you are ready I have provided some tips for avoiding overload, check out your tool box.

Let me just say too for the record, working overtime or taking on extra hours is okay from time to time, but not every week, and not if you're not getting enough sleep.

Balance Is The Key!

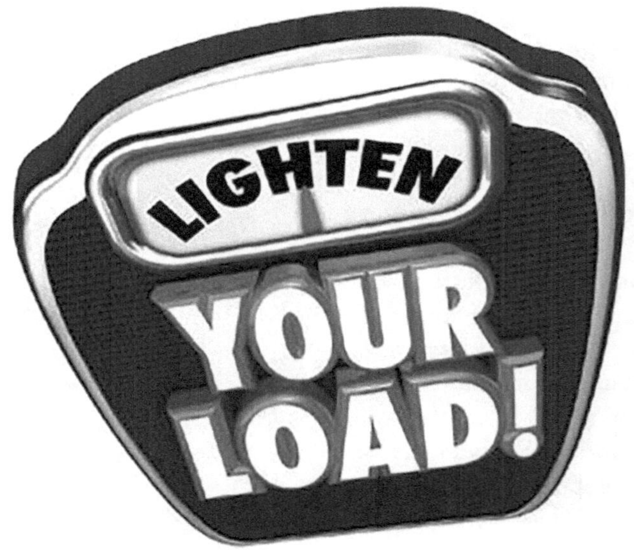

Overtime? "Not Today", No!

The Importance of Sleep

The bible says it is in vain that you rise up early and go late to rest, eating the bread of anxious toil; for he gives the beloved sleep. **Psalms 127:2**

"Caregiver's" I know working overtime allow you to catch up on some of your financial responsibilities or provide a way to enjoy the finer things in life. Absolutely nothing wrong with that, here's the problem, some of you can't give it up, you won't stop working overtime. All you do is work, let me ask you this, what about Jesus, what about our creator too, you know He's a jealous God, when are you going to spend time with him, hum?

A lot of us just need to get our priorities straight some of that work can wait!

It is recommended that people get at least eight or more hours of shut-eye each night. If you don't and continue to disrespect the blessing of rest and sleep, you will live to regret it someday. Because there are nightmare inducing truths on what can happen to a person who takes rest and sleep for granted, one expert put it like this, and I like it,

"Lose Sleep, Lose Your Mind and Health!"

I Hope This Helps!

No Sleep, No Good!

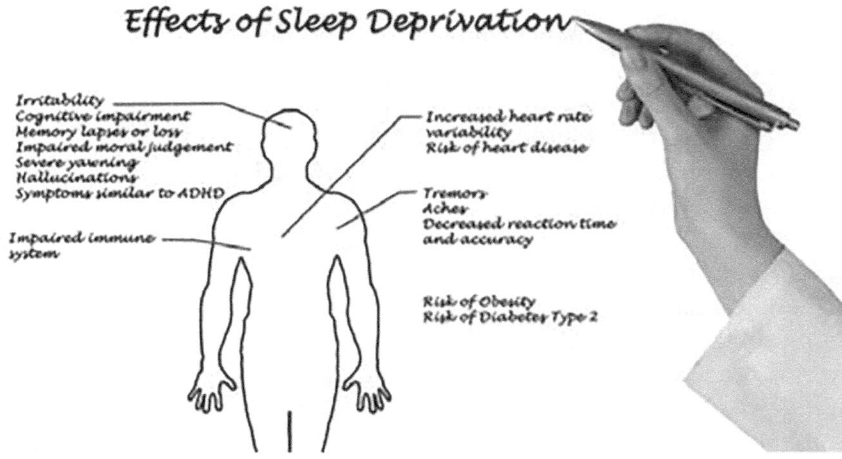

Caregivers don't let work and money rob you of your most precious asset,

'Long Life and Good Health!

 Miss Asondra StarN'air

Sleep For Good Health and Success!

When You Don't Sleep, You Slumber!

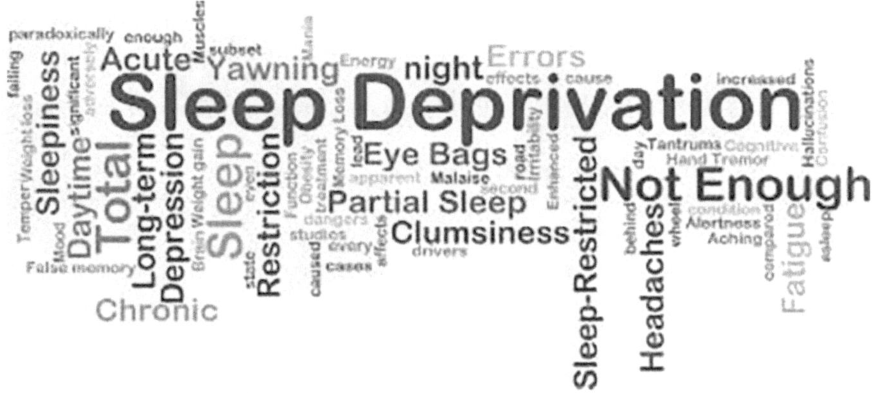

And Some Go Under..

Transfers & Turns

One or two person transfers are often determined by the Register Nurse it's an assessment determining the abilities of that individual and it also helps the risk of injury to both the caregiver and the other person.

But something is happening in long term care and assistant living facilities more and more caregivers have back problems that won't go away. Some caregivers just can't do their jobs anymore, they have to quit. too bad, what a shame.

What's going on? I'll tell you what's going on because I have been there.

In many of these facilities and also in some home-care setting, care-giver are on their own. But in facility setting it's bad, it's real bad. A lot of these places are short staffed, caregivers are loaded down with too many residence and when these residence need you, some of them expect us to come right away, but many of them can't move, they are two persons assist and transfers. **What about my back? Where is my help?** (street version) You ain't got no help! Where the nurses at? Repeat,

New Set of Rules

BACK INJURY RESOLVED

1. Everyone is a two person turn or transfer; caregiver decides that per situation.
2. Be skillful with all transfers.
3. Master pivoting for weight bearing individuals.
4. Don't work at places that do not care about your backs. "No help", "crank beds", Shake the dust off your feet and go to the next town!
5. Take nice long hot baths 3 times a week. Add relaxer to your water, e.g 'epson salt' works well.
6. Exercise regularly, and do back stretches.
7. Cut back on overtime, show more respect to the body.
8. Report caregivers that refuse to help with transfers.
9. Work where you are taken care of and valued. Your physical body matters!
10. Remember this everybody, **"Your Back Out, You're Out"**!

"YOU GOT NO HELP, AND YOU AIN'T GETTING NO HELP! And you are not alone, your co-worker is going through the same thing. **"Overload", Short Staffed!** So these caregivers do what they think they have to do to keep their jobs. They move them or use **'Hoyer Lifts'** by themselves, so now, not only are these caregivers damaging their backs but their jeopardizing their state license too. And for that person also, that's a two person transfer, well, that caregiver can't find help, so they say to themselves "forget it!" I've got twenty -two or more rooms, and seven get -ups, before I can leave, so then that caregiver lifts and transfers those people themselves, that's what's going on in America. Am I right about that caregivers? You **"Betcha By**

Golly Wow" I am! Oh, I hear a melody, I need a mic, I tell you Caregivers, as I write this book, 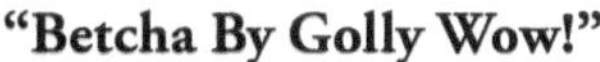 you're the one that I am praying for, forever, and ever will my fight for you keep growing strong, keep growing strong. If I could, I'd help change some of the laws, that would protect you from any damages or falls, I'd make it mandatory that nurses helped you with your residence, patients and all, I'd make them put all the rules up on the wall....anything ask, caregivers just call... **I Betcha by Golly Wow,** the back problems we're facing would be once and forever solved.

"Betcha By Golly Wow!"

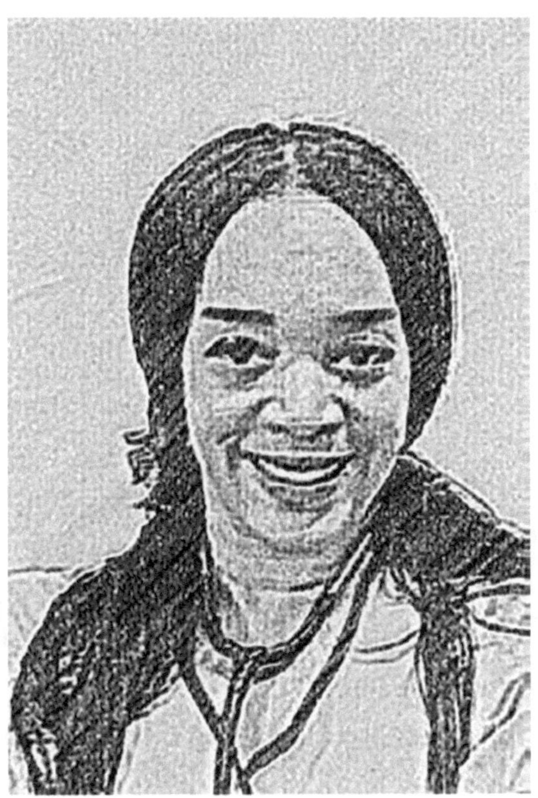

The Interview

- Never ever wear jeans to an interview.
- Arrive at least fifteen minutes early.
- Make sure your cell phone is turned off.
- Stand until asked to be seated.
- Have a business greeting. Example, you can say something like this: "Hello, my name is. ________________
- Thank you so much for this interview. I am so glad to be here."
- Don't forget to SMILE!
- Let the interviewer lead, not you.
- Limit your response, but make it an excellent one.
- If asked, if you have any questions, always say yes.

It is very important you show some real interest in the organization you'll be working for. I always ask a few questions—just a few, two or three. For example, "Are you a franchise, or do you have other affiliates you partner with? What is your company's policy on harassment/ bullying in the workplace?" Here's another one: "Do you welcome new ideas, and are their opportunities for advancement?"

Those are some examples of mine. You can ask other questions, but have some. Intelligent individuals always have questions because we understand that we are not just going for a job but establishing relationships of understanding and respect—a partnership. Just like they have an expectation of us, the caregiver, we also want to be assured we will have an overall good experience working for them as well.

- Carry an organized business case of some sort that has copies of everything I listed over there to the right, in your tool box.
- Have an 'Exit Greeting'. The first and last impressions normally seals the job!

Sample Exit: "I can't tell you enough how grateful I am that you took the time to see me. I really love being a caregiver, and I hope you can tell as well. I like what your agency/ company has to offer. I would love to work for you, and hope the feeling is mutual. It was a pleasure meeting you. Again, thank you for seeing me today. Enjoy the rest of your day!"

That's mine. You can use this one or one of yours, just **"Exit Well"!**

Work Attire

Caregiver, Watch What YOU Wear!

Caregivers it is very important that we watch what we wear to work especially if you are not always required to wear scrubs. Some of you wear attire you have no business ever wearing to work. And may be setting yourself up for sexual advances, I'm talking to the women, I don't care how old your male subject may be, men still have eyes. Dress Appropriately!

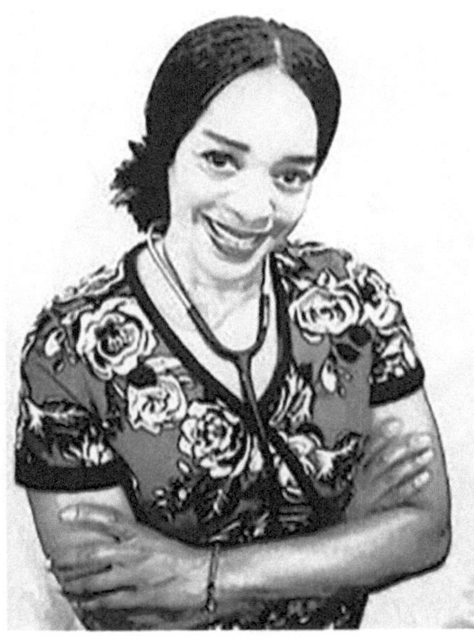

Tools You Can Use!

WATCH WHAT YOU WEAR TO WORK!

➤ Do not ever wear low cut tops to work. Those in your care ladies should never see any parts of your breast even when you bend over to pick up something, if you can see it, so can they, don't wear that top, STOP! Turn around, Take it off!

➤ Leggings are out too, oh, don't even think about it! They show everything and things we don't want to see. Leggings are too, too seductive and very inappropriate for any job unless you wear a dress length top with it.

➤ Listen, tight fitting anything at work is a no, no instead, wear medium loose fitting clothes, be comfortable when you sit and work, why be restricted?

➤ Consider the spouse or other family members too. In other words Caregivers, show some respect!

➤ **Dress Your Title**, okay, caregivers, lets reverse it, **Title Your Dress.** Do I look Professional, Or like 'Street Mess'?

Check out the tool box, it will help you stay in compliance with dress codes. Remember, there is a time and place for everything, so caregivers,

'Let's Dress Appropriately'!

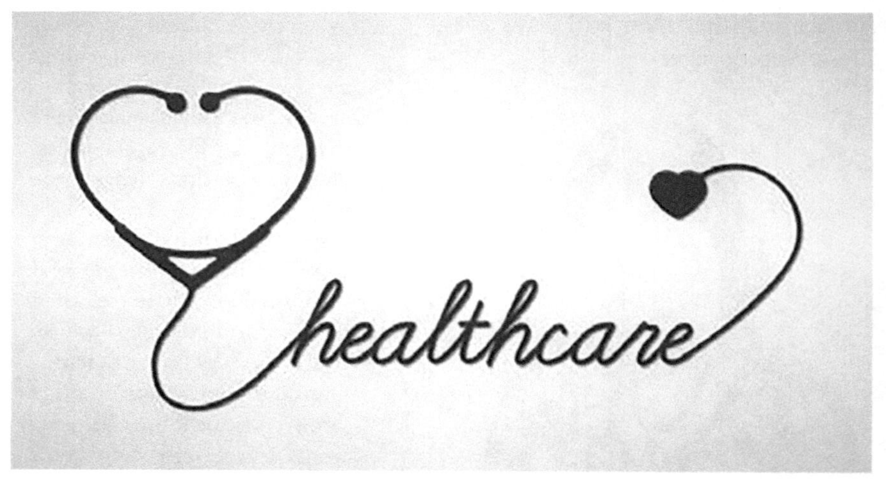

 Miss Asondra StarN'air

SECTION V

Medical Terminology and More!

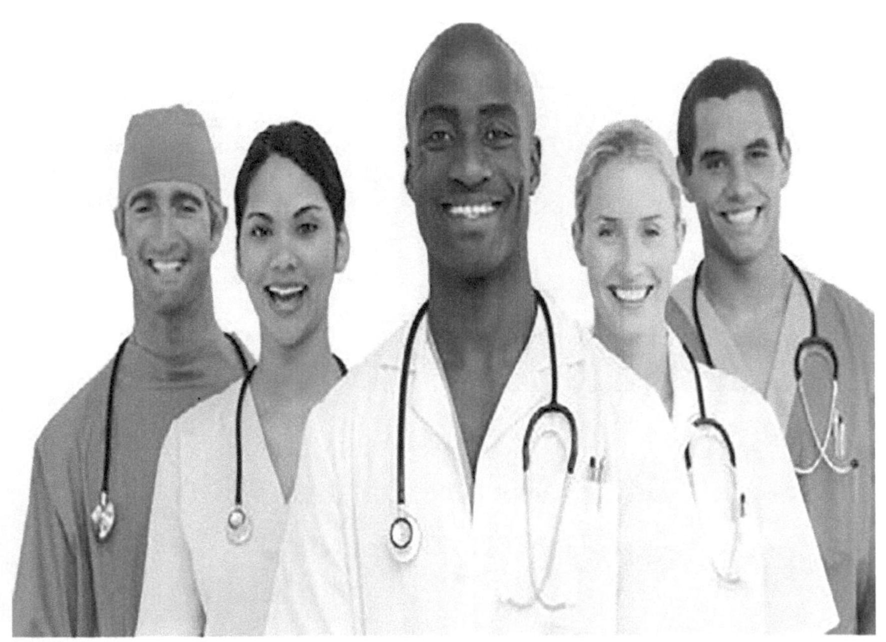

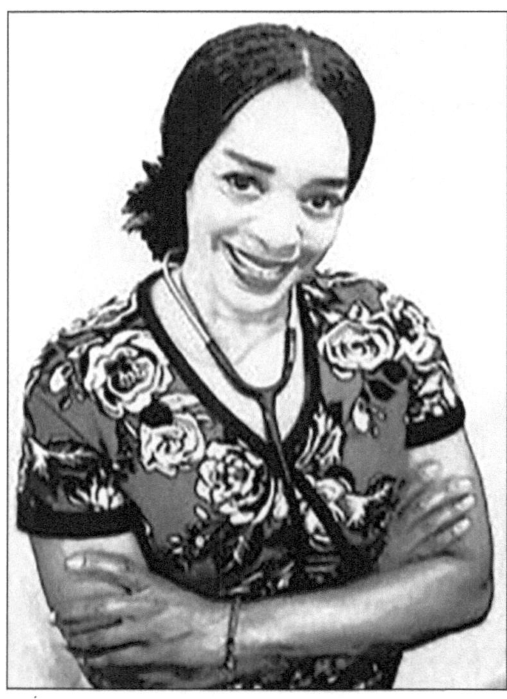

This Book Was Created For "YOU"!

Make It Do What It Do!

MEDICAL TERMINOLOGY ABBREVIATIONS

The following list contains some of the most common abbreviations found in medical records. Please note that in medical terminology, the capitalization of letters bears significance as to the meaning of certain terms, and is often used to distinguish terms with similar acronyms.

@—at
A & P—anatomy and physiology
ab—abortion
abd—abdominal
ABG—arterial blood gas
a.c.—before meals
ac & cl—acetest and clinitest
ACLS—advanced cardiac life support
AD—right ear
ADL—activities of daily living
ad lib—as desired
adm—admission
afeb—afebrile, no fever
AFB—acid-fast bacillus
AKA—above the knee
alb—albumin
alt dieb—alternate days (every other day)
am—morning
AMA—against medical advice
amal—amalgam
amb—ambulate, walk
AMI—acute myocardial infarction
amt—amount
ANS—automatic nervous system
ant—anterior
AOx3—alert and oriented to person, time, and place
Ap—apical

AP—apical pulse

approx—approximately

aq—aqueous

ARDS—acute respiratory distress syndrome

AS—left ear

ASA—aspirin

asap (ASAP)—as soon as possible

as tol—as tolerated

ATD—admission, transfer, discharge

AU—both ears

Ax—axillary

BE—barium enema

bid—twice a day

bil, bilateral—both sides

BK—below knee

BKA—below the knee amputation

bl—blood

bl wk—blood work

BLS—basic life support

BM—bowel movement

BOW—bag of waters

B/P—blood pressure

bpm—beats per minute

BR—bed rest

34 MEDICAL TERMINOLOGY ABBREVIATIONS

BRP—bathroom privileges

BS—breath sounds

BSI—body substance isolation

BSO—bilateral salpingo-oophorectomy

BUN—blood, urea, nitrogen levels

BVM—bag-valve-mask

bx—biopsy

c—with

C & S—culture and sensitivity

c-spine—cervical spine

CA—cancer

CAD—coronary artery disease

 MISS ASONDRA STARN'AIR

cal—calorie

CAT—computerized axial tomography

cath—catheter

CBC—complete blood count

cc—cubic centimeters

CC—chief complaint

CCU—coronary care unit, critical care unit

CHD—coronary heart disease

CHF—congestive heart failure

CHO—carbohydrate

chol—cholesterol

circ—circumcision

cl liq—clear liquid

CNS—central nervous sysyem

c/o—complains of

COPD—chronic obstructive pulmonary disease

CPK—creatine phosphokinase

CPR—cardiopulmonary resuscitation

CPT—chest physical therapy

CS—central supply

CSF—cerebrospinal fluid

CT—computer tomography

CVA—cerebrovascular accident (stroke)

CVU—cardiovascular unit

cx—cervix or complaint of

CXR—chest X ray

cysto—cystography

d/c—discontinue

D & C—dilation and curettage

DAT—diet as tolerated

DC—discontinue or discharge

del—delivery

Del. Rm.—delivery room

diff—differential

DNA—deoxyribonucleic acid

DNR—do not resuscitate

DOA—dead on arrival

DOB—date of birth
DPT—diphtheria, pertussis, tetanus
DRG—diagnosis-related grouping
D/S—dextrose in saline
DT's—delirium tremens
DW—distilled water
D5W 5%—dextrose in water
Dx—diagnosis

MEDICAL TERMINOLOGY ABBREVIATIONS 35

EBL—estimated blood loss
ECG—electrocardiogram
ED—emergency department
EEG—electroencephalogram
EENT—eyes, ears, nose, throat
EKG—electrocardiogram
EMG—electromyogram
EOA—esophageal obturator airway
ESR—erythrocyte sedimentation rate
est—estimated
ER—emergency room
ET—endotracheal
ETA—estimated time of arrival
etiol—etiology
ETOH—ethyl alcohol, intoxicated
exam—examination
exp—exploratory
ext—external, extract, extraction
FBOA—foreign body obstructed airway
FBS—fasting blood sugar
FBW—fasting blood work
(F. Fl)—force fluids
FH—family history
FHS—fetal heart sounds
FHT—fetal heart tone
FIFO—first in, first out
FSH—follicle-stimulating hormone
ft—foot

 Miss Asondra StarN'air

FUO—fever of undetermined origin

Fx—fracture

GB—gallbladder

GI—gastrointestinal

GU—genitourinary

GTT—glucose tolerance test (pancreas test)

gtt(s)—drop(s)

gyn—gynecology

& H—hemoglobin and hematocrit

HCG—human chorionic gonadotrophin

hct—hematocrit

HDL—high-density lipoprotein

hgb—hemoglobin

HOB—head of bed

hr (h)—hour

HIV—human immunodeficiency virus

H&P—history and physical

HR—heart rate

hs—hour of sleep, bedtime

ht—height

Hx—history

hypo—hypodermic injection

hyst—hysterectomy

IBS—irritable bowel syndrome

I & D—incision and drainage

I & O—intake and output

36 MEDICAL TERMINOLOGY ABBREVIATIONS

ICP—intracranial pressure

ICU—intensive care unit

IM—intramuscular

ing—inguinal

inj—injection

IPPB—intermittent positive pressure breathing

irrig—irrigation

IS—intercostal space

isol—isolation

IT—inhalation therapy

IUD—intrauterine device
IV—intravenous
IVF—in vitro fertilization
IVP—intravenous pyelogram
K+—potassium
KCl—potassuim chloride
KUB—kidney, ureter, bladder
L—lumbar
L & D—labor and delivery
lac—laceration
lab—laboratory
lap—laparotomy
lat—lateral
LD—lethal dose
LDH—lactic dehydrogenase
LDL—low-density lipoprotein
liq—liquid
LLQ, LLL—left lower quadrant (abdomen), lobe (lung)
LMP—last menstrual period
LOC—level of consciousness
LP—lumbar puncture
lt—left
LUQ, LUL—left upper quadrant (abdomen), lobe (lung)
MA—mental age
MAST—medical antishock trousers
MCI—mass casualty incident
meds—medications
MI—myocardial infarction
MICU—mobile intensive care unit
min—minute
MN—midnight
MOM—milk of magnesia
MRI—magnetic resonance imagery
MS—morphine sulfate, multiple sclerosis
MVA—motor vehicle accident
NVD—nausea, vomiting, diarrhea **Na+**—sodium
NaCl—sodium chloride

      MISS ASONDRA STARN'AIR

N/C—nasal cannula
no—complaints
neg—negative
neuro—neurology
NG—nasogastric
NGT—nasogastric tube
nitro—nitroglycerine
NKA—no known allergies
noc (t)—night
NPO—nothing by mouth
MEDICAL TERMINOLOGY ABBREVIATIONS 37
NS—normal saline
nsg—nursing
NSR—normal sinus rhythm
NVS—neurological vital signs
O—oxygen
OB—obstetrics
OD—right eye, overdose
oint—ointment
OOB—out of bed
OPD—outpatient department
OR—operating room
ord—orderly
ORTH—orthopedics
ortho—correct, right (bones)
os—mouth
OS—left eye
OT—occupational therapy
OU—both eyes
oz—ounce
p—after
P—pulse
& A—percussion and auscultation
PAC—premature atrial contraction
palp—palpation
PAR—post-anesthesia room
PAT—paroxysmal atrial tachycardia**

pc—after meals

pCO2—partial pressure of carbon dioxide

PDR—physician's desk reference

PE—physical exam, pulmonary embolism

PEDS—pediatrics

per—by or through

PERL(A)—pupils equal and reactive to light (and accommodation)

PET—positron emission tomography

PH—past history

pH—hydrogen ion concentration

PID—pelvic inflammatory disease

PKU—phenylketonuria

pm—between noon and midnight

PNS—peripheral nervous system

po—by mouth

post (pos)—posterior

postop, PostOp—postoperative

(p.p.)—postprandial (after eating)

pO2—partial pressure of oxygen

PPD—purified protein derivative (TB test)

preop, PreOp—before surgery

prn—as needed, whenever necessary

pro time—prothrombin time

pt—patient, pint

PT—physical therapy

PTT—partial prothrombaplastin time

PVC—premature ventricular contraction

Px—physical exam, prognosis

q—every

qd—every day

qh—every hour

q2h, q3h,...—every two hours, every three hours,...

38 MEDICAL TERMINOLOGY ABBREVIATIONS

qhs—every night at bedtime

qid—four times a day

qns—quantity not sufficient

qod—every other day

 MISS ASONDRA STARN'AIR

qs—quantity sufficient

r (R)—rectal

R (resp)—respirations, rectal

RAIU—radioactive iodine uptake study

RBC—red blood cell/count

reg—regular

Rh—rhesus

RK—radial keratomy

RL—ringer's lactate

RLQ, RLL—right lower quadrant (abdomen), lobe (lung)

RML—right middle lobe (lung)

RO—reality orientation

R/O—rule out

ROM—range of motion

R.R.—recovery room

RUQ, RLL—right upper quadrant, lobe

rt—right

RV—residual volume

Rx—take (prescription)

s—without

S & S—signs and symptoms

ss—1/2

Sats—oxygen/blood saturation level

SA—sinoatrial

SB—small bowel

sc—subcutaneous

SGOT—serum glutamic oxaloacetic transaminase

SGPT—serum glutamic pyruvic transaminase

SIDS—sudden infant death syndrome

Sig:—label/write

SL—sublingual

SMAC—sequential multiple analysis computer

SOB—shortness of breath

spec—specimen

sp. gr.—specific gravity

SQ, sub q—subcutaneous

SSE—soap suds enema **stat**—immediately

STD—sexually transmitted disease
STH—somatotropic hormone
SVD—spontaneous vaginal delivery
SVN—small volume nebulizer
SVT—supraventricular tachycardia
Sx—symptoms
T—temperature, thoracic
T & A—tonsillectomy and adenoidectomy
tab—tablet
tachy——tachycardic
TAH—total abdominal hysterectomy
TB—tuberculosis
TCDB—turn, cough, deep breath
temp (T)—temperature
TH—thyroid hormone
TIA—transient ischemic attack

MEDICAL TERMINOLOGY ABBREVIATIONS 39

tid—three times a day
TMJ—temporomandibular joint
tol—tolerated
TPN—total parenteral nutrition
TPR—temperature, pulse, respirations
tr—tincture
trach—tracheotomy, tracheostomy
TSH—thyroid-stimulating hormone
TT—tetanus toxiod
TUR—transurethral resection
TV—tidal volume
TVH—total vaginal hysterectomy
TX—traction
UA—urinalysis
umb—umbilicus
unc.—unconscious
ung—ointment
unk—unknown
ur—urine
URC—usual, reasonable, customary

URI—upper respiratory infection
US—ultrasonic
UTI—urinary tract infection
fib—ventricular fibrillation
V tach—ventricular tachycardia
vag—vaginal
VC—vital capacity
VD—venereal disease
vit—vitamin
vo—verbal order
vol—volume
V/S—vital signs
WA—while awake
WBC—white blood cell/count
w/c—wheelchair
WNL—within normal limits
wt—weight
y/o—year(s) old

40 MEDICAL TERMINOLOGY ABBREVIATIONS

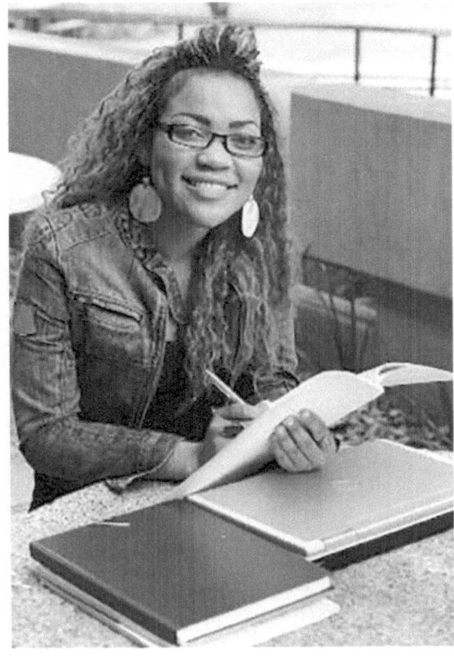

Human Anatomy (Male & Female)

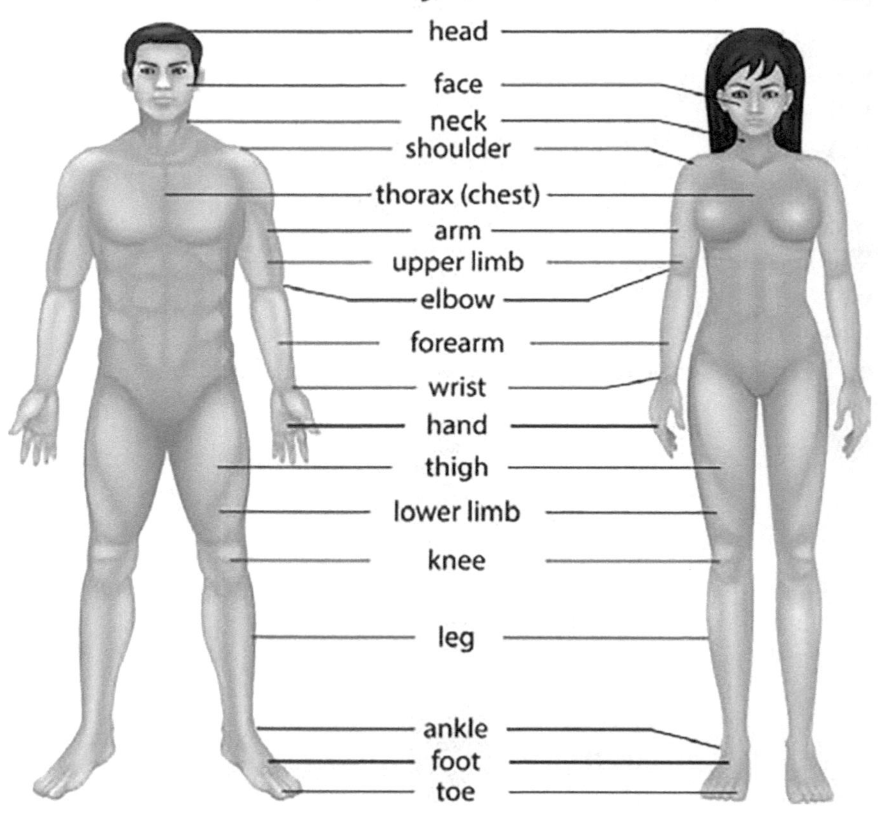

Stay In The Know!

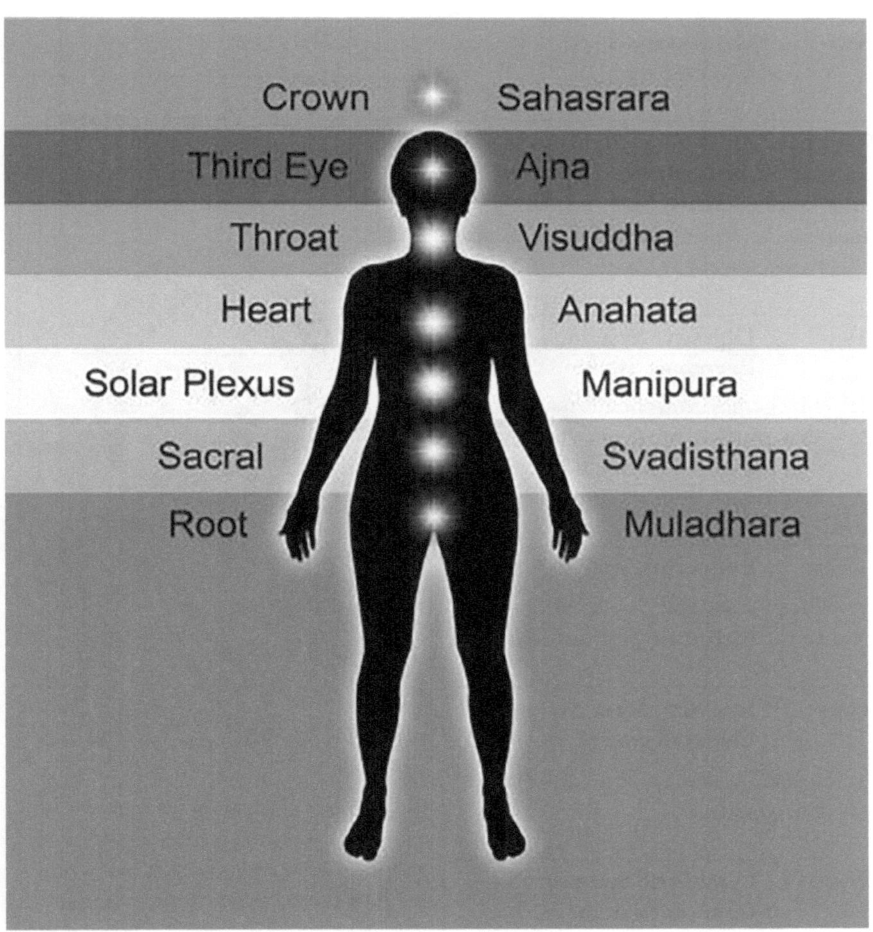

The Main Systems of the Human Body

Two   **Cardiovascular / Circulatory**

This part of the body circulates blood around the body via the heart, arteries and veins, delivering oxygen and nutrients to organ and cell then carries their waste products away.

Two   **Digestive System / Excretory System**

1. Mechanical and chemical processes that provide nutrients via mouth, esophagus, stomach and intestines.
2. Eliminates from the body

Three   **Endocrine System**

Provides chemical communication within the body using hormones.

Four   **Integumentary System / Exocrine system**

Skin, sweat, nails, hair and other exocrine glands.

Five   **Lymphatic System/ Immune System**

1. This system is made up of a network of lymphatic vessels that carry clear fluids called lymph.
2. Defends the body against disease-causing agents.

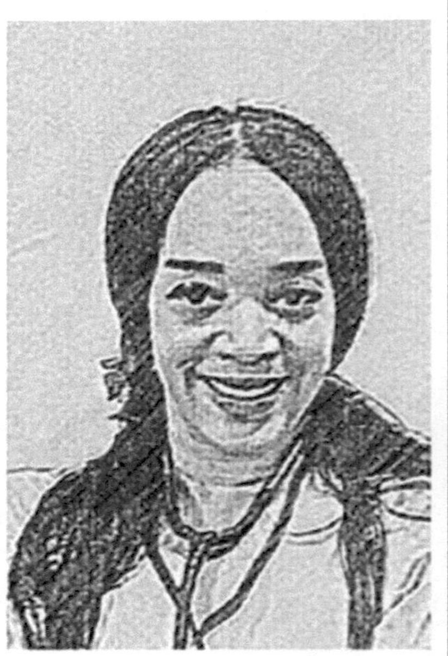

Study to Make Thyself Approved!

Caregivers, the more we know, the more we grow, the more we grow, the more we have to show. Let the world see how far we've come and can go!

Miss Asondra StarN'air
'The Lady With The Heart

Six   **Muscular System /Skeletal System**

1. Enables our bodies to move using muscles
2. Skeletal, made up of bones, that support the body and its organs.

Seven   Nervous System

Collects and processes information from the senses via nerve and the brain and tells the muscles to contract to cause physical action.

Eight   Renal System/Urinary Track System

The system where the kidneys filter blood.

Nine   Reproductive System

The sex organs required for production of offspring.

Ten   Respiratory System

The lungs and the trachea that bring air into the human body.

There you have it, the main systems of the human body, spend more time learning all you can about each one of the body systems on your own, you can never stop learning.

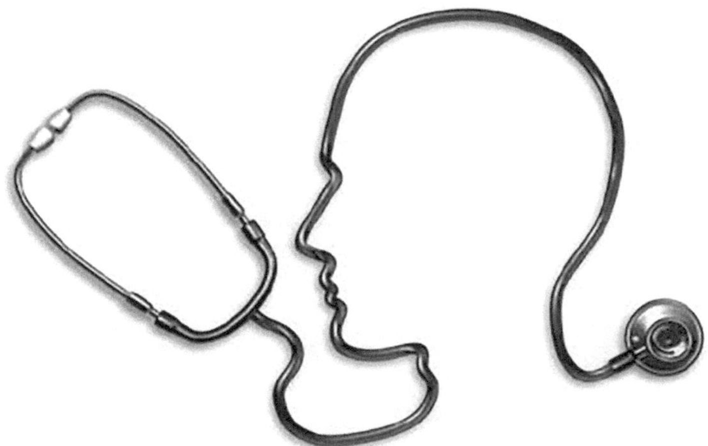

Stay In The Know, Grow!

Body Part	Medical Name
Head	Cranium
Forehead	Frontalis
Eyeball	Globe
Eye Socket	Orbit
Eye Whites	Cornea
Eye Color Ring	Iris
Eye Hole	Pupil
Ears	Pinna
Ear Canal	External Meatus
Ear Drum	Tympanic Membrane
Nose Bridge	Nasal bones
Nostrils	Nares
Cheeks	Malar region
Cheek Bone	Zygomatic arch
Lips	Labia
Tongue	Lingulus
Mouth	Oral Cavity
Gums	Gingiva
Upper Jaw	Maxilla
Lower Jaw	Mandible
Chin	Mentis
Teeth	Dentition
Voice Box	Larynx
Adam's Apple	Thyroid Cartilage
Pit of Throat	Manubrial Notch
Swallow Pipe	Esophagus
Collar Bones	Clavicles
Shoulder Blade	Scapula
Chest Bone	Sternum
Ribs	Costal

Rib Joints	Costochondral joints
Pit of Stomach	Epigastrium
Navel	Umbilicus
Loins	Flank
Bladder Area	Suprapubic
Bird, Twat, Puss-, Cun-, Beaver	Vagina
Womb	Uterus
Bird, Junk, Weiner, Dic-	Penis
Foreskin	Prepuce
Balls, Nuts	Testicles
Bum, Butt, As-	Gluteus
Neck Spine	Cervical or C-spine
Mid Back Spine	Thoracic or T-spine
Lower Back Spine	Lumbar or L-spine
Spine Bones	Vertebrae
Tailbone	Coccyx
Shoulder	Deltoid
Armpit	Axilla
Upper Arm Bone	Humerus
Elbow	Olecranon
Funny Bone	Ulnar Nerve
Forearm Outter Bone	Radius
Forearm Inner Bone	Ulna
Wrist	Metacarpals
Hand	Carpals
Fingers	Phalanges
Hips	Pelvis
Upper Leg Muscles	Quadriceps
Upper Leg Bone	Femur
Knee Cap	Patella
Shin Bone	Tibia
Ankle	Malleoli
Heel	Calcaneus

Foot Arch	Metatarsals
Toes	Phalanges
Great Toe	Hallux
Trunk	Torso
Breasts	Mammaries
Nipples	Areola
Brain	Cerebrum
Heart	Myocardium
Lungs	Pulmonary system
Liver	Hepatic system
Kidneys	Renal system
Digestive Tract	Alimentary Canal
Skin	Integumentary System
Baldness	Alopecia

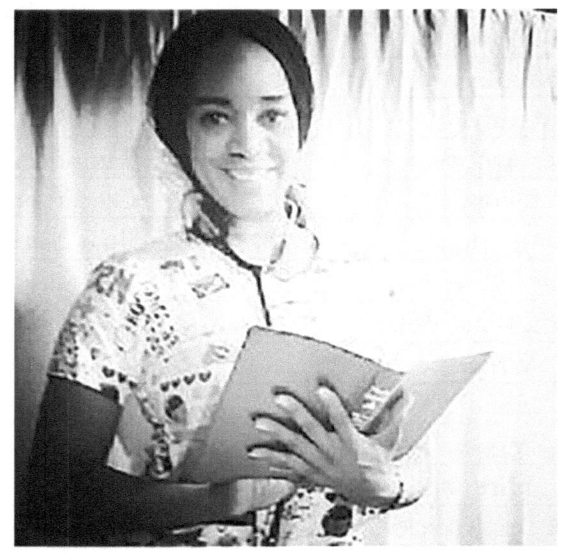

We're No Longer 'Aides', Time To Get Paid!

Stay In The Know "Grow"!

Signs and Symptoms to Report.

Evaluate the situation, is it safe? Do I call 911 or can I handle it within my scope?

Educate, tell the individual /family why you are doing what you are doing.

Keep records, make sure they are neat, accurate, concise and complete. Documentation is a must!

Help the person relax.

Eye and ears open, "Caregivers" watch out for changes in breathing, sounds of destress or pain.

Lay down slowly or sit up whichever is preferred and most comfortable to the person.

Position them comfortably and keep them warm, do not allow a chill to occur.

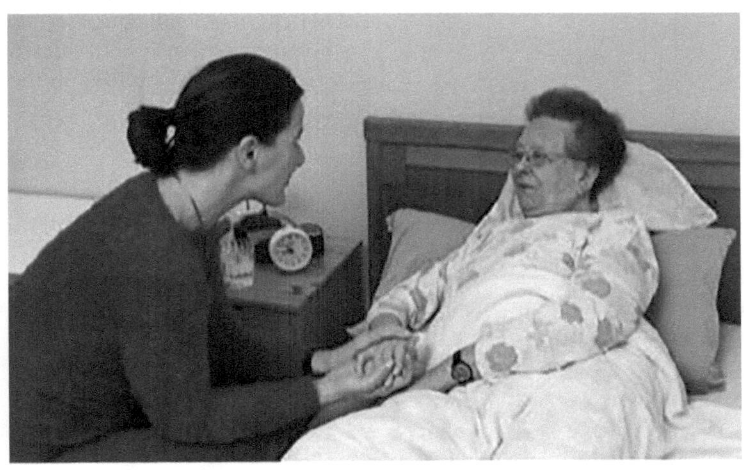

Signs and Symptoms Cont..

Signs and Symptoms, please take note that some situations may not be urgent, however it is very important to recognize and report signs and symptoms of disease and /or side effects of medication so that proper treatment can be carried out.

State Tested Nurse Assistants (**STNA**) caregivers, please remember we are the eyes and ears of the Doctor's and Nurses. Our role is vital to the healthcare team, report what you hear and see promptly.

If you are someone caring for a loved one, and they have these signs and symptoms below as well, call the doctor.

General Body Systems	**Vitals: TPR & BP**
. Dehydration	. Low temperature
. Shaking chills	. Elevated temperature
. Loss of appetite	. Weak, trendy pulse
. Allergic reaction	. Fast or slow pulse
. Rapid weight gain	. Irregular pulse
. Abnormal posture, movement or gait	. Noisy respirations
. Dizziness, weakness, fainting	. Difficulty breathing
. Frequent or severe headache	. Painful breathing
. Swelling in any part of the body	. Shallow/deep respirations
. Weight loss without dieting	. Not Breathing (CPR) quick, call 911

Skin	**Eyes**
. Burns	. Profuse tearing
. Too dry/moist	. Discharge or bleeding
. Yellowing of skin	. Loss of sight (full or partial)
. Rash, moles, open sores	. Redness of eyes or eyelids
. Unusual bruising or bleeding	. Twitching, sensitivity to light
. Wounds or sores that do not heal	. Dullness, brightness, dark circles
	. Dilated/ big/ small contracted pupils
	. Foreign body in eye, scratchy/pain
	. Change in color, swelling in the lids

Signs and Symptoms

Arm and Legs	**Feet**
. Deformities	. Swelling, pain
. Varicose veins	. Corns or bunions
. Lumps, bruises	. Thick discolored nails
. Swelling or pain	. Ingrown toenails
. Wounds or sores that do not heal	. Deformities
. Unusual weakness in arm or legs	
. Inability to move arms or leg or hand	
. Broken bones	
. Strains or injuries	

 MISS ASONDRA STARN'AIR

More Signs and Symptoms to Report

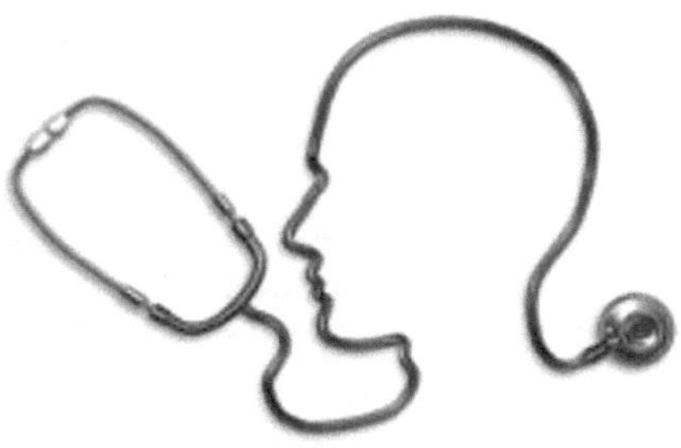

Mental State

. Fatigue
. Agitation
. Sudden change in behavior
. Drowsiness
. Unusual confusion or disorientation
. Comatose or unconscious
. Nearly unconscious /semi-conscious
. Bereavement
. Up-set
. Not feeling well
. Alzheimer's / Dementia behavior

Know the Mental States

Awake Alert and Oriented **(AAO)** Orientation is a function of mind it's used by nurses and doctor as a mental state test.

AAO x 1 = Awareness of Person. sometimes a person is oriented to himself. That means can't recall or recognize anyone else.

AAO x 2= Knowledge of Place.
e.g. such as hospital, room, city and state.

AAO x 3= Knowledge of Time and Date. may include awareness of time of day and seasons.

AAO x 4= Knowledge of Events event may include what just happened or why he's at the hospital or nursing home.

Caregivers, note, when you hear that a person is oriented x 3, altogether that means the individual is awake and responsive, and oriented to all 3, **Person, Place and Time.**

Stop and Notice!

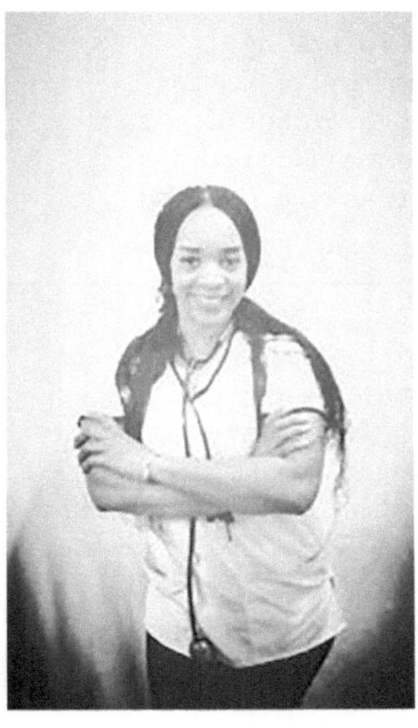

Being as pain free as possible is what we all want right! But that's not always the case, again, as caregivers it is our responsibility to pay attention to what's going on with individuals in our care, and document. Anytime a client, patient or resident tells you they are in pain, **"ACT"**, tell your charge nurse, don't ignore, or assume they are just seeking attention, that's not for us to decide. And to family care providers, act like a professional caregiver, although you may not be and follow these guide lines too. You never know, that person may be in real trouble and need medical attention.

Remember
Document

Sign and Symptoms to Report Continues....

Ears

. Loss of hearing
. Discharge or bleeding
. Pain in ear or back of ear
. Profuse harden ear wax
. Foreign body in the ear

Nose

. Sneezing
. Breathing difficulties
. Repeated nose bleed
. Foreign body in the nose
. Runny nose /not chronic
. Chronic discharge

Mouth

. Hoarseness
. Jaw swelling
. Tongue coated, red, pale
. Swollen and /or discolored lips
. Teeth, sharp, broken, toothache
. Difficulty in swallowing, talking
. Pain in the mouth
. Gums, swelling, bleeding, ulcer sores that do not heal
. Rash or blister in or outside of mouth
. Soar throat
. Uncontrollable Coughing or choking when eating
. Coughs that will not go away
. Inflammation of the lips, Severe dry lips, chapped and peeling. Swelling of the lips

Neck

. Stiffness or pain in neck
. Swelling or lump in neck

Document

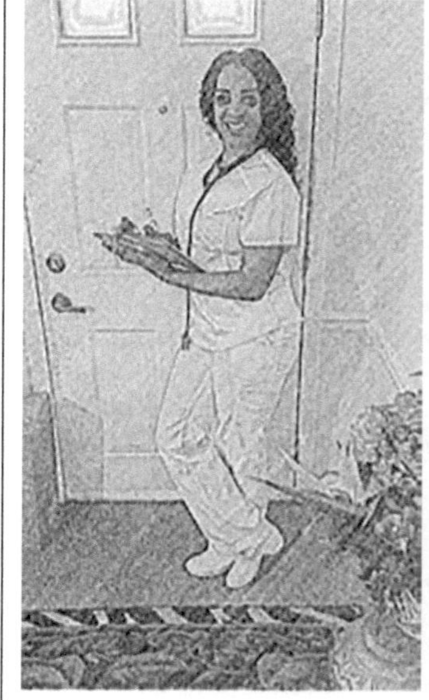

Nurse Assistant StarN'air

  MISS ASONDRA STARN'AIR

Sign and Symptoms To Report Continues........

Abdomen

. Rigid abdomen
. Nausea or vomiting
. Pain in abdomen
. Any swelling or lumps
  in abdomen or groin

Chest

. Pain in the chest
. Coughing up blood or pus
. Lump in breast or under arm
. Chronic or congested cough
  lasting more than a week
. Shortness of breath (SOB) or
  difficulty breathing

Rectum

. Hemorrhoids
. Bleeding or drainage from rectum
. Abnormal bowel movement (blood,
  Mucous, worms, diarrhea, fluid)
. Chronic constipation (dry hard stool)

Genitals

. Itching
. Redness
. Swelling
. Discharge
. Pain or difficulty in urination
. Unable to void
. Void frequently
. Incontinence, unusual for the person
. Sharp pain and burning
. Discomfort during urination, sore
. Foul color or smell
. Blood or blood in stool or urine

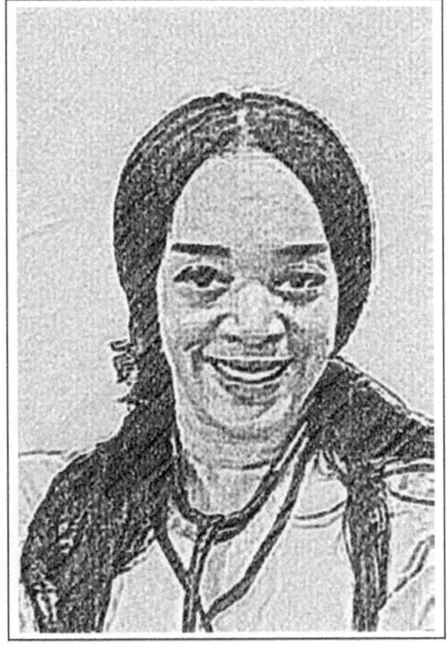

Check us out, We are not the aides of
past generations, We are Skilled
Professional Caregivers Now'!
We are a vital part of the healthcare
team. We are Professional Care
Providers, not aides.

Diabetes Mellitus

Commonly called Diabetes, people with this disease either cannot produce enough insulin or cannot effectively use the insulin they do have to produce or control their blood sugar (glucose) level.

Yet it's still on the rise here in the United States. Everyone should be aware of this potentially fatal disease according to 2014 statistic report CDC 29.1 million people here in the united states alone has diabetes and 27.8% which is about 8.1 million people have it and don't know they have it. There are two types of diabetes:

Type 1 and Type 2

Type 1: also called **Juvenile Diabetes** or insulin dependent the pancreas produces little or no insulin. It's a chronic condition/ongoing, cannot be cured, but treatment and special diet along with exercise makes this disease manageable can last for years or lifelong.

Type 2: also called, **Adult Onset Diabetes,** it's very common, more than 3 million people are diagnosed with type 2 diabetes. It is characterized by high blood sugar, insulin resistance and relative lack of insulin. This type is treatable by a medical professional, however, chronic and can also last for years or be lifelong.

DM GUIDE FOR CAREGIVERS

Signs and Symptoms

- Hunger
- Fatigue
- Blurry vision
- Extreme thirst
- Frequent urination
- Unexplained weight loss
- Soars that don't heal
- Frequent infections

Caregivers Care Plan

- Encourage dental checks.
- Never put lotion between the toes.
- All meals served as scheduled do not skip meals.
- Encourage shoes or slippers when up on the floor.
- Encourage physical daily activities and exercise.
- Wash feet and thoroughly dry between the toes
- Do not cut toe nails.
- Report any lesions found on body to nurse or supervisor.

Give insulin if directed by nurse and certified to do so.

Lastly, when checking blood sugar apply lancet to the chosen finger, never the pad. Rotate finger to avoid callus formation.

Diabetes

Caregiver, know your the blood sugar levels, what's normal what's not. Normally, blood sugar level should fall between 70-110. It's too high when it's above 120, this is called "Hyperglycemia". When blood sugar is too low (below 70) it is called "Hypoglycemia

Signs and Symptoms

Hyperglycemia

. Feels weak

. Drowsy, sleepy

. Pain in abdomen

. Nausea, vomiting

. Dehydration, dry mouth and skin

. Spuporous, not alert

. Skin flushed, red and warm

. Slow and lethargic movements

. Rapid respirations

Hypoglycemia

. Nausea,

. Headache

. Fast pulse

. Feel hungry

. Blurred vision

. Unsteadiness

. Tingling in the hands, feet or face

. Feels too hot or cold

. Tremors, shakiness

. Feels dizzy, light headedness, heart pounding

. Excessive sweating, slurred speech

Normal Vital Signs Guidelines for EMS, by Age Group

Compiled using Emergency Care and Transportation of the Sick and Injured, EMS Field Guide and Journal of Emergency Medical Services.

You will find it extremely valuable in the field to memorize these vital signs guidelines. To help you memorize them, I have organized them by type and by age group. You can decide which will be easier to remember.

Vital Signs by Type

Pulse	
Description: regular, irregular, strong or weak	
Adult	60 to 100 beats per minute
Children - age 1 to 8 years	80 to 100
Infants - age 1 to 12 months	100 to 120
Neonates - age 1 to 28 days	120 to 160

Blood pressure		
	Systolic	Diastolic
Adult	90 to 140 mmHg	60 to 90 mmHg
Children - age 1 to 8 years	80 to 110 mmHg	
Infants - age 1 to 12 months	70 to 95 mmHg	
Neonates - age 1 to 28 days	>60 mmHg	

Respirations	
Description: normal, shallow, labored, noisy, Kussmaul	
Adult (normal)	12 to 20 breaths per minute
Children - age 1 to 8 years	15 to 30
Infants - age 1 to 12 months	25 to 50
Neonates - age 1 to 28 days	40 to 60

Vital signs by age

Adult vital signs

Stay In The Know

Pulse	60 to 100 beats per minute
Blood pressure	90 to 140 mmHg (systolic) 60 to 90 mmHg (diastolic)
Respirations	12 to 20 breaths per minute
Child vital signs (age 1 to 8 years)	
Pulse	80 to 100 beats per minute
Blood pressure	80 to 110 mmHg systolic
Respirations	15 to 30 breaths per minute
Infant vital signs (age 1 to 12 months)	
Pulse	100 to 140 beats per minute
Blood pressure	70 to 95 mmHg systolic
Respirations	25 to 50 breaths per minute

Neonatal vital signs (full-term, ≤28 days)	
Pulse	120 to 160 beats per minute
Blood pressure	>60 mmHg systolic
Respirations	40 to 60 breaths per minute

Other references

Lung sounds	
Crackles or rales	crackling or rattling sounds
Wheezing	high-pitched whistling expirations
Stridor	harsh, high-pitched inspirations
Rhonchi	coarse, gravelly sounds

Stay In The Know

Pulse oximetry

Range	Value	Treatment
Normal	95 to 100%	None or placebo
Mild hypoxia	91 to 94%	Give oxygen
Moderate hypoxia	86 to 90%	Give 100% oxygen
Severe hypoxia	≤85%	Give 100% oxygen w/ positive pressure

Glasgow Coma Scale

ADULT	E	INFANT
Eye opening	E	**Eye opening**
Spontaneous	4	Spontaneous
To speech	3	To speech
To pain	2	To pain
No response	1	No response
Best motor response	M	**Best motor response**
Obeys verbal command	6	Normal movements
Localizes pain	5	Localizes pain
Flexion - withdraws from pain	4	Withdraws from pain
Flexion - abnormal	3	Flexion - abnormal
Extension	2	Extension
No response	1	No response
Best verbal response	V	**Best verbal response**
Oriented and converses	5	Coos, babbles
Disoriented and converses	4	Cries but consolable

Stay In The Know!

Inappropriate words	3	Persistently irritable
Incomprehensible sounds	2	Grunts to pain/restless
No response	1	No response

$$E + M + V = 3 \text{ to } 15$$

- 90% less than or equal to 8 are in coma
- Greater than or equal to 9 not in coma
- 8 is the critical score
- Less than or equal to 8 at 6 hours - 50% die
- 9-11 = moderate severity
- Greater than or equal to 12 = minor injury

Coma is defined as not opening eyes, not obeying commands, and not uttering understandable words.

Additional information: Traumatic Brain Injury Resource Guide and House of Defrance.

Apgar Scale (evaluate @ 1 and 5 minutes postpartum)			
Sign	**2**	**1**	**0**
A — Activity (muscle tone)	Active	Arms and legs flexed	Absent
P — Pulse	>100 bpm	<100 bpm	Absent
G — Grimace (reflex irritability)	Sneezes, coughs, pulls away	Grimaces	No response
A — Appearance (skin color)	Normal over entire body	Normal except extremities	Cyanotic or pale all over
R — Respiration	Fast, crying	Slow, irregular	Absent

Pain Scale

The 0-10 pain scale is becoming known as the "fifth vital sign" in hospital and pre-hospital care. Adults can usually quantify their pain on a numeric scale, however children may need help in articulating their pain.

Time after Time

Military Time to Regular Time Conversion Chart

Military Time	Regular Time	Military Time	Regular Time
0100	1:00 AM	1300	1:00 PM
0200	2:00 AM	1400	2:00 PM
0300	3:00 AM	1500	3:00 PM
0400	4:00 AM	1600	4:00 PM
0500	5:00 AM	1700	5:00 PM
0600	6:00 AM	1800	6:00 PM
0700	7:00 AM	1900	7:00 PM
0800	8:00 AM	2000	8:00 PM
0900	9:00 AM	2100	9:00 PM
1000	10:00 AM	2200	10:00 PM
1100	11:00 AM	2300	11:00 PM
1200	Noon	0000 or 2400	Midnight

Minutes	Decimal	Minutes	Decimal	Minutes	Decimal	Minutes	Decimal
1	0.02	16	0.27	31	0.52	46	0.77
2	0.03	17	0.28	32	0.53	47	0.78
3	0.05	18	0.3	33	0.55	48	0.8
4	0.07	19	0.32	34	0.57	49	0.82
5	0.08	20	0.33	35	0.58	50	0.83
6	0.1	21	0.35	36	0.6	51	0.85
7	0.12	22	0.37	37	0.62	52	0.87
8	0.13	23	0.38	38	0.63	53	0.88
9	0.15	24	0.4	39	0.65	54	0.9
10	0.17	25	0.42	40	0.67	55	0.92
11	0.18	26	0.43	41	0.68	56	0.93
12	0.2	27	0.45	42	0.7	57	0.95
13	0.22	28	0.47	43	0.72	58	0.97
14	0.23	29	0.48	44	0.73	59	0.98
15	0.25	30	0.5	45	0.75	60	1

SECTION VI

Caregiver's Lifelong Learning & Adult Education Center

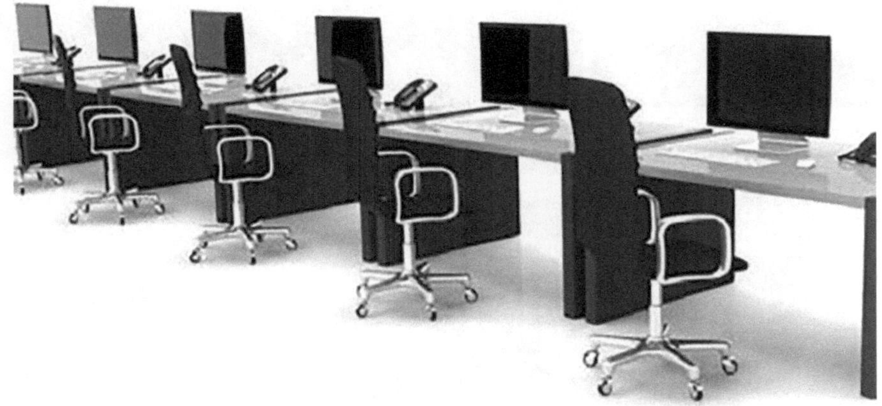

Welcome, New Day Caregivers!

21st Century CareGivers, Hello, It's A New Day!

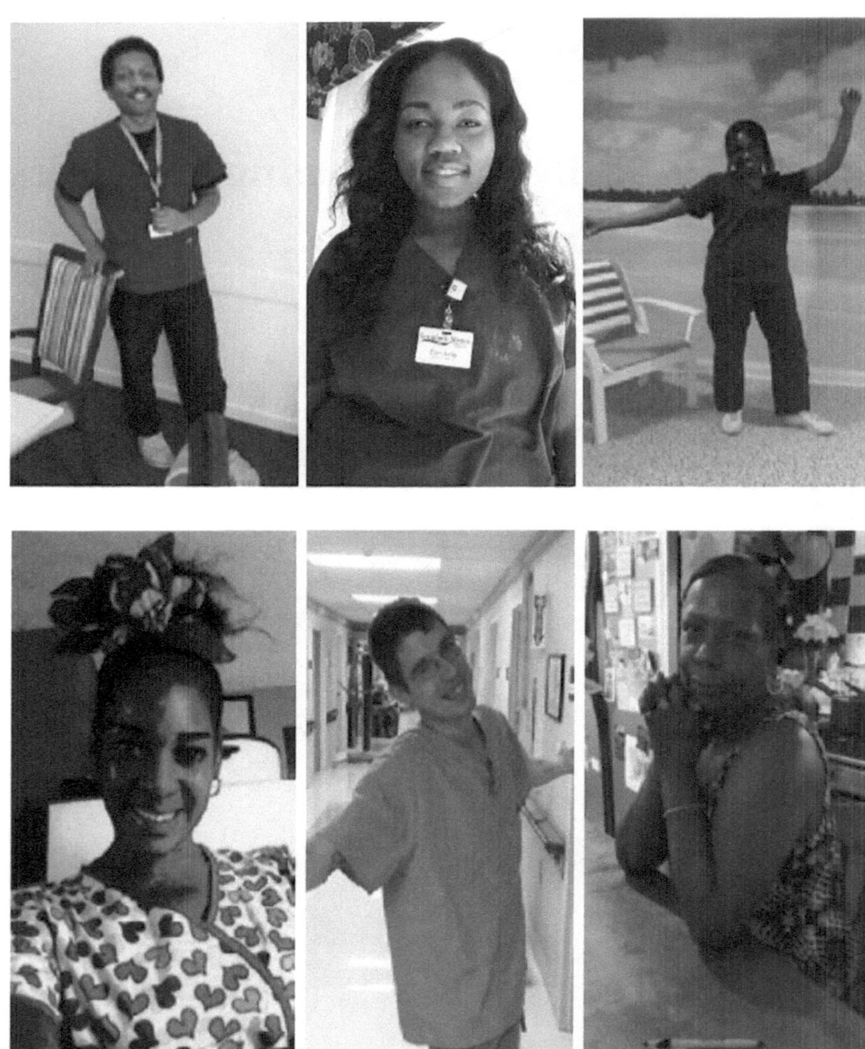

  MISS ASONDRA STARN'AIR

New Day Caregivers

When it comes to finding a job in the health care industry it is very important caregivers choose the right Company or Agency. It's not just about landing a job it's about landing the right one. Ask questions, like what does this company offer me and my family? Today Caregiver must not settle, we must began to set high standards for ourselves. If the employer doesn't offer adequate wages and benefits, **"Move On."**

Trust In God! He is our main source, our daily bread comes for him, he will provide everything we need while we weed out employers who just want to keep us "aides" and underpaid. Research shows Caregivers are in such high demand, that's power in our hands so let's stop setting for crumbs. Keep going on interviewing until you find the right fit. When companies and agencies pay us and treat us like professionals, then that's it! Join the team, until then, don't settle for poor. **We Are More, We Do More, We Deserve More.** So Caregivers, join me, **'Let's Fight for More!'**

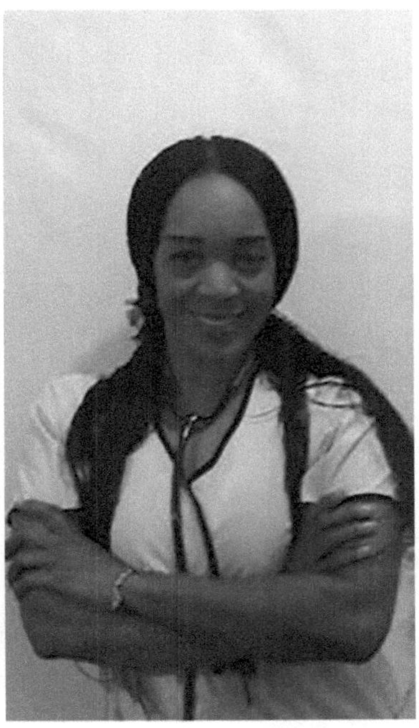

Get Ready!

Remember

Education

Always

Delivers Success

So, READ!

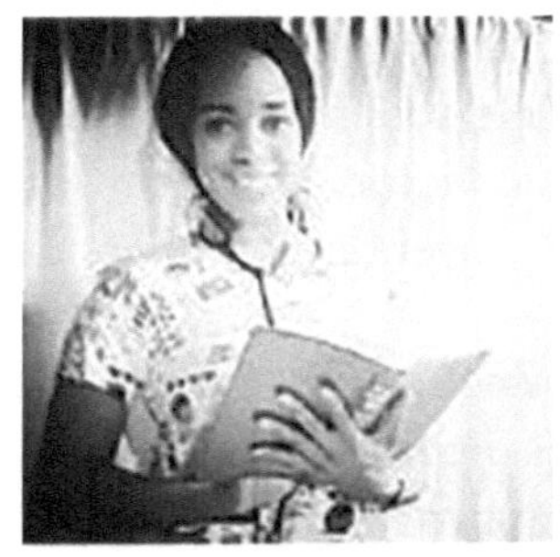

1. Read Daily
2. Welcome, 'Tea Time' reading
3. Make your time reading enjoyable.
4. Choose your material carefully
5. Own your own bibles
6. Take classes
7. Go back to school, it's never too late.
8. Read on your lunch breaks instead of gossiping.
9. Read to those in your care
10. Go to the library more often,
11. Sit, **Read and Relax!**
12. Learn also to read between the lines, if you know what I mean.
13. Read the fine print, before you sign.
14. Read to grow, to know, to show you are competent!
15. Read about things you don't know, that's how we get intelligent and grow.
16. Keep a book with you at all times.
17. Read what saith the **LORD!**
18. Read **'A Caregiver's Bible to Excellence'** often.
19. Read for others!
20. Read my lips, **"I Love You!"**

Ombudsman

What is an Ombudsman?

An Ombudsman is a legal representative often appointed by a governmental or organization to investigate complaints made by individuals in the interest of the citizen or employees.

Usually this is a state official appointed to oversee an investigation of complaints about improper government activity against citizens. One do not have to be part of a union to contact an Ombudsman.

"We The People Matters!"

- Student
- Seniors
- Employees
- Caregivers

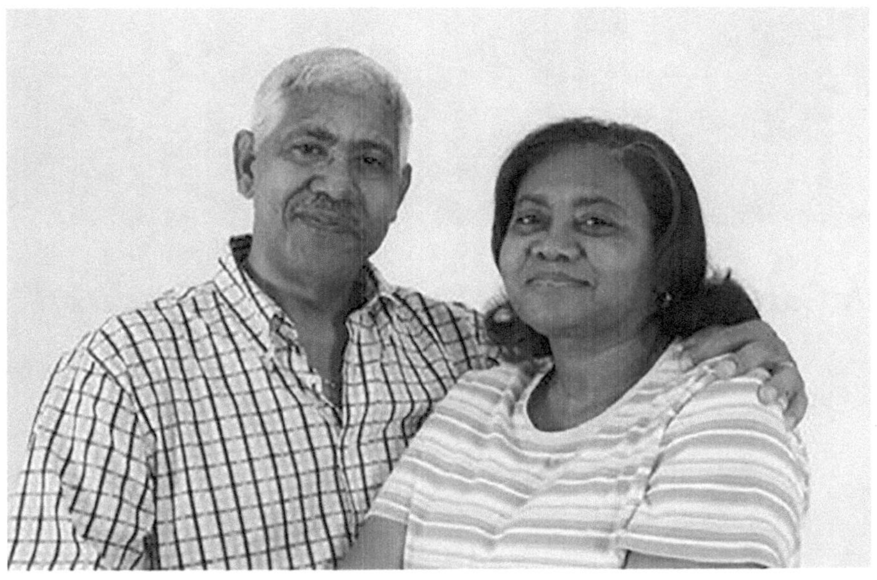

How We're Treated Matters Too!

Nursing Home Bill of Rights

Hello Star, I'm So Proud of You!

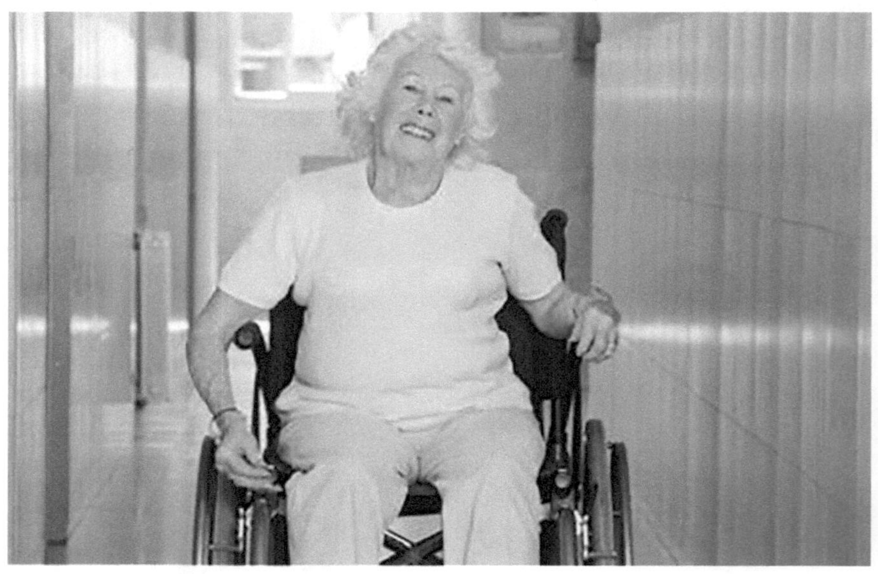

A Caregiver's Bible To Excellence, *"Is Excellent!"*
Thanks for Including Us "Star"!

Nursing Home Resident's **Bill of rights**

Under federal regulations, all nursing homes must have written policies that describe the rights of residents. The nursing home is required by law to make this policy statement - the **"Nursing Home Resident's Bill of Rights"** - available to any resident who requests it. The following outlines the issues that should be covered in the bill of rights.

1. **The Right To Be Informed Of Your Rights And The Policies Of Time**

   The nursing home must have written policies about your rights and responsibilities as a resident. You must sign a statement saying that you have received and understood these rights and the rules of the home when you are admitted.

2. **The Right To Be Informed About The Facility's Services And Charges**

   Every resident has the right to be fully informed of the services available in the facility and of the charges related to those services. This includes charges for services not covered under Medicare or Medicaid and charges that are not covered by the facility's basic rate.

3. **The Right To Be Informed About Your Medical Condition**

   Every resident has the right to be fully informed of his/her medical condition, unless the physician notes in the medical record that it is not in the patient's interest to be told.

4. **The Right To Participate In The Plan Of Care**

   Every resident must be given the opportunity to participate in the planning of his/her medical treatment. This includes the right to refuse treatment.

5. **The Right To Choose Your Own Physician**

   Every resident has the right to choose his/her own physician and pharmacy. Residents do not have to use the nursing home's physician or pharmacy.

6. **The Right To Manage Your Own Personal Finances**

   You can either manage your own funds or authorize someone else to manage them for you. If you authorize the home to handle your funds, you have the right to:

   - Know where your funds are and the account number
   - Receive a written accounting statement every 3 months
   - Receive a receipt for any funds spent
   - Have access to your funds within 7 banking days

7. **The Right To Privacy, Dignity And Respect**

Every resident has the right to be treated with consideration, respect, and with full recognition of his/her dignity and individuality, including privacy in treatment and in care for his/her personal needs.

8. **The Right To Use Your Own Clothing And Possessions**

Every resident may retain and use his/her personal clothing and possessions as space permits, unless to do so would infringe upon rights of other patients, or constitute a hazard to safety.

9. **The Right To Be Free From Abuse And Restraints**

Every resident has the right to be free from mental and physical abuse, and free from chemical and physical restraints except as authorized in writing by a physician for a specified and limited period of time, or when necessary to protect the patient from injury to him/herself or to others.

10. **The Right To Voice Grievance Without Retaliation**

Every resident should be encouraged and assisted to exercise his/her right to voice grievances and recommend changes in policies and services to facility staff and/or outside representatives of his/her choice without fear of coercion, discrimination, or reprisal.

11. **The Right To Be Discharged Or Transferred Only For Medical Reasons**

Residents may only be discharged or transferred for medical reasons, or for his/her welfare or that of other residents. You must be provided with 30-days advance written notice of the transfer or discharge. The law gives you the right to appeal your discharge or transfer.

12. **Your Rights Of Access**

Residents may receive any visitor of their choosing and may refuse a visitor permission to enter their room or may end a visit at any time

- Residents have the right to immediate access by family and reasonable access to others
- Visiting hours of at least 8 hours must be posted in a public place
- Members of community organizations and legal services may enter any nursing home during visiting hours
- Communication between the resident and visitor are confidential
- Visitors may talk to all residents and offer them personal, social, and legal services
- Visitors may help residents claim their rights and benefits through individual assistance, counseling, organizational activity, legal action, or other forms or representation.

If you feel any of these rights have been violated, call your local state Ombudsman.

PHASES OF AGING

In the United States all people over the age 18 are considered adults but there is a very large difference between say an 21 year old and a 50 year old wouldn't you agree, most people would. So we separate them. **"Young Adults" and "Middle Adults".**

But what some of you caregivers may not know is the elderly population, have been divided in to what is called **'Life Stage Subgroups.'**

- **The Young Old.**   65-74
- **The Middle Old.**   75-84
- **The Old Old.**   85 and older

Reason for this is because today's seniors are not the seniors of their generation these seniors are living a lot longer. And thriving too, especially **'The Young Old'**. Many in this subgroup need very little help or none at all. They still drive and live relatively normal and independent lives. Some of these movers and shakers however, live in assistant living communities, downsizing and preparing for the time they will need help, but until then this age group is still having a good time living life to the fullest. The next subgroup **'Middle Old'** is starting to need some assistance, may not be ready for long term care (**LTC**) facilities, but still, very important caregiver keep close eyes on changes that may be taking place. This group is more prone to falls and may show some early signs of memory care impairments such as Dementia and Alzheimer's Disease but not all, just keep close watch on this group.

Now we have the last Sub group **'The Old, Old'** I think that says it all! This Group is **old, old,** and very frail and venerable.

It is our responsibility as Caregivers to help love and take care of the sick, elderly, poor, widowed and anyone else that is in need of care. Whether Formal or Informal we must step in and lend a helping hand. *Leviticus 19:32 you shall stand up before the gray head and honor the face of the old man. and you shall fear god: I Am the Lord.*

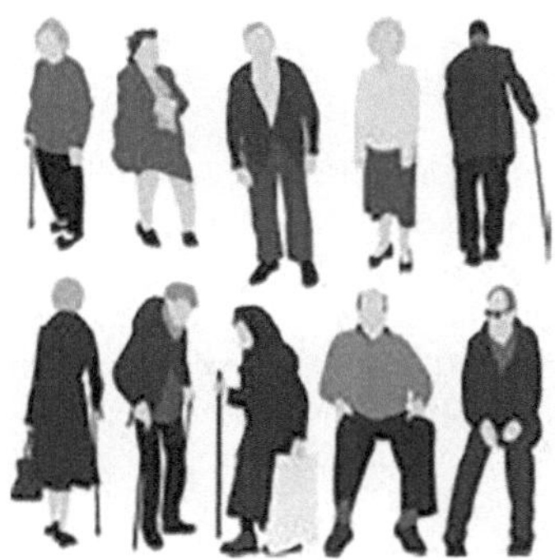

Help The Seniors, The Poor and Very Old, 'Jump On Board!'

Declaration of Independence

IN CONGRESS, July 4, 1776.

The unanimous Declaration of the thirteen united States of America,

When in the Course of human events, it becomes necessary for one people to dissolve the political bands which have connected them with another, and to assume among the powers of the earth, the separate and equal station to which the Laws of Nature and of Nature's God entitle them, a decent respect to the opinions of mankind requires that they should declare the causes which impel them to the separation.

We hold these truths to be self-evident, that all men are created equal, that they are endowed by their Creator with certain unalienable Rights, that among these are Life, Liberty and the pursuit of Happiness.--That to secure these rights, Governments are instituted among Men, deriving their just powers from the consent of the governed, --That whenever any Form of Government becomes destructive of these ends, it is the Right of the People to alter or to abolish it, and to institute new Government, laying its foundation on such principles and organizing its powers in such form, as to them shall seem most likely to effect their Safety and Happiness. Prudence, indeed, will dictate that Governments long established should not be changed for light and transient causes; and accordingly all experience hath shewn, that mankind are more disposed to suffer, while evils are sufferable, than to right themselves by abolishing the forms to which they are accustomed. But when a long train of abuses and usurpations, pursuing invariably the same Object evinces a design to reduce them under absolute Despotism, it is their right, it is their duty, to throw off such Government, and to provide new Guards for their future security.-- Such has been the patient sufferance of these Colonies; and such is now the necessity which constrains them to alter their former Systems of Government. The history of the present King of Great Britain is a history of repeated injuries and usurpations, all having in direct object the establishment of an absolute Tyranny over these States. To prove this, let Facts be submitted to a candid world.

He has refused his Assent to Laws, the most wholesome and necessary for the public good.

He has forbidden his Governors to pass Laws of immediate and pressing importance, unless suspended in their operation till his Assent should be obtained; and when so suspended, he has utterly neglected to attend to them.

He has refused to pass other Laws for the accommodation of large districts of people, unless those people would relinquish the right of Representation in the Legislature, a right inestimable to them and formidable to tyrants only.

He has called together legislative bodies at places unusual, uncomfortable, and distant from the depository of their public Records, for the sole purpose of fatiguing them into compliance with his measures.

 MISS ASONDRA STARN'AIR

He has dissolved Representative Houses repeatedly, for opposing with manly firmness his invasions on the rights of the people.

He has refused for a long time, after such dissolutions, to cause others to be elected; whereby the Legislative powers, incapable of Annihilation, have returned to the People at large for their exercise; the State remaining in the mean time exposed to all the dangers of invasion from without, and convulsions within.

He has endeavoured to prevent the population of these States; for that purpose obstructing the Laws for Naturalization of Foreigners; refusing to pass others to encourage their migrations hither, and raising the conditions of new Appropriations of Lands.

He has obstructed the Administration of Justice, by refusing his Assent to Laws for establishing Judiciary powers.

He has made Judges dependent on his Will alone, for the tenure of their offices, and the amount and payment of their salaries.

He has erected a multitude of New Offices, and sent hither swarms of Officers to harrass our people, and eat out their substance.

He has kept among us, in times of peace, Standing Armies without the Consent of our legislatures.

He has affected to render the Military independent of and superior to the Civil power.

He has combined with others to subject us to a jurisdiction foreign to our constitution, and unacknowledged by our laws; giving his Assent to their Acts of pretended Legislation:

For Quartering large bodies of armed troops among us:

For protecting them, by a mock Trial, from punishment for any Murders which they should commit on the Inhabitants of these States:

For cutting off our Trade with all parts of the world:

For imposing Taxes on us without our Consent:

For depriving us in many cases, of the benefits of Trial by Jury:

For transporting us beyond Seas to be tried for pretended offences

For abolishing the free System of English Laws in a neighbouring Province, establishing therein an Arbitrary government, and enlarging its Boundaries so as to render it at once an example and fit instrument for introducing the same absolute rule into these Colonies:

For taking away our Charters, abolishing our most valuable Laws, and altering fundamentally the Forms of our Governments:

For suspending our own Legislatures, and declaring themselves invested with power to legislate for us in all cases whatsoever.

He has abdicated Government here, by declaring us out of his Protection and waging War against us.

He has plundered our seas, ravaged our Coasts, burnt our towns, and destroyed the lives of our people.

He is at this time transporting large Armies of foreign Mercenaries to complete the works of death, desolation and tyranny, already begun with circumstances of Cruelty perfidy scarcely paralleled in the most barbarous ages, and totally unworthy the Head of a civilized nation.

He has constrained our fellow Citizens taken Captive on the high Seas to bear Arms against their Country, to become the executioners of their friends and Brethren, or to fall themselves by their Hands.

He has excited domestic insurrections amongst us, and has endeavoured to bring on the inhabitants of our frontiers, the merciless Indian Savages, whose known rule of warfare, is an undistinguished destruction of all ages, sexes and conditions.

In every stage of these Oppressions We have Petitioned for Redress in the most humble terms: Our repeated Petitions have been answered only by repeated injury. A Prince whose character is thus marked by every act which may define a Tyrant, is unfit to be the ruler of a free people.

Nor have We been wanting in attentions to our British brethren. We have warned them from time to time of attempts by their legislature to extend an unwarrantable jurisdiction over us. We have reminded them of the circumstances of our emigration and settlement here. We have appealed to their native justice and magnanimity, and we have conjured them by the ties of our common kindred to disavow these usurpations, which, would inevitably interrupt our connections and correspondence. They too have been deaf to the voice of justice and of consanguinity. We must, therefore, acquiesce in the necessity, which denounces our Separation, and hold them, as we hold the rest of mankind, Enemies in War, in Peace Friends.

We, therefore, the Representatives of the united States of America, in General Congress, Assembled, appealing to the Supreme Judge of the world for the rectitude of our intentions, do, in the Name, and by Authority of the good People of these Colonies, solemnly publish and declare, That these United Colonies are, and of Right ought to be Free and Independent States; that they are Absolved from all Allegiance to the British Crown, and that all political connection between them and the State of Great Britain, is and ought to be totally dissolved; and that as Free and Independent States, they have full Power to levy War, conclude Peace, contract Alliances, establish Commerce, and to do all other Acts and Things which Independent States may of right do. And for the support of this Declaration, with a firm reliance on the protection of divine Providence, we mutually pledge to each other our Lives, our Fortunes and our sacred Honor.

   MISS ASONDRA STARN'AIR

October 30, 2015

Presidential Proclamation --
National Family Caregivers Month, 2015

NATIONAL FAMILY CAREGIVERS MONTH, 2015

BY THE PRESIDENT OF THE UNITED STATES OF AMERICA

A PROCLAMATION

Day in and day out, selfless and loving Americans provide care and support to family members and friends in need. They are parents, spouses, children, siblings, relatives, and neighbors who uphold their unwavering commitment to ensure the lives of their loved ones shine bright with health, safety, and dignity. During National Family Caregivers Month, we rededicate ourselves to making sure our selfless caregivers have the support they need to maintain their own well-being and that of those they love.

One of the best measures of a country is how it treats its older citizens and people living with disabilities, and my Administration is dedicated to lifting up their lives and ensuring those who care for them get the support and recognition they deserve. Earlier this year, older Americans and caregivers, as well as their advocates, came together at the White House Conference on Aging, which provided an opportunity to discuss ways to identify and advance actions to improve quality of life for our Nation's elderly. Through the Affordable Care Act, we are providing more options to help older Americans remain in their homes as they age, and the law is giving caregivers the peace of mind of having access to quality, affordable health insurance. Additionally, I will keep pushing to make paid family leave available for every American, regardless of where they work -- because no one should have to sacrifice a paycheck to care for a loved one.

When our men and women in uniform come home with wounds of war seen or unseen -- it is our solemn responsibility to ensure they get the benefits and attentive care they have earned and deserve. Caregivers in every corner of our country uphold this sacred promise with incredible devotion to their loved ones, and my Administration is committed to supporting them. We have extended military caregiver leave to family members of eligible veterans dealing with serious illness or injury for up to 5 years after their service has ended, and we remain dedicated to providing greater flexibility for our military families and for the members of our Armed Forces as they return home and handle the transition to civilian life.

For centuries, we have been driven by the belief that we all have certain obligations to one another. Every day, caregivers across our country answer this call and lift up the lives of loved ones who need additional support. During National Family Caregivers Month, let us honor their contributions and pledge to continue working toward a future where all caregivers know the same support and understanding they show for those they look after.

NOW, THEREFORE, I, BARACK OBAMA, President of the United States of America, by virtue of the authority vested in me by the Constitution and the laws of the United States, do hereby proclaim November 2015 as National Family Caregivers Month. I encourage all Americans to pay tribute to those who provide for the health and well-being of their family members, friends, and neighbors.

IN WITNESS WHEREOF, I have hereunto set my hand this thirtieth day of October, in the year of our Lord two thousand fifteen, and of the Independence of the United States of America the two hundred and fortieth.

BARACK OBAMA

A Change Is Going To Come!

Table 1.4 Occupations with the most job growth, 2014 and projected 2024 (Numbers in thousands)

2014 National Employment Matrix title and code		Employment		Change, 2014–24		Median annual wage, 2015
		2014	2024	Number	Percent	
Total, all occupations	00-0000	150,539.9	160,328.8	9,788.9	6.5	$36,200
Personal care aides	39-9021	1,768.4	2,226.5	458.1	25.9	$20,980
Registered nurses	29-1141	2,751.0	3,190.3	439.3	16.0	$67,490
Home health aides	31-1011	913.5	1,261.9	348.4	38.1	$21,920
Combined food preparation and serving workers, including fast food	35-3021	3,159.7	3,503.2	343.5	10.9	$18,910
Retail salespersons	41-2031	4,624.9	4,939.1	314.2	6.8	$21,780
Nursing assistants	31-1014	1,492.1	1,754.1	262.0	17.6	$25,710
Customer service representatives	43-4051	2,581.8	2,834.8	252.9	9.8	$31,720
Cooks, restaurant	35-2014	1,109.7	1,268.7	158.9	14.3	$23,100
General and operations managers	11-1021	2,124.1	2,275.2	151.1	7.1	$97,730
Construction laborers	47-2061	1,159.1	1,306.5	147.4	12.7	$31,910
Accountants and auditors	13-2011	1,332.7	1,475.1	142.4	10.7	$67,190
Medical assistants	31-9092	591.3	730.2	138.9	23.5	$30,590
Janitors and cleaners, except maids and housekeeping cleaners	37-2011	2,360.6	2,496.9	136.3	5.8	$23,440
Software developers, applications	15-1132	718.4	853.7	135.3	18.8	$98,260
Laborers and freight, stock, and material movers, hand	53-7062	2,441.3	2,566.4	125.1	5.1	$25,010
First-line supervisors of office and administrative support workers	43-1011	1,466.1	1,587.3	121.2	8.3	$52,630
Computer systems analysts	15-1121	567.8	686.3	118.6	20.9	$85,800

A Change Is Going To Come!

2014 National Employment Matrix title and code		Employment		Change, 2014–24		Median annual wage, 2015
		2014	2024	Number	Percent	
Licensed practical and licensed vocational nurses	29-2061	719.9	837.2	117.3	16.3	$43,170
Maids and housekeeping cleaners	37-2012	1,457.7	1,569.4	111.7	7.7	$20,740
Medical secretaries	43-6013	527.6	635.8	108.2	20.5	$33,040
Management analysts	13-1111	758.0	861.4	103.4	13.6	$81,320
Heavy and tractor-trailer truck drivers	53-3032	1,797.7	1,896.4	98.8	5.5	$40,260
Receptionists and information clerks	43-4171	1,028.6	1,126.3	97.8	9.5	$27,300
Office clerks, general	43-9061	3,062.5	3,158.2	95.8	3.1	$29,580
Sales representatives, wholesale and manufacturing, except technical and scientific products	41-4012	1,453.1	1,546.5	93.4	6.4	$55,730
Stock clerks and order fillers	43-5081	1,878.1	1,971.1	92.9	4.9	$23,220
Market research analysts and marketing specialists	13-1161	495.5	587.8	92.3	18.6	$62,150
First-line supervisors of food preparation and serving workers	35-1012	890.1	978.6	88.5	9.9	$30,340
Electricians	47-2111	628.8	714.7	85.9	13.7	$51,880
Maintenance and repair workers, general	49-9071	1,374.7	1,458.1	83.5	6.1	$36,630

Table 1.4 Occupations with the most job growth, 2014 and projected 2024 (Numbers in thousands)

Footnotes:
Data are from the Occupational Employment Statistics program, U.S. Bureau of Labor Statistics.
Source: Employment Projections program, U.S. Bureau of Labor Statistics

Job Growth Resources For Caregivers

Horrible, **'Modern Day Slavery'**. All over the world, Caregivers **MUST**, say no to low poverty wages like these. Today, right now, it's time to take to the streets and march, fight for equality and fair business practices. We are not the aides of past generations. **We Are More, We Do More, We Deserve More So "WE" are Asking For More!**

The HCAHPS

When it comes to **"Quality Care",** hospitals make every effort to ensure patients are receiving the best care possible by hiring good and Qualified Staff to help build a top rating performance. It is very important caregivers going into hospital setting for employment become aware of what's expected of them. Because most hospitals demands **"High Quality Care"** for their patients. As I see it, that should be the goal everywhere, not just in hospitals, Home-care, Assistant Living, Private Care, and at home, **"Everywhere."**

So, exactly what is **HCAHPS?** it is a consumer assessment questionnaire hospitals use to monitor quality of care received by staff given to patients for evaluation.

HCAHPS stands for: **Hospital Consumer Assessment Of Healthcare Provider and Systems**

It's a survey also known as the **"Voice of the Patient"**

It gives Massachusetts General Hospital (**MGH**) a view into patients perception of whether they are happy with the care and service in hospitals.

The scores are open for public viewing via internet.

The survey is important for 4 reasons:

1. The patient has a voice and can let that voice be heard regarding the quality of care received.
2. Hospital gets to read and make changes to improve performance.
3. Everyone including the public can assess what's being shared.
4. Those that score high in quality care, **"Get Rewarded",** they get reimbursements! **"Everybody Wins!!!!"**

Here are the list of questions asked on the survey:

- Doctors conversation / communication
- Nurse conversation / communication.
- Staff responsibility/communication
- Hospital Environment
- Pain Management & Medical Conversation
- Food Service

Rated on scale 1-10
10 being the highest!

Caregivers, keep this in mind, not only do we want the high rating for our organization, the employers we work for but, also we want the high rating of excellence to show the world that Christ still lives, he lives in us and it shows in our work ethics and performance, remember, we really work for God, not man. Therefore, **"Be Excellent!"**

Acute Care

What is Acute Care? Acute Care is a branch of secondary health care where a patient receives active but short term treatment for a severe injury or episode of illness, an urgent medical condition, or during recovery from surgery. In medical terms, care from acute health conditions is the opposite from chronic care, or longer term care.

So for you caregivers, who chooses to work in acute care setting, let me tell you, you have more responsibilities as well as opportunities for advancements. Because you not only serve the patients you also are expected to communicate well with the entire medical health care team. And you must be able to use medical terminology well because you'll be using them on a daily bases.

Not only that, there's more, **STNA'S** are given a little more extra training, than those who work primary in setting like nursing homes, home health, assistant living and private care.

A lot of Hospital's have their own extra training programs for their employ-ees at no cost and also, they will help fund your healthcare education too if you want to advance further with them. There is so much opportunity out there for caregivers today especially for the State Tested Nursing Assistants (**STNA's**). I say go for it, but, become a **'Caregiver for Christ'!**

Let him show you what His **"Caregivers"** looks like, walk like, talk like, works like and act like.

Right now, is a great time to be a caregiver! We have so much more opportunities in this generation than ever before, take advantage of it! Let's not blow it on meritocracy.

Step Up to Quality, Be a Five Star! ★ ★ ★ ★ ★

In Jesus name **Amen!**

Facility Healthcare Workers

For those caregivers who work in hospitals, nursing homes, or healthcare facilities it is very important too, that you become familiar with its structure and ways. There is more to it than just going to work a whole lot more.

There are systems put in place to ensure an overall safe and quality of care experience, not only for those we provide care for but for **"All of Us"** the entire health care team, that includes you and me **"Caregivers"**!

Because this is confidential information, not for pubic reading or use, I cannot go into detail but I will say, if you are working in a facility or want to you can request what is known as **"The Environment of Care"** (EC) packet "I have mine". This packet breaks down the foundation on which they build their name and repetition on and it is a joint commission by the entire healthcare industry. Inside this EC packet there are three basic components and eight programs that are required of the healthcare organization, their role, departments and our role as employee's.

It is very important that caregivers realize and keep in mind always that, we don't go to work every day just to care for the sick, we also go to care for each other and the organization too, remember what I told you "Caregivers", **"Team Work Makes The Dream Work"**! And that message is so appropriate here because you need to know, it take all of us to run the show!

We do this by making sure daily that we help maintain a loving and friendly environment for our co-workers, patients and their families. We take care of **"Everyone"** coming and going. Matched up with skills, quality care and topped off with, love and compassion, with this kind a Environment Of Care we are sure to receive five star ratings individually and collectively. So no, we don't just **'Go To Work'** oh no! Reverse that one too, **'We' 'Work To Go'** to the **Top!** ★ ★ ★ ★ ★

We can get there, read **'A Caregivers Bible To Excellence'** don't stop!

Hospice

Hospice is a special concept of care designed to help provide comfort and support to patients who have been diagnosed with a terminal illness.

Hospice care neither prolongs life nor hasten death.

Hospice care focuses on comfort and quality of life rather than a cure. The goal of hospice is to make sure the individual have an alert and pain-free life. Relieve all suffering as much as possible and to live each day as fully with dignity and respect.

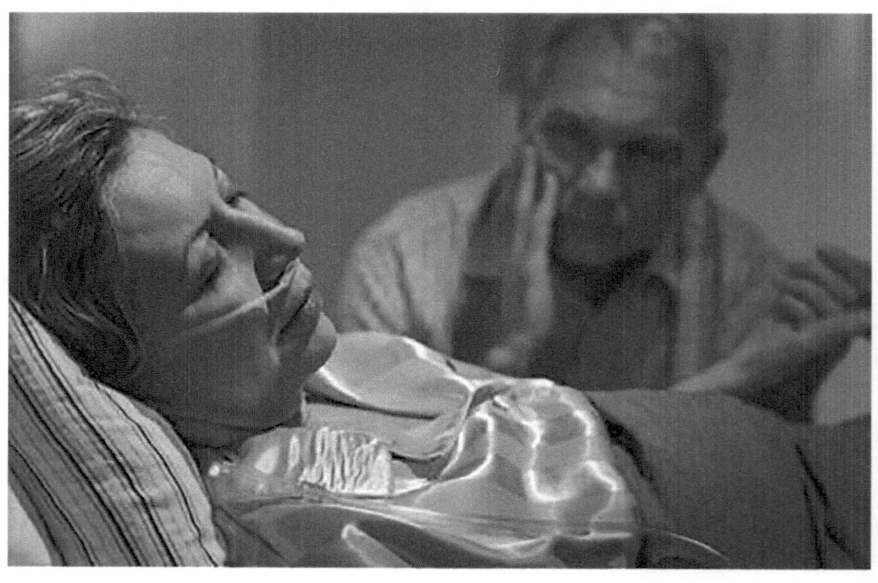

What could be better than that!

For we believe that Jesus died and rose again, and so we believe that God will bring with Jesus those who have fallen asleep in him.

1 Thessalonians 4:14

 MISS ASONDRA STARN'AIR

Stages of Dying

The stages, popularly known by the acronym **DABDA**, include:

1. **Denial** – The first reaction is denial. In this stage individuals believe the diagnosis is somehow mistaken, and cling to a false, preferable reality.
2. **Anger** – When the individual recognizes that denial cannot continue, they become frustrated, especially at proximate individuals. Certain psychological responses of a person undergoing this phase would be: "Why me? It's not fair!"; "How can this happen to me?"; "'Who is to blame?"; "Why would this happen?".
3. **Bargaining** – The third stage involves the hope that the individual can avoid a cause of grief. Usually, the negotiation for an extended life is made in exchange for a reformed lifestyle. People facing less serious trauma can bargain or seek compromise.
4. **Depression** – "I'm so sad, why bother with anything?"; "I'm going to die soon, so what's the point?"; "I miss my loved one, why go on?"

During the fourth stage, the individual despairs at the recognition of their mortality. In this state, the individual may become silent, refuse visitors and spend much of the time mournful and sullen.

5. **Acceptance** – "It's going to be okay."; "I can't fight it, I may as well prepare for it."

In this last stage, individuals embrace mortality or inevitable future, or that of a loved one, or other tragic event. People dying may precede the survivors in this state, which typically comes with a calm, retrospective view for the individual, and a stable condition of emotions.

Bereavement, Grief and Loss

Losing a love one is hard, it seems no one can fully understand your loss, your pain, not even you. No amount of comforting will do. When that persons gone, part of you is gone too, I've been there. Losing my dad was the hardest thing I ever had to endure. But we must go on "We Must!"

After a serious loss we want something to ease the pain, but we must be careful not to harm ourselves in the process; we must be strong and choose healthy and Godly ways to cope.

Cry, and keep crying if you have to but, at some point stop and realize that life goes on... We all have to leave this place too one day, so we have to learn to embrace life and death as it comes.

The best place to turn to when this happens is to Jesus, He will get you through it all, He will heal you completely if you let him, but the more you resist his loving and comforting arms the more you stay stuck in that grief, we don't want that. God wants you healed, up and going again.

If there is anybody else out there experiencing a loss of any kind, a job loss, death of a marriage, a dear friend or have loss a pet, whatever your losses are God can help and He wants to. He's known for healing the broken-hearted, and binding up all kinds of wounds. In fact, the bible says

COME TO ME ALL YOU WHO ARE WEARY AND BURDENED AND I WILL GIVE YOU REST
Matthew 11:28

- Turn to God!
- Read scriptures on healing.
- Keep embracing your faith.
- Do uplifting activities.
- Be with family members and close friends.
- Turn to your pastor /church family
- Prayer works so keep praying for your healing, everyday pray!

Stay Close to God!

- Keep a healthy lifestyle.
- Don't over eat, incorporate exercise during this time it will take the edge off the physical symptoms of grief giving you better control over your body and emotions.
- Give yourself all the time you need to grieve. Cry it's okay.
- Men, it's okay too for you to cry. **'Real Men Do Cry'**, Jesus wept. John 11:35
- Get away for a while if you can, if not find a special place in your home to be in spirit with that person you loss. It's perfectly fine to still talk to the deceased, and celebrate the good times shared, go for it, whatever helps.

Other types of losses,'Life Stuff':

- Accept the things you can't change.
- Trust God to work things out in your favor.
- Wait on God because He has the perfect person for you.
- God gives, God takes away, trust him, listen, do what he say!
- When God closes one door, He always opens another, you're on your way!

Some Loses Are Good For Us!
"In God We Trust!"

He is closer to the broken hearted, and saves those who are crushed in spirit. ***Psalms 34:18.***

So if there's anybody out there, that has had a lost, or hurting in any way, call on the name of Jesus. Let him care for you, after all, He is the **"Ultimate Caregiver"** Yes indeed, He is **'The Greatest Caregiver Of All!'** He will heal you, put you back together again. Make you whole and give you new life with purpose if you let Him. Just know that, healing takes time so be patient, keep reading his word and allow the master to do his thing.

Again, don't rush the healing by settling for quick fixes such as alcohol, substance abuse, overindulgence on foods or sinful pleasures. Jesus cares about what happens to you, don't do that! Just try to take things one day at a time and you'll be fine.

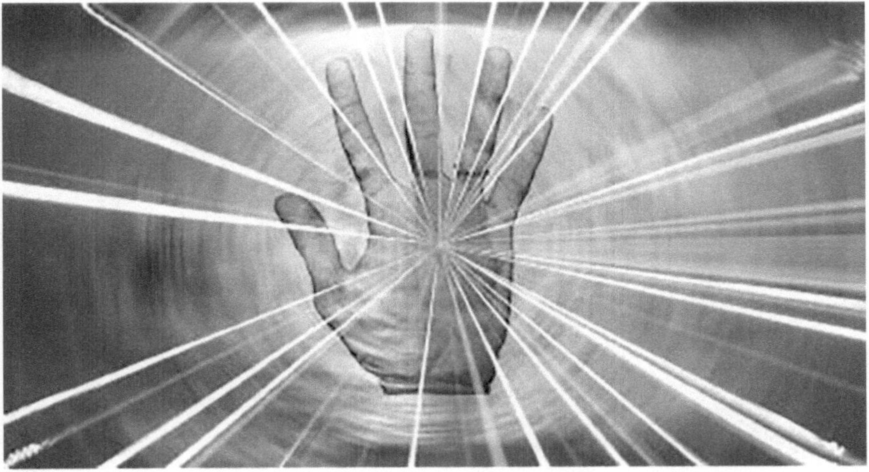

Have mercy on me, Lord for I am faint; heal me, **LORD**, for my bones are in agony. My soul is in deep anguish. How long, **LORD**, how long? Turn, **LORD** and deliver me; save me because of your unfailing love. Psalms 6:2-4

A Sitter

Sitters also sometimes are referred to as companion care providers. They are used a lot by many employers and families as comfort care or prevention care or both depending on the individuals need. See, a lot of families don't want their love ones left alone, so they use a sitter, a companion care provider to be there when they can't be. And sitters are used too, as prevention like I said, because there are those patients that are high risk for injuries due to falls, pulling out of Iv's or other tubes.

Today 'Sitters' are in high demand as well, families and other staffing places need someone to go in and sit, however many times sitter do more than sit if they are STNA's like myself, we can help out with other things if we want too, I want to.

Another reason for the demand of sitter too, **'Suicide Watch'** some people just do not want to live anymore. We are there to make sure they don't succeed at taking their own life. We are there to love on them and give them hope. Each life matters to us. **"In God We Trust!"**

These kinds of cases many times require 24 hours, seven day a week staffing. **Caregivers Are Needed Everywhere!**

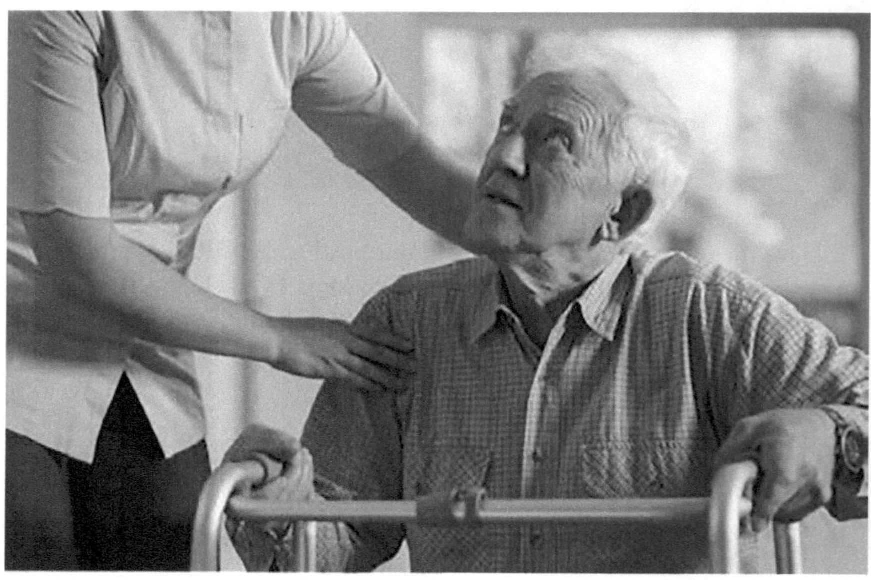

We are there also to help redirect and stop accidents before they happen!

  Miss Asondra StarN'air

Department Of Developmental Disabilities
DODD

Those working with the developmental disable are under the Protocol and guidelines of each state, California, has theirs, Ohio has theirs, each state has their own local numbers but all are under the authority of our united states government.

More than that, the Government sets all the rule and cuts the checks too; they have their own system put in place, with all the Do's and Don'ts. Plus the pay scale rates for both the consumer (the disabled person) and the caregiver.

Warning, caregivers. be advised. when you work for a disabled consumer that's receiving benefits and subsidies from the government, know that not only are you working for that consumer but you are working for the government as well, so you'd better cross your I's and dot your T's. But no worries, The DODD Administration has

put together a wonderful packet for caregivers from how too's to where to go get everything you need to become a certified provider. Once you are certified, you will be given a license number, I have one, get yours too. If interested, just call or go online to start the application process.

Let me share this, working with the mentally challenged or disabled has some unique yet satifying rewards of it's own. Consumer can be out in the community with the caregiver doing normal everyday stuff. Shopping, having fun and eating out, things like that.

Caregivers Information Center

- Surprise consumers with something new to do or eat.
- Give the individual time and space in-between the day to spend a little quite time alone if ISP (individual Service Plan) allows it, don't over crowd them.
- Take them shopping at fun thrift shops, or just window shop.
- Plan inexpensive outing and trips take them to the Zoo.
- Have an outdoor or indoor picnic
- Read their ISP, get to know all you can about that consumer.
- Observe, and see what the individual can and cannot do, then make the necessary adjustments.
- Get your med pass license, agency will pay for it. Many consumers take meds.
- Offer to take them to church. Never force.
- Love and care for the disabled as if you are taking care of Jesus and all will go well for you.

In fact, many of them work themselves, our job is to make them feel welcome and as normal a possible. How do we do this? Caregiver we do this when we love and spend quality time with them, that's how we do it!

But be advised, there will be some behavior challenges, however, once you complete all the necessary training you will be fine. We are professionals we can handle it.

I have worked with many consumers and it leaves me with a good feeling knowing that I can Care-Give to anyone forward and backwards. **Care-Give, Give-Care,** you won't find a better provider anywhere! New caregivers I wish you all the success, go out there too and become one of the best!

Universal Precautions

Universal Precaution refers to the practice of medicine. Those working in acute care setting such as hospitals, medical centers anywhere there is high risk of exposer to blood and body fluids.

Healthcare workers, caregivers, everybody, listen up, we are at high risk, that's why we **MUST** protect ourselves by means of wearing Personal Protective Equipment **(PPE)** such as medical gloves, goggles, gowns and face shields when necessary.

It is recommend in the united states now that all **"Health Care"** setting including Home health Care organizations and agencies practice Universal Precautions by making sure employees are provided with Personal Protective Equipment **(PPE)** when needed. Home-care employees, listen, next time you are in the area or you stop by the office ask for a universal precaution kit. You might not know this but home-care by law are now required to have them, if they don't have them, ask them to get you one. And when they hand you one, keep it in your Florence Nightingale Bag **(FNG Bag)** hey, you never know when you might need it, this way you'll already have it.

I'll say it again, Caregivers must protect themselves, don't ever think you are immune to catching diseases. You catch colds, and flus, you can catch fatal diseases too.

Use both Universal and Standard Precaution **(Hand Washing)** always to help greatly reduce your chances of becoming infected.

EVERYBODY, EVERYWHERE
BEWARE
"WASH YOUR HANDS"

SECTION VII

Roots/Culture

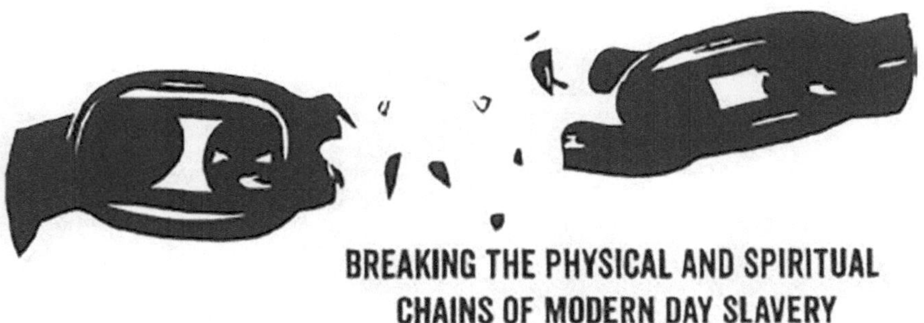

Movement Toward Freedom
There's a Boat, Caregiver's There's a Boat!

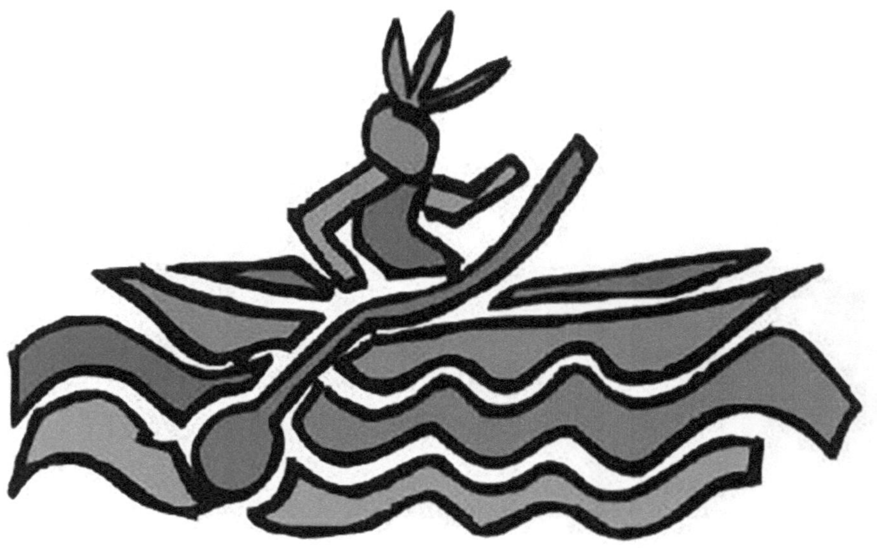

Roots

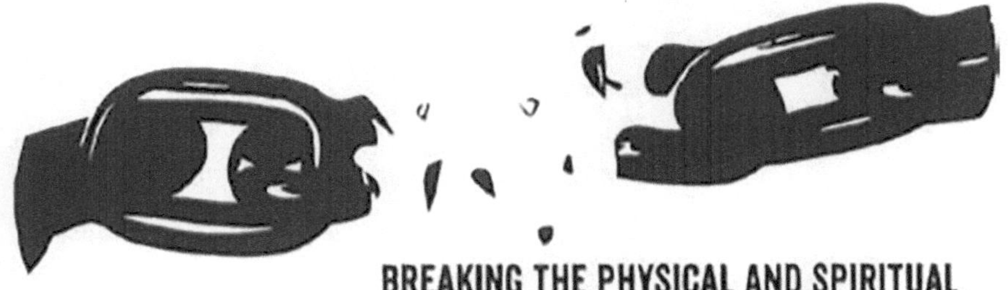

BREAKING THE PHYSICAL AND SPIRITUAL CHAINS OF MODERN DAY SLAVERY

African American's have been working overtime, double hard, ever since we laid foot on American soil. Yes things have gotten better, but our pay as caregivers in particular is insulting. Again we are part of the health care team, yet paid like slaves. Mistreated too if we speak up about the inequality. Well a **New Day** is dawning, Success is calling!

First let's start by giving "Aides" a new name. How about 'Home Health Associates' (HHA) no more Home Health Aides, to me, calling us aides links us with maids and slaves. And it makes us feel worthless, unappreciated,downgraded, underpaid and stereotyped. For example, niggers, dumb, poor, down and out, fat, bastards, uneducated, stupid and

lazy, animals, you people, work horse, cheap labor, slaves. There I said it! "Slaves". Giving us a more professional title like the one I just spoke of has more respectability don't you think? Yes it does, more it has more and love. So caregivers, **"FIGHT"** after today, don't let people call you aides anymore, tell them you are a caregiver, not an aide. You are an associate of the healthcare team.

Home Health Associates base rate by now, 2018 should be at 12.00 an hour with full benefits and yearly raises. State Tested Nurse Assistants (STNA) 15.00 an hour with full benefits and yearly raises for both, But it's not. Why not? **We are more, We do more, We deserve More, Pay us More!** Caregiver we cannot continue to sit back and do nothing anymore, how long do you want to struggle of be poor? Let's fight! If you're with change, then say no more. Today we have to come together, "break the silence, and speak up." Look, I know they say "Some Things Never Change",but I say **"Some Things Must!"**

In God We Trust!

Time to March for Change!

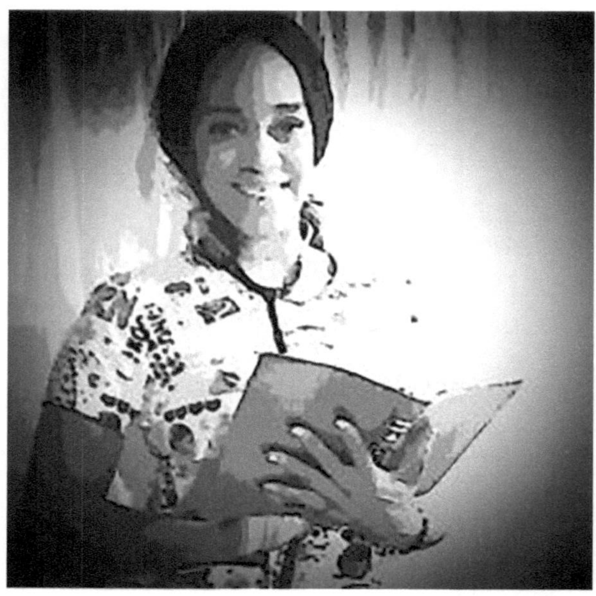

March for freedom and equality, walk together and don't grow weary, we must secure our future not only for us but for our children and their children's children. White supremacy and economic inequality of women especially toward the black female or male must end on planet earth, the very future of humankind depends on it. Crumbs are for Dogs, Not for Black People!

The World Needs To Become "ONE"

1 Corinthians 12:12

Black People Matter, All People Matter!

 MISS ASONDRA STARN'AIR

History Lesson 101
"Those Who Do Not Learn From History Are Doomed To Repeat It"

Over here, over here, come on over here!!!! We have niggers for sale! Here's a nigger right here, a black female slave, can we get our first bid? You can get a lot of work out of this nigger, you'll get your money's worth. This nigger is strong and is able to do whatever you want, you don't have to pay these niggers nothing if you don't want too. They work for cheap. Let them scrub your floors and wash your sheets. Do we have another bid? Going once, twice, **SOLD!** to the business owner in the back for **'Nine Dollars'**.

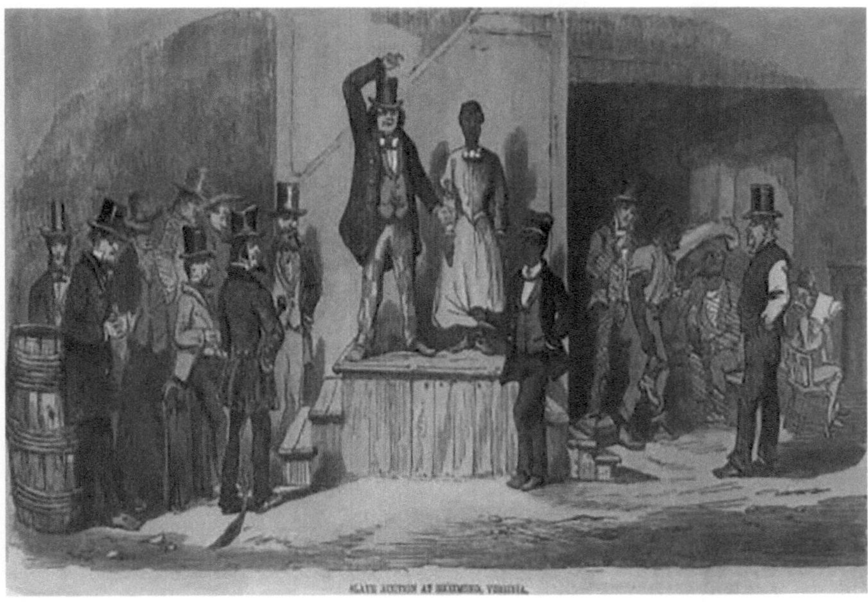

The late great Marvin Gaye ask the question decades ago in a song, What's Going On? Tell Me What Going On? But, hey I'll Tell You What's Going On, and I don't have to hide it in a song, but I wouldn't mind a nice drum beat! Especially if we have to go back boycotting and marching in the streets. Like I said, oh I can see, exactly what's going on. What's happening is most Blacks in this county are still being ruled over by whites. We're on the bottom, they're on the Top! Will this injustice over my people ever be stopped?
Modern Day Slavery or Slavery Day Modern
Forward or Backward what difference does it make,
Black people still come up with empty plates.

Don't buy into all those smiles and chatter, in some of their hearts
Black Lives Still Don't Matter!

Many who are first will be last, and many who are last will be first!
Matthew 19:30

Caregivers of all Ethnicity Matters! Women Matter!
The Poor and Oppressed Matter!
A Caregiver's Bible to Excellence Matter like it or not,
'THIS BOOK MATTERS!'

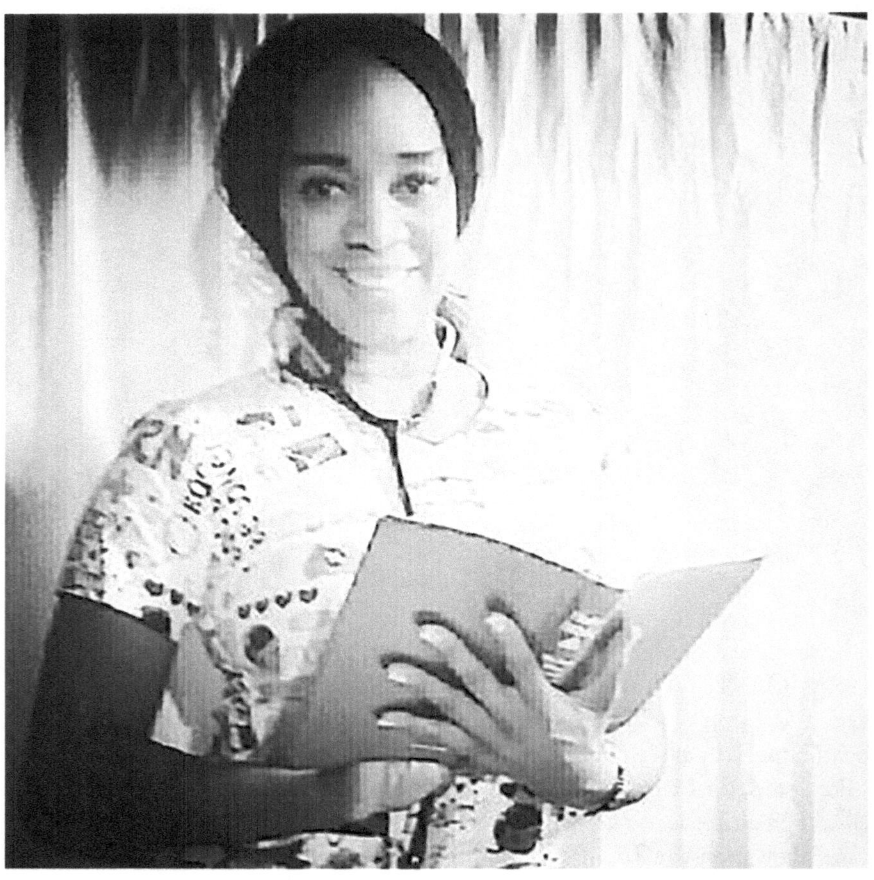

If some of **'YOU'** feel convicted in your hearts, **"Change"**, stop
thinking you have the right to rule over another race, **"You Don't!"**

         Miss Asondra StarN'air

Prejudice and 'The Great Depression' of the 1930's

(Matthew 19:30)

Prejudice a preconceived opinion that is not based on reason or actual experience. Prejudice in any form is **WRONG.** Does prejudice still exist?

"You bet it does" for far too long now black caregivers all over the world has experienced mistreatment, not only from some of the clients they serve also from the healthcare industry. Why is this and why too, are black care-givers paid so little when they are such a vital part of the healthcare industry? Why?

Along with that, it seems to be a disproportionate amount of black women to white women or any other race working home care cases today and are still struggling to make ends meet, why is that?

Too many unanswered questions, so I did some digging, "know your history so you don't have to repeat it'! What I am about to share with you will not only wake you up if you are a caregiver or thinking about becoming one. But let's deal with the word **'Aide'** first, I've been a caregiver for quite some time now and still, I can't take being called an aide, you have to call me a caregiver or by my name. Something about the title **'Aide'** has always bothered me from day one. And I never really knew why? It just felt degrading, and made me feel worthless as a person.

So I asked God about it, I asked Him, Lord, please tell me why does the word aide make me feel so bad, everybody else seems to be fine with it 'except me'? Why do I hate it so? He said to me, "when people don't know their history, it is true, they are doomed to repeat it, start there." So I did, I researched and found what I'm about to share with all of you. Some of you, that are not black, will be offended and may feel threatened too because I am getting to the truth, and the truth is "Black Women" in home care are still nothing but slaves for white America. Black people, don't take my word for it, do the research, I did. What I am about to share with some of you aides should make you rebel from ever being called aides again. Aides has been stereotyped to mean ugly things to some, like black, poor, troubled, down and out, poverty stricken people, and worse, slaves. Uneducated people who can't find "Real" jobs. Therefore the system is doing us a favor in hiring us, we are a desperate people so, 'White American' can pay us what it wants to. And guess what, "They Do!" they're still doing that today. And too, before we get started, I am also aware that some of my own people could care less about what I found out in my research. Some of you may say this, so what at least "We Got a Job!" That's right, a lot of you, if you are black, may feel that way. Because many of you have become comfortable with the way things are. You don't want to speak out, or risk being fired or black balled off future cases. Well, I say to all of you who are in bondage to fear and what others can do to you, "I ain't scared", I'm not a slave, I'm breaking free, and Christ is going to lead me. Why don't come too, Blacks, Hispanic's, Chinese, Poor and Whites that haven't been treated right, everybody, everywhere I don't care. Time to get paid well for all the hard work we do. To the rest, stay in chains remain slaves, keep settling for crumbs, barely making it, living impoverished lives like bums. No thank you, I got work to do! We got work to do caregivers. No more being "Just Over Broke!' Slaving for Money Hungry Folks! Now for all those who are interested in what I have dug up from the past, then pull up a chair, grab your water bottles you are about to see what I see, some things have not changed 'White America' still holds the key. I call it 'Modern Day Slavery' because it's more discrete and more sophisticated then ever before. I want to talk to black aides in America right now, all of us, who work in home-care in-particular. I want to talk to you about **'The Great Depression' of the 1930's** Franklin D. Roosevelt was president at the time.

Back in the 1930's during the **"Great Depression"** era, it was one of the worst economic downturn in the history of the industrialized world. It began after the stock market crashed and wiped out millions of investors. Suddenly just like that, they were all broke! It was horrific and frightening too, leaving the country in a great depression hence the name. Soon after that, the economy took a turn too, people in the united states were losing their jobs, especially men, these were industrial jobs, factory and manufacturing jobs. Back then known as sex jobs, meaning men did this kind of work and woman did that kind of work. For example, women could be in clerical, work as telephone operators, become teachers, become nurses, anything that had to do with service, we could do; but not manufacturing or industrial jobs. No, that was for men and men only. That's what they meant back then by, 'Sex Jobs' women do this and men do that! Get it? Got it! Then let's move on....

Well, during that time, **Franklin D, Roosevelt** was president he was elected in 1933, But the effects of the stock market crash of 1929 still left the economy in bad shape. So, something had to be done, and done it was. Because people were panicking, individuals were becoming desperate for any opportunity to work men and women alike, black and white. Everybody, Everywhere, including their Mama, that's how bad it was. But, wait a minute, check this out, because of the sexious mentally of that era, men 'found

 MISS ASONDRA STARN'AIR

themselves out of work' manufacturing, industrial jobs all shut down, like a broken down railroad track, taking no more passengers, **NONE!**

But women, on the other hand, were still working, so they became the "Bread Winners" during that time. Yes the adult females were the ones bring home the bacon and frying it up in a pan sort of speak.

Women were out there working very long hours; they were exhausted, worn out, tired, up all day on their feet helping to make sure their families eat.

Caregivers as you can see, things were tough, people were really, really struggling. So much so, that "The Federal Law" is what they called the Government back then, stepped in and enforced new and stick laws on what women could and could not do. They came up with a law in 1932 – 1937 which made it illegal for more than one person per family to find employment with the federal civil service. Therefore, causing more strain on families forcing some to find work elsewhere.

Hold on keep reading "Aides"… I hate that word with a passion but it's relevant here, just wait. The federal law or government as we know it back then also formed a policy against women. This policy was called **"The New Deal"** these programs were developed and approved by the government to stereotype women and cast women into traditional "Housekeeping Roles".

"WHAT" (like a liberty mutual commercial,) the government did what, (and the church choir say), "StarN'air" "shurr, hush," shut your mouth!" Help me Jesus! See, people, when you read, the truth is never far behind, but I had to dig and dig, they kept it hidden well, sounds like a Madonna song! Live to Tell! Yes believe it or not, the government came up with our title 'Aides'. Oh but hold on, wait a minute, our kind of Aide is different from the dictionaries version, which says: an aide is an assistant to an important person especially to a political leader 'a president aide' or a right hand man, you get the gist of it, I'm sure. Let's see if you get the gist of this, keep reading. This **"New Deal"** back then was called the **(FERA)Federal Emergency Relief Administration.**

It was this **"New Deal"** that hurt women all over the world especially black aides, So to help boost the economy, the people in power (Our Government along with **President Roosevelt** came up with a plan. They were about to put women to work because jobs was scarce, times were hard, no work in sight for men. And during that time also, the federal law started enforcing it's perception of women onto the masses. They said, in so many words that all women were good for was service type jobs. (and you know what else but, they dared not come out and say that publicly) Therefore, women back then, were all forbidden to do man like jobs, the government made it against the law and president Franklin D. Roosevelt, was cool with it. Now what?

So, the **"New Deal"** came up with something women could do, **Housekeeping!** Yes **"Housekeeping"!** Go out and clean homes. I suppose the thinking behind this was, it would be another way to help put many more women to work. So that they could help the men out, with bills, and keep food in the house. Remember, men weren't working, factory and industrial jobs were all shut down. So, I guess something was better than nothing. I would have done it, how about you? I think you would have too. We are women, we do what we have to do. Right!

Nevertheless, it worked, females went in and started cleaning other people's homes, but they started making black woman cook too. So, caregivers, there you have it, that's the history, how we became known as '**Aides /Maids!** And soon you will find out too, **SLAVES**. Pause here for a minute, lets fast forward, to now, right now, 2018. Can somebody please tell me, how we turn "Home Care' housekeeping /maid into 'Health Care'? **Hello?** How we do that and still get paid like maids, impoverished wages? Something's not right, Can I get ah Amen? All I can say is, let those who have eyes see, and those with ears, hear.

Let's, move on.. because you ain't seen or heard nothing yet. Just keep on reading, soon you'll connect the dots, but right now I'm on a roll I can't stop.

Sorry I went on and on but, something has to give, it's time for a change. Every day, I'm praying caregivers, that, change will come. We will be highly favored, respected and paid like the professionals we've become.

Okay Let's leave 2018 and go back to the 1930's and pick up where we left off shall we, '**The New Deal'** so, where was I? We were talking about 'Aides' yes, housekeeping aides, so the law, which was the government, they are the ones who created that negative downgrading name "Aides" for us, along with all the prejudices and stereotypes that goes along with that job. And now it's up to **"US"**, you and me, **"We The People"** to say no to such a degrading name like '**Aide'.** We are Health Care Professionals now, not maids or slaves.

Meanwhile, let's get back to what was happening with this '**New Deal'** stuff. Oh no, now **"Huston We Got a Problem"?** What's the problem? Caregivers, here's the problem(better start connecting the dots) a lot of those well to do white women with the white gloves and fancy hats on didn't want white aides, their own kind, coming in their homes, scrubbing and cleaning for them, no, they wanted black female niggers. Yelp, just like the one you saw on the auction block at the beginning of this chapter. Connect the dots! How are you feeling now? The well do do white folks/ mainly the white women of the house wanted niggers, blacks. They believed in their hearts that we are their slaves, and mistreated like ah dog begging for food, we get their scraps, their crumbs. I have a question for you, if you work in home care, how much do you make an hour out of the 25 to 35 dollars per hour they take in. 8, 9 or 10 an hour, am I right? And do you thinks that fair or right? We do 95% of the work, they keep most of the money and give us the leftovers, 8 to 10 dollars an hour. This I say is '**Modern Day Slavery**, at its most sophisticated level. Some things never change, but today, some things must. Shocking hum, but in my gut, when I first heard the name aide I new it was something dark and ugly, and of course I'm most certainly not talking about blacks, we are one of the most beautiful, powerful and strongest people who ever walked plant earth. Don't believe it read your real your history, blacks were kings and queens. My people are beautiful! Again, Learn from your history or you're doomed to repeat it! Sorry to say, but we're repeating it! Aides are Slaves, all colors alike, black and white. We are not being respected or economically treated right! **We Have To Fight!**

Let's get ready to wrap up this **'New Deal'** crap, because that **New** so called Deal, hurt black people all over the world. We are still feeling it's effect today. We are still paid degradingly. And also too, to keep us suppressed, down and out, we are still stuck with that horrible name **"AIDE"**. That name alone, will never be respected or get us paid, never! Calling us aides is the same as calling us slaves. As you can see, I am very troubled by all the injustice done to Aides, blacks in particular. Our struggles are far from over. White women in the 1930's wanted the black female for their workers/slaves. (take a look around today, 2018 whose running the home care agency? Mostly white women, and who are the aides? I'll let you all answer that one. Oh and here's another thing, white aides make more than black aides in home care.) One, because she was black and two because she was cheap.

But it doesn't stop there, the federal law, said **OK** we will give these rich whites people what they want and find these high class white folks some black female niggers. So they got involved some more and started looking for locations throughout the cities to gather female niggers so that white women could have their picking as if they were at a fruit or meat market; except "black women" **'WE'** were the prime cut. "Shut up"! No it's true! If you want to keep being called an aide,that's you. So the **Federal Law** /also known as the **The Government** today went on a search to do just that, gather female niggers for white women. So that white women/people could come have a look at us, and see how we were built and if they liked what they saw then these white women would offer us the job. And if the going rate was a quarter and hour they paid white aides that and paid us a nickel, how unfair and fickle. And here's something else black people need to know, sit down, brace yourself, what I just shared with you about these various location they set up to pick out **"AIDES"** well, aides, that too became known as a form of **'The Slave Market'** and the slave market happened on **"BLACK FRIDAY"** hence the name today as you head out to Walmart. As long as I live this black queen will never shop on a "Black Friday." We Want Change!" Question, how long will **"YOU"** be scared to fight back for your right to be free? "March with me!" Bottom line, 100 years later, 88 to be exact, Black lives still don't matter! And it won't until we fight, for what's fair and right. Today there is no way I will ever accept being called an Aide, Aides don;t get respected or paid! And we are not maids. We are Healthcare Professionals. Don't get it twisted! **We Are More, We Do More, We Deserve More, Pay us More!**

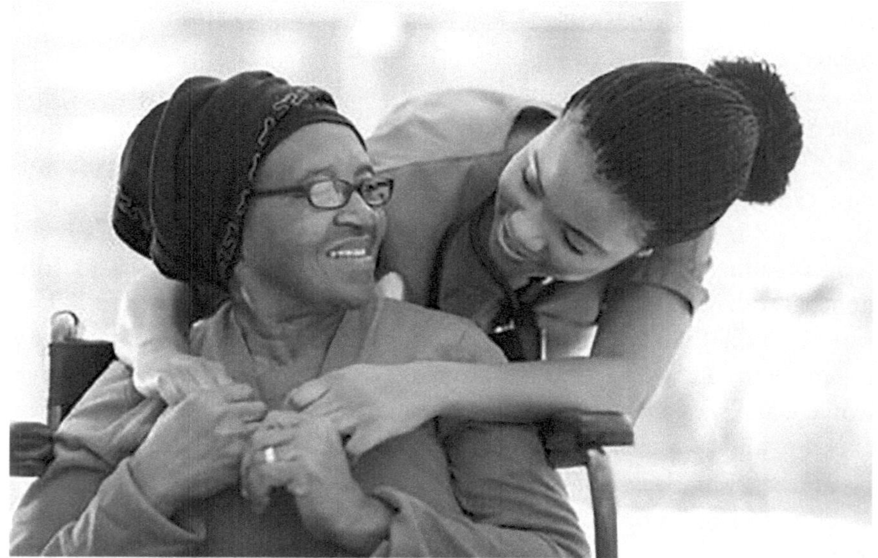

   Miss Asondra StarN'air

"Ebony Eyes"

Black Friday' is us, and a bet you didn't know that **'Ebony Eyes!'** This is a shout out to all black People, You are loved and appreciated "**Ebony Eyes!** Keep your head up to the sky! A change is gonna come. Believers will see the salvation of the Lord!

Meanwhile lets continue to make stride and celebrate Black pride! Furthermore, lets us always forgive those who persecute and hurt us.

As we move forward to a new day let us also move beyond the divides of black and white thinking and began to come together as one, what was done was done. Now it's time to move on....

And first on the agenda is our **"Caregivers"** we want the following:

- Respectable Wages and Yearly Raises
- Health Care Coverage
- A Caregivers/ Nursing Assistant Association **"Worldwide"**.
- Paid Vacations, 401K

I do hope that after learning about the history of aides that major changes are made. Our government owe it to black people and all people who have been left out and oppressed a fair chance at the **American Dream**. Our constitution, is no constitution at all if one race rules over another. Let's unite and love one another like sisters and brothers!

Today is a new day for caregivers all over the world, God is about to do something amazing. He's going to put an end to all prejudices, stereotyping and bigotry, He wants all people free. I hope you are with me, together we can help build a better tomorrow!

Right now, we say peace and love to all those who has a changed heart. it's time for you too, to speak out for fairness, love and equality, make your mark!

'Never Stop fighting for Change' in Jesus name,

Amen!

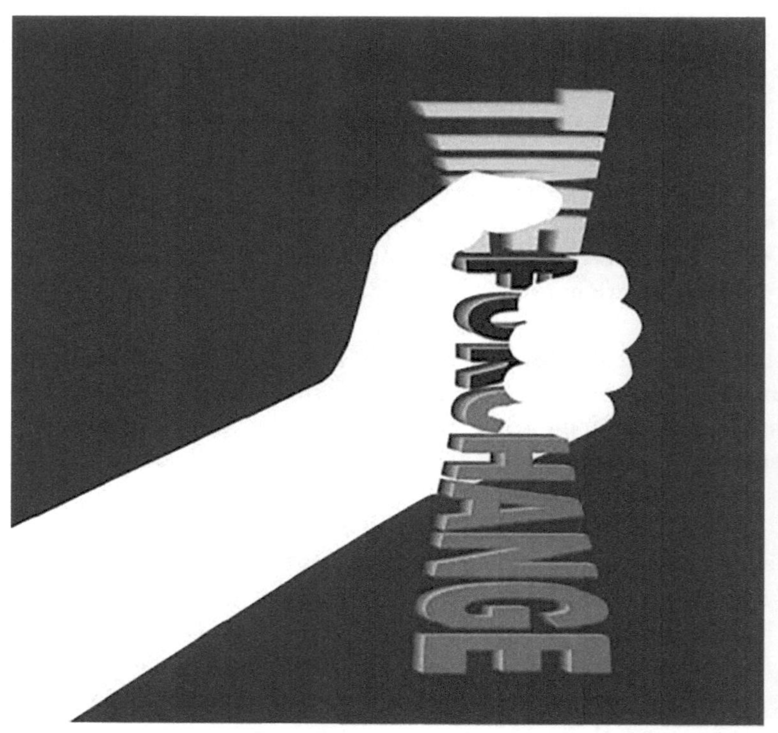

Miss Asondra StarN'air

I Am Not an Aide/Slave

I'm ah, New Day Care Giver

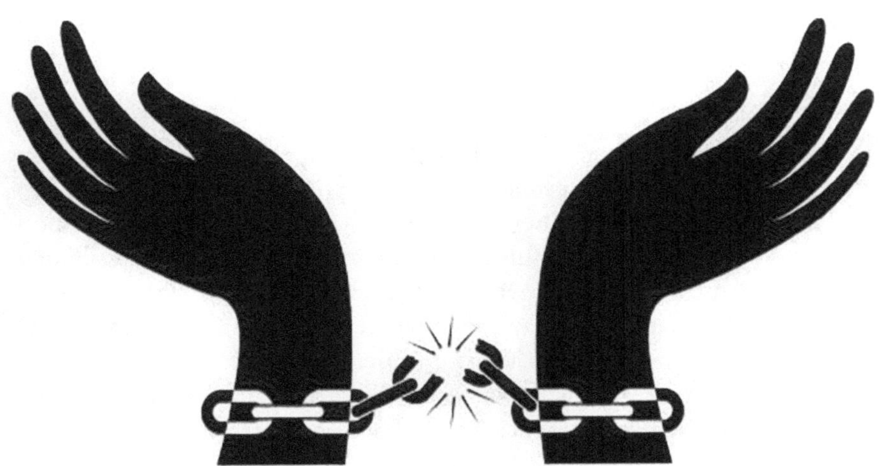

No More Chains!

Respect

"R E S P E C T find out what it means to me" **Aretha Franklin** said it best but I want to take it a step further and break it down from a "Caregiver prospective"

Realize

Everyone

Shines

Professional Caregiver's

Everywhere

Can

Too

'Home Care Workers' should be called 'Home Care Providers', we are more than workers, we are people just like everyone else.

We demand to be taken seriously and will no longer tolerate disrespect because we wear scrubs. Our future is bright and full of endless possibilities too. We are not aides of old generation, they cooked and cleaned, we do more than that. Caregiver today are now part of the entire healthcare team. Without us there would be no hands on care. We are also the eyes and ears for the doctors and nurses, when there is a change in condition, or something just don't seem right many times it's the hands on caregivers that does the reporting, why? because **"WE"** are the ones who spends the most time with the person and **"WE"** are the ones who develop the ongoing relationship that sometimes can last for many, many years depending on situation. Bottom line, **"WE"** are the Florence Nightingale's of our time. **Respect Us!** And if you Respect us, **Pay Us!** Give home care providers what we deserve too, things like, health care, yearly raises, 401K's, paid holidays, bonuses, opportunities to advance, maternity leave and anything else you give the rest of the health care team, we want that too! The fact is Home Care has become one of the fastest growing occupations in the united states according to the U.S Census

 Miss Asondra StarN'air

Bureau **"WE"** are becoming America's bread and butter. Well, where is our slice? Respect us don't play games, be fair, be nice!

R E S P E C T, find out what it means to Caregivers **R E S P E C T.**

All we are asking people, is for a little respect when we clock in, some re, re, re, respect when we get to work and clock in, Lord have mercy now... all we want is a little **RESPECT!** Sing it Caregiver's and put your hands up, high-five to MS. Franklin, sing that song, we want a little respect, all over this world caregivers want a little respect, tell everybody in the white house and our government too, caregivers want a little respect. **Re, re, re, RESPECT!** All colors of the world black, red, white and blue; oh just acknowledge and pay us well for all the dedicated hard work **"WE"** do! **R E S P E C T** us, we're all talkin' to you! **R**ealize **E**veryone **S**hines **P**rofessional Caregivers **E**verywhere **C**an **T**oo!

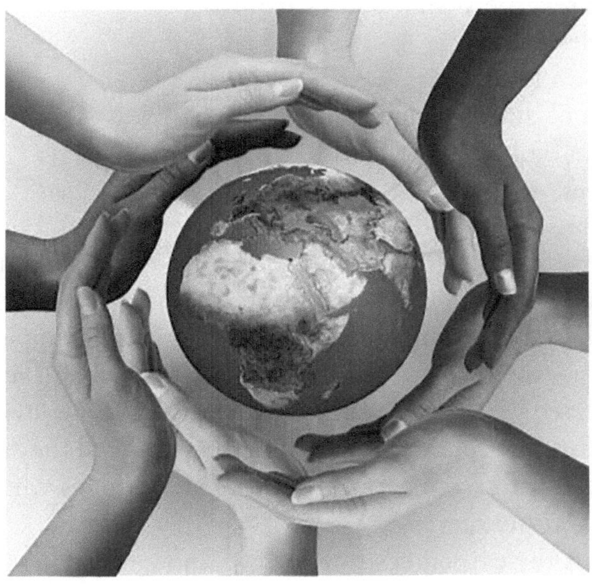

R- E -S- P- E- C- T find out what it means to me,
R- E- S -P -E -C -T take care of **T-C-B!**

Stereotype

Sterotype is a widely held but fixed and oversimplified image or idea of a particular type of person or thing. Healthcare workers **"AIDE"** is a perfect example.

Here are some of the common Sterotypes of black **"AIDES"** in America

- Black, single and uneducated
- Dumb that's all they can do
- Fat/Obese
- Poor/poverty stricken/on welfare
- Housekeepers/Maids/Aunt Jemima's
- Useless/Aides
- Have a lot of kids
- Lots of drama, troubled lives.
- From broken down homes
- Slaves, will work for cheap.

Of course none of this could be further from the truth but the stereotyping remains in this world if you are not a Doctor or Registered Nurse/LPN. You're just an aide, kind of like what the uppity folks did with Jesus too, they scoffed at him. You know when you really look at his life you'll see Jesus was a caregiver too, he went about loving, healing and caring for the people. Just like caregivers do. Well they stereotyped him also, read it for yourself in Matthew 13:55 this is what people of means said and I quote:

"He's just the carpenter's son and we know Mary his mother and his brothers, James, Joseph, Simon and Judas. In other words, they're nobodies, they're common, they ain't nothin!"

That's classic stereotyping right there, so just like they scoffed at Jesus what do you think the world is going to do to you and me, the caregiver," The Aide"? Like Our Lord, to them (and you know who you are), we ain't nothin but AIDES That's what we are and that's all we'll ever be. Oh, but not after this book comes out! Caregiver all over the world are about to reach newer and higher ground. We are about to turn this world upside down.

Miss Asondra StarN'air

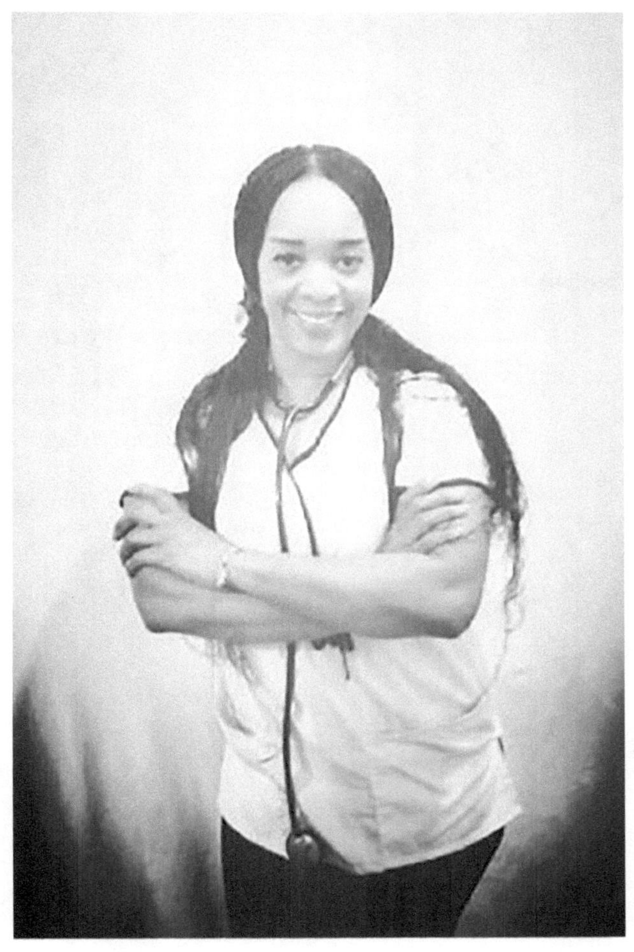

Look At Me "NOW!" Do I Look Like A Slave? "No"
"We've Come a Long Way Baby!"

Can't say this enough, READ, learn your history or you are doomed to repeat it. We are not the aides of the 1929-30 depression, we are
'The New Day Caregivers'
We Are More, We Do More, We Deserve More, Pay Us More!

C.A.R.E G.I.V.E.R.S

Christ

Almighty

Reaches out to

Everybody, everywhere

Gives

Individuals

Varieties of gifts

Each person

Received

Something Special

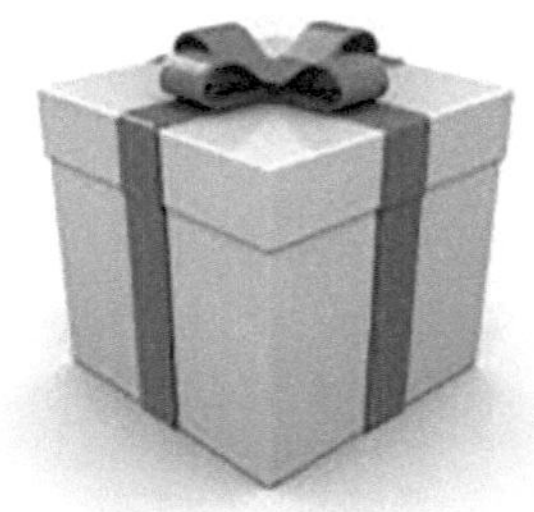

Caregivers We are Blessed!

Remember

- Caregivers, God has a plan for each and every one of us.
- So no need to be jealous or envy. What is for you, is for you. No one else can have it.

God has set you apart from anyone else. He has restored and made you whole. He has given you a special gift perhaps more than one. It is now up to you to do something with it.

Everybody's Got A Gift
If You Look Inside, You'll Find It!

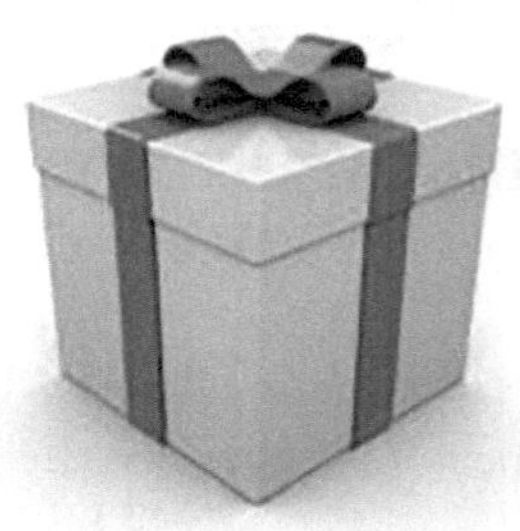

Caregiver Abuse

Caregiver abuse is real! Caregivers still get mistreated and abused all the time, from some clients, sometimes the office and from other co-workers too. Why does this happen? And what's being done about it? Nothing!

Why are caregivers dealing with so much disrespect still, I still hear horrible stories about female caregivers getting beat up on the job. Scratched, kicked and punched in the face by senior citizens, yet they want protection against us, What about the caregiver? Why aren't we being protected? Over and over again a lot of caregiver on a daily bases in America are being abused by the elderly and nothing is being done about it. One day in a home-care setting I walked in on this 90 year old woman spitting and hitting a black pregnant caregiver and calling her nigger. We called management, they listened, but nothing was done about that either, it was back to work as usual.

What's going on? If that caregiver were to spit back on that abusive senior she'd be fired or on her way to court, this is not right. So what, I say, that she was 90 years old, and of course, we wouldn't hit or spit back, we are caregivers, it still does not give that 90 years old the right to abuse caregivers.

What message are we sending? That once we get sick or old we can start abusing others? Or is the message too, like it was in the 1930's "Theirs Aides" niggers, do to them what you want to. Personally, that's exactly what I suspects going on. 'Aides' have always been used and abuse especially black ones.

I have been in this business now for a very long time and it feels like we have no rights at all. People can do and say whatever they want to us and we've better just deal with it or find another job. That attitude or mindset from business owner MUST change!

Abuse of any kind is wrong and mustn't be tolerated!

Fortunately, most of my experiences with seniors have been awesome. Because of God, He gave me the gift of care-giving, I knew how to work with the most difficult ones and win them over one by one. But I did get tested and treated like a nigger several times too, I will admit that, but after they saw how good I was at loving and forgiving their awful and terrible prejudice behavior and how professional I still performed and carried myself, like I said, I had them eating out of the palm of my hands. I won every last one of them over; and I have Jesus to thank for all that. Most of my caregiver abuse experiences came from other caregivers, nurses, and upper management and not from the customer. All of them were intimidated by my professionalism, each used it to their advantage though, They gave me some of the difficult cases. And wicked and trouble making co-workers took advantage of my trouble shooting skills and my naiveness, they'd smile and talk with me, but they were gathering personal information so that they could use to spread roomers and lies. All of this stuff was happening because I was different and fit none of the horrible, negative stereotypes, and I was very attractive too, that only made things worse for me. In the facilities all the residence and a lot of the other STNA's thought I was a RN. I was humble, I was about the business of care-giving each time I went in. I was wholeheartedly there for those residence that's why they thought I was a RN. But, once they discovered I was an STNA, I got stereotyped right away, "AIDE". Next thing I knew, caregiver bullies came after me. Caregivers, nurses, you name it. I won't get into what all they tried to do to me here, but I will say God kept his angels around me.

Nevertheless

Reader, can I tell you this, this section of my book hurt it still bring tears. I want out of this section, quick, fast and in a hurry! Oh, if only you knew all the hell I've been through. When you have a great heart and really, really love what you do, people come after you. I have been lied on, set up, blackballed by agencies, and watched management protected their bullies. Yes, I've seen it all! So caregiver, if you are experiencing any of this, **"Me Too"**. This book is for you, you are the one God wanted me to find, I've been where you are. You are not alone, there are others out there being abuses by this industry. Trust GOD, he will protect you and make a way for you I promise you. If things get too hard where you are at, get out of there, shake the dust off your feet and move to the next town/ workplace. **Matthew 10:14** "Enough is Enough!"

"Caregivers Matters"!

We Have Niggers For Sale

Today are we still being sold as slaves? If not, 'White America' tell us why, in a multi -billion dollar industry, home-care now being the leader in those huge profits, black people and other aides are still struggling to make ends meet and are without benefits and health care? It's 2018, we are still the riches county in the world, We want to know, **HOW IS THIS POSSIBLE?** Don't be quite. "We Deserve More" answer us!

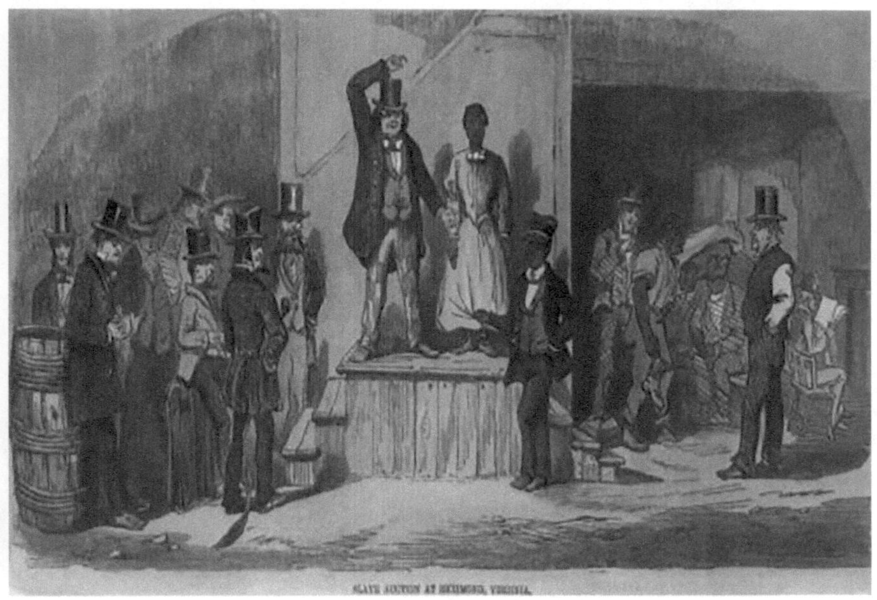

Modern Day Slavery
Enough is Enough!

Caregivers of all Ethnicity Matters! Women Matter! The Poor and Oppressed Matter! A Caregiver's Bible to Excellence Matter
Like it or not, "This Book Matters!"

Mediocracy

What is *Mediocracy*? According to Oxford dictionaries, it is a dominant class of people or a system in which mediocrity is rewarded. And there I was, so naïve—a caregiver ready to take on the world. I invested time, money, education, and lots of love too for everybody. I set out to give my employers all of my heart and dedication to becoming one of the most loyal and reliable caregivers ever. The vision God set before me was to love everywhere I go, not only take care of the patients but my coworkers too. **I did that!** I still do but I found out quickly **"Mediocrity Rules",** I was the fool!

There are more mediocre people in the world and in the work place, than there are great people. People who come to this planet to really love and serve human kind have become so rare to find!

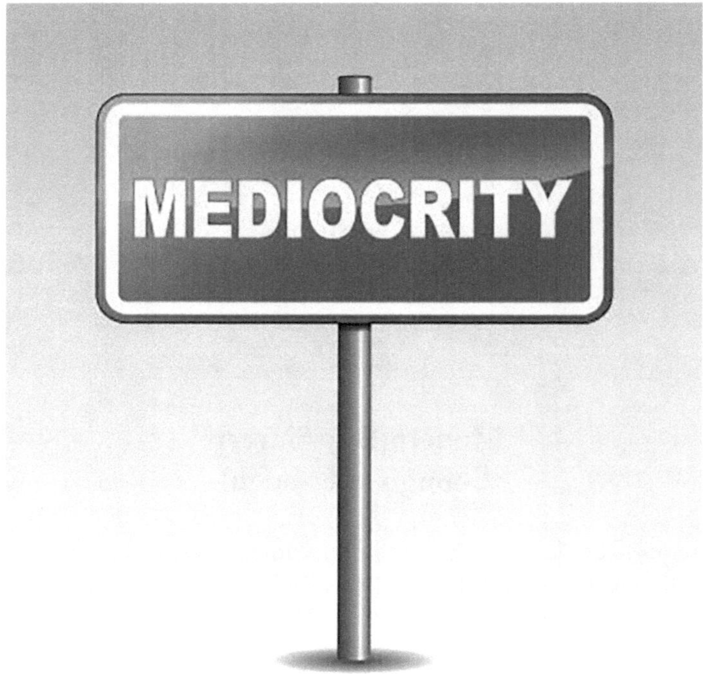

A Road to No Where!

Culture

Culture refers to the characteristics and knowledge of a particular group of people. They are defined by everything from language, religion, cuisine, social habits, music, and art.

Culture is the invisible bond that ties people together.

The importance of culture lies in its close association with the way of thinking and living. Difference in cultures have led to a diversity in people from all parts of the world.

Culture influences how we approach living; it also helps shape our thinking, behavior, and personality.

Caregivers all over the world needs to take into account the culture and customs of the people in their care and everywhere, realizing not everyone share the same views or beliefs. As caregivers (especially those working in home settings), we need to find out what makes that person comfortable. We do this by asking questions and show sincere interest in others.

Here Are Some Examples:

- What would you like me to call you?
- How would you like me to prepare your meals?
- Is there anything you want me to know about you or how you want things done?
- Do you want service on holidays? (Some don't believe in holidays.)
- If you are caring for the Jewish community, have them give you a list of what's allowed and what's not. Learn all you can about their culture and customs, share that knowledge with others.
- If you are not sure about something or how to do what is being asked, go back and ask for clarification, do not assume. Especially if you do not fully understand how to do or work with their equipment and devices. Caregivers, it's okay and encouraged to ask for a hands on demonstration of what's being asked of you.
- Read, Read, Read, find out about other cultures, that's how we grow, that's how we know about the many wonderful things in life.

Embrace Other Cultures and Other Cultures Will Embrace "YOU"!

Jewish Culture for Caregivers

Caregiver,"Stay in the Know" when working in Jewish settings study the culture. There are a variety of Jewish beliefs and practices, which therefore make it difficult to provide detailed guidance for the caregiver.

Within the culture, there are many classifications: Hasidic, Orthodox, Conservative, Reconstructed, and Reform. Each group has its own beliefs on certain issues. It is imperative that caregivers ask before assuming anything. For example, regarding nursing care, some will not accept caregivers of the opposite gender.

Therefore, male caregivers will not be permitted to care for some of these Jewish women. So you see, there is a lot here— not to mention all the dietary practices and celebrations within each group.

Find out the following:

- History, background so you can do your job well.
- Religious beliefs, facilities practices, etc.
- Culture and Celebrations
- Beliefs related to "Healthcare'
- Nursing care
- Spiritual care
- Diet/food preferences and practices.
- Personal care/ ADLs, routines and customs.

Stay informed. Learn all you can about different cultures and their practices. Stay diversified too, that's what smart caregivers do!

Jewish Snapshot!

- ➤ **Hasidic:** Arose as a spiritual revival movement back in the eighteenth century.
- ➤ **Orthodox:** Subscribes to a tradition, applications of the laws and ethics of the Torah.
- ➤ **Conservative:** Traditional Judaism without the fundamentals, which means they may not go along with everything, more open-minded.
- ➤ **Reconstructed:** More modern and American-based because of an evolving civilization.
- ➤ **Reform:** Also known as **Liberal** or **Progressive Judaism,** which emphasizes the superiority of its ethical aspects compared to ceremonial ones. Also, it believes in a revelation that goes beyond the theophany at Mount Sinai

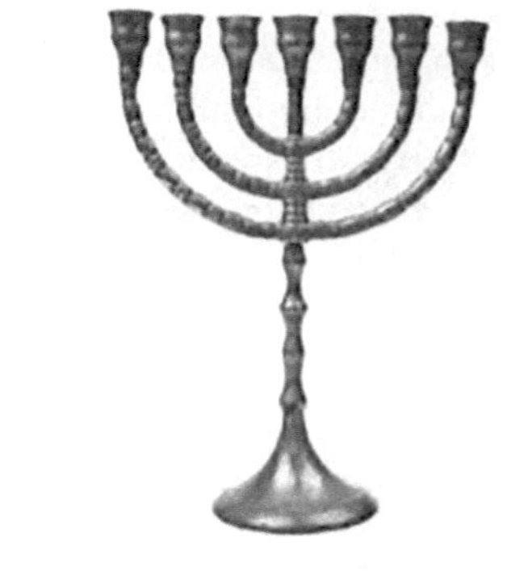

SECTION VIII

Inspiring Conversations for the Mind, Body and Soul!

Relax, it's just You and Jesus now!

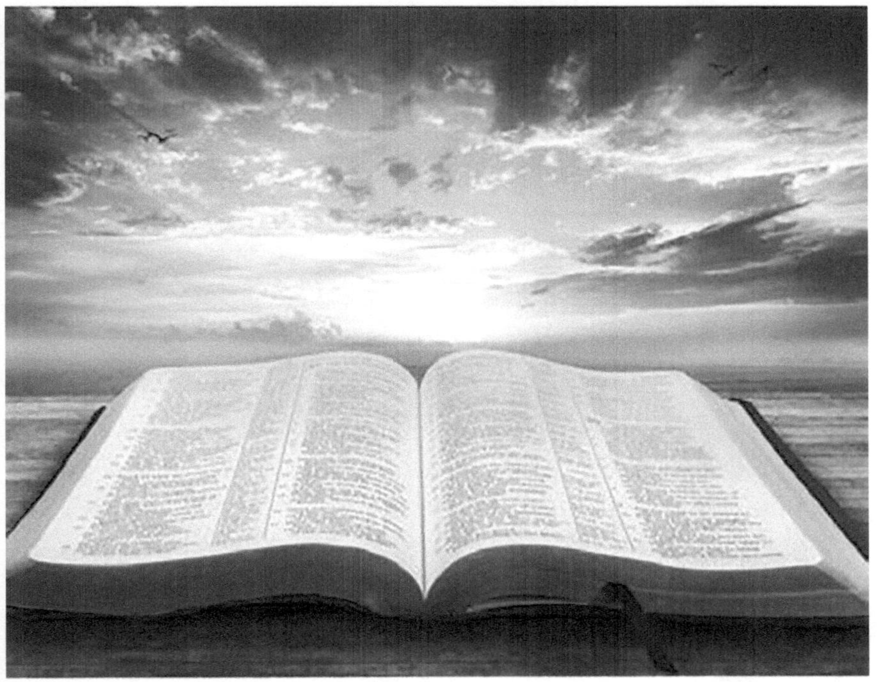

"The teaching of God's word gives light,
so even the simple can understand"!
Psalms 119:130

The Vine and the Branches

John 15:1-17 (NIV)

"I am the true vine, and my Father is the gardener. He cuts off every branch in me that bears no fruit, while every branch that does bear fruit he prunes so that it will be even more fruitful. You are already clean because of the word I have spoken to you. Remain in me, as I also remain in you. No branch can bear fruit by itself; it must remain in the vine. Neither can you bear fruit unless you remain in me.

"I am the vine; you are the branches. If you remain in me and I in you, you will bear much fruit; apart from me you can do nothing. If you do not remain in me, you are like a branch that is thrown away and withers; such branches are picked up, thrown into the fire and burned. If you remain in me and my words remain in you, ask whatever you wish, and it will be done for you. This is to my Father's glory, that you bear much fruit, showing yourselves to be my disciples.

"As the Father has loved me, so have I loved you. Now remain in my love. If you keep my commands, you will remain in my love, just as I have kept my Father's commands and remain in his love. I have told you this so that my joy may be in you and that your joy may be complete. My command is this: Love each other as I have loved you. Greater love has no one than this: to lay down one's life for one's friends. You are my friends if you do what I command. I no longer call you servants, because a servant does not know his master's business. Instead, I have called you friends, for everything that I learned from my Father I have made known to you. You did not choose me, but I chose you and appointed you so that you might go and bear fruit—fruit that will last—and so that whatever you ask in my

name the Father will give you. This is my command: ***"Love" Each Other."***

 Miss Asondra StarN'air

The World Hates the Disciples

John 15:18-25

"If the world hates you, keep in mind that it hated me first. If you belonged to the world, it would love you as its own. As it is, you do not belong to the world, but I have chosen you out of the world. That is why the world hates you. Remember what I told you: 'A servant is not greater than his mas-ter.' If they persecuted me, they will persecute you also. If they obeyed my teaching, they will obey yours also. They will treat you this way because of my name, for they do not know the one who sent me. If I had not come and spoken to them, they would not be guilty of sin; but now they have no excuse for their sin. Whoever hates me hates my Father as well. If I had not done among them the works no one else did, they would not be guilty of sin. As it is, they have seen, and yet they have hated both me and my Father. But this is to fulfill what is written in their Law: 'They hated me without reason.

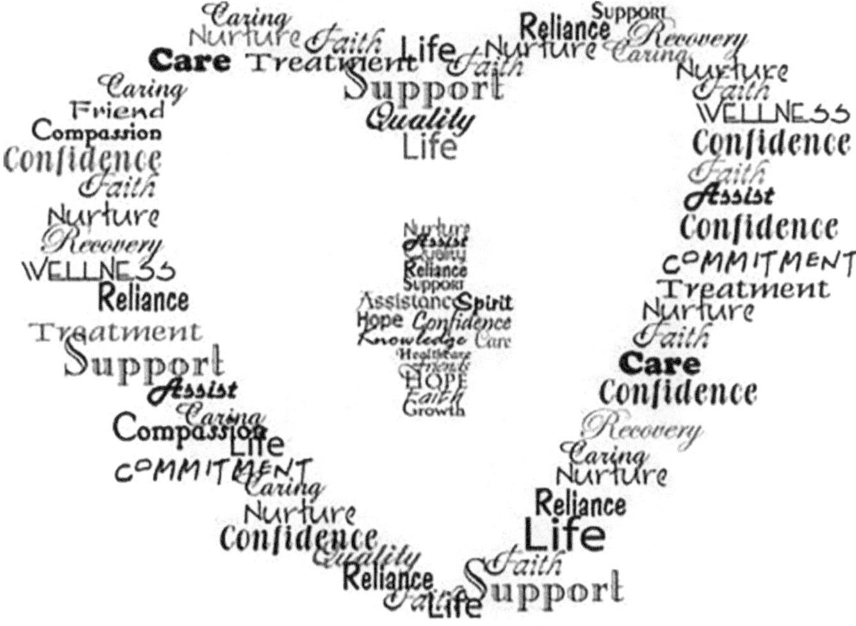

The Work of the Holy Spirit

John 15:26-27

"When the Advocate comes, whom I will send to you from the Father—the Spirit of truth who goes out from the Father—he will testify about me. And you also must testify, for you have been with me from the beginning.

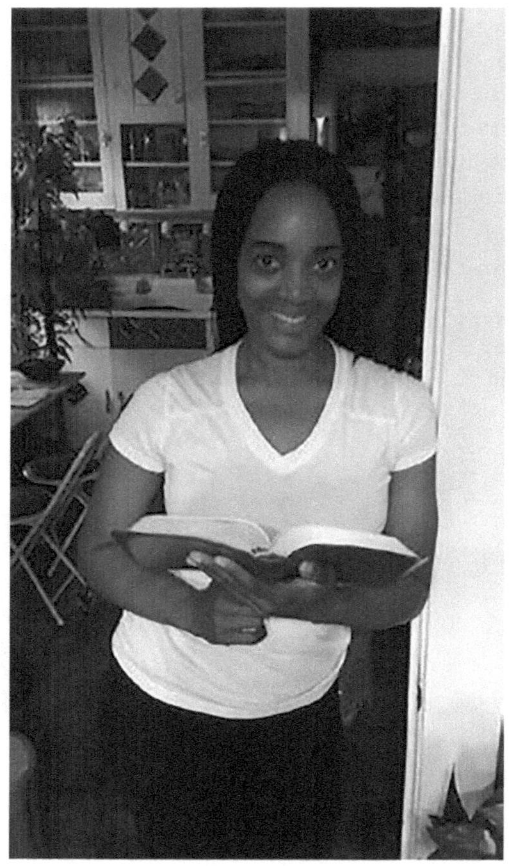

So, if you are a **"Me Too"** been attacked and mistreated, hang in there, stay focus on serving Jesus, he went through even worse. Remember, no weapons formed against true and faithful Christian will ever prosper. **I'm Still Standing!**

Matthew 5:13-16 New International Version (NIV)

Salt and Light

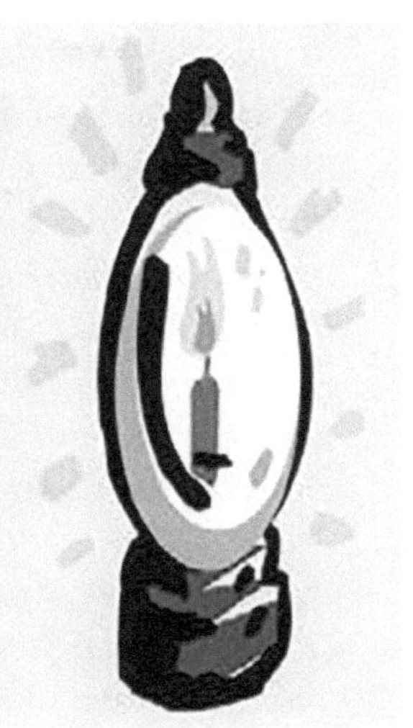

[13] "You are the salt of the earth. But if the salt loses its saltiness, how can it be made salty again? It is no longer good for anything, except to be thrown out and trampled underfoot.

[14] "You are the light of the world. A town built on a hill cannot be hidden. [15] Neither do people light a lamp and put it under a bowl. Instead they put it on its stand, and it gives light to everyone in the house. [16] In the same way, let your light shine before others, that they may see your good deeds and glorify your Father in heaven.

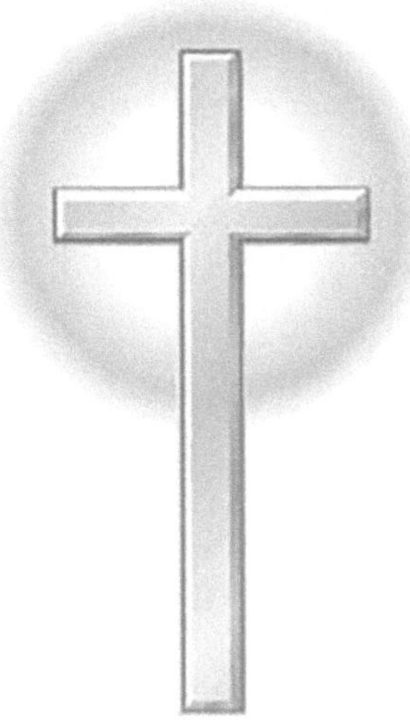

The Ten Commandments *(Exodus 20:2-17 NKJV)*

1. "I am the Lord your God, who brought you out of the land of Egypt, out of the house of bondage. You shall have no other gods before Me.

2. "You shall not make for yourself a carved image, or any likeness of anything that is in heaven above, or that is in the earth beneath, or that is in the water under the earth; you shall not bow down to them nor serve them. For I, the Lord your God, am a jealous God, visiting the iniquity of the fathers on the children to the third and fourth generations of those who hate Me, but showing mercy to thousands, to those who love Me and keep My Commandments.

3. "You shall not take the name of the Lord your God in vain, for the Lord will not hold him guiltless who takes His name in vain.

4. "Remember the Sabbath day, to keep it holy. Six days you shall labor and do all your work, but the seventh day is the Sabbath of the Lord your God. In it you shall do no work: you, nor your son, nor your daughter, nor your male servant, nor your female servant, nor your cattle, nor your stranger who is within your gates. For in six days the Lord made the heavens and the earth, the sea, and all that is in them, and rested the seventh day. Therefore the Lord blessed the Sabbath day and hallowed it.

5. "Honor your father and your mother, that your days may be long upon the land which the Lord your God is giving you.

6. "You shall not murder.

7. "You shall not commit adultery.

8. "You shall not steal.

9. "You shall not bear false witness against your neighbor.

10. "You shall not covet your neighbor's house; you shall not covet your neighbor's wife, nor his male servant, nor his female servant, nor his ox, nor his donkey, nor anything that is your neighbor's."

I Will Bless the Lord at All times!

His Praise Shall Continually Be In My Mouth!!!

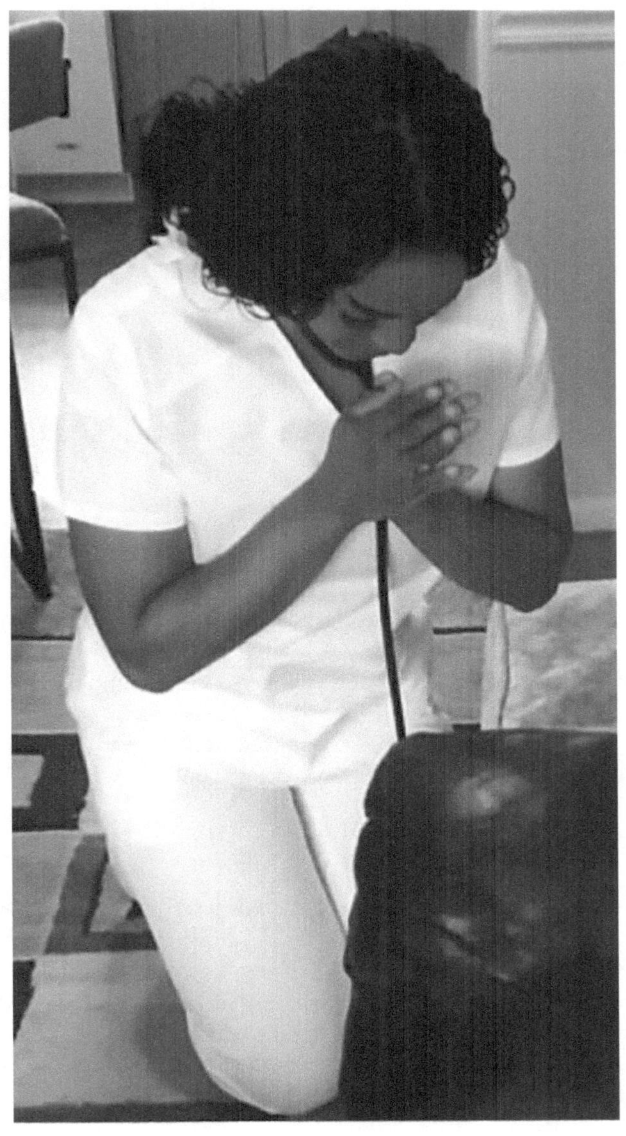

Matthew 5

Introduction to the Sermon on the Mount

5   Now when Jesus saw the crowds, he went up on a mountainside and sat down.
    His disciples came to him,
2   and he began to teach them.

The Beatitudes

He said:

3   "Blessed are the poor in spirit,
    for theirs is the kingdom of heaven.
4   Blessed are those who mourn, for they will be comforted.
5   Blessed are the meek,
    for they will inherit the earth.
6   Blessed are those who hunger and thirst for righteousness, for they will be filled.
7   Blessed are the merciful,
    for they will be shown mercy.
8   Blessed are the pure in heart, for they will see God.
9   Blessed are the peacemakers,
    for they will be called children of God.
10 Blessed are those who are persecuted because of righteousness, for theirs is the
    kingdom of heaven.
11 "Blessed are you when people insult you, persecute you and falsely say all kinds
    of evil against you because of me.
12 Rejoice and be glad, because great is your reward in heaven, for in the same way
    they persecuted the prophets who were before you.

Salt and Light

13 "You are the salt of the earth. But if the salt loses its saltiness, how can it be
    made salty again? It is no longer good for anything, except to be thrown out and
    trampled underfoot.
14 "You are the light of the world. A town built on a hill cannot be hidden.
15 Neither do people light a lamp and put it under a bowl. Instead they put it on
    its stand, and it gives light to everyone in the house.
16 In the same way, let your light shine before others, that they may see your good
    deeds and glorify your Father in heaven.

The Fulfillment of the Law

17 "Do not think that I have come to abolish the Law or the Prophets; I have not come to abolish them but to fulfill them.

18 For truly I tell you, until heaven and earth disappear, not the smallest letter, not the least stroke of a pen, will by any means disappear from the Law until everything is accomplished.

19 Therefore anyone who sets aside one of the least of these commands and teaches others accordingly will be called least in the kingdom of heaven, but whoever practices and teaches these commands will be called great in the kingdom of heaven.

20 For I tell you that unless your righteousness surpasses that of the Pharisees and the teachers of the law, you will certainly not enter the kingdom of heaven.

Murder

21 "You have heard that it was said to the people long ago, 'You shall not murder,[a] and anyone who murders will be subject to judgment.'

22 But I tell you that anyone who is angry with a brother or sister[b][c] will be subject to judgment. Again, anyone who says to a brother or sister, 'Raca,'[d] is answerable to the court. And anyone who says, 'You fool!' will be in danger of the fire of hell.

23 "Therefore, if you are offering your gift at the altar and there remember that your brother or sister has something against you,

24 leave your gift there in front of the altar. First go and be reconciled to them; then come and offer your gift.

25 "Settle matters quickly with your adversary who is taking you to court. Do it while you are still together on the way, or your adversary may hand you over to the judge, and the judge may hand you over to the officer, and you may be thrown into prison.

26 Truly I tell you, you will not get out until you have paid the last penny.

Adultery

27 "You have heard that it was said, 'You shall not commit adultery.'[e]

28 But I tell you that anyone who looks at a woman lustfully has already committed adultery with her in his heart.

29 If your right eye causes you to stumble, gouge it out and throw it away. It is better for you to lose one part of your body than for your whole body to be thrown into hell.

30 And if your right hand causes you to stumble, cut it off and throw it away. It is better for you to lose one part of your body than for your whole body to go into hell.

Divorce

31 "It has been said, 'Anyone who divorces his wife must give her a certificate of divorce.'[f]

32 But I tell you that anyone who divorces his wife, except for sexual immorality, makes her the victim of adultery, and anyone who marries a divorced woman commits adultery.

Oaths

33 "Again, you have heard that it was said to the people long ago, 'Do not break your oath, but fulfill to the Lord the vows you have made.'

34 But I tell you, do not swear an oath at all: either by heaven, for it is God's throne;

35 or by the earth, for it is his footstool; or by Jerusalem, for it is the city of the Great King.

36 And do not swear by your head, for you cannot make even one hair white or black.

37 All you need to say is simply 'Yes' or 'No'; anything beyond this comes from the evil one.

Eye for Eye

38 "You have heard that it was said, 'Eye for eye, and tooth for tooth.'[h]

39 But I tell you, do not resist an evil person. If anyone slaps you on the right cheek, turn to them the other cheek also.

40 And if anyone wants to sue you and take your shirt, hand over your coat as well.

41 If anyone forces you to go one mile, go with them two miles.

42 Give to the one who asks you, and do not turn away from the one who wants to borrow from you.

Love for Enemies

43 "You have heard that it was said, 'Love your neighbor[i] and hate your enemy.'

44 But I tell you, love your enemies and pray for those who persecute you,

45 that you may be children of your Father in heaven. He causes his sun to rise on the evil and the good, and sends rain on the righteous and the unrighteous.

46 If you love those who love you, what reward will you get? Are not even the tax collectors doing that?

47 And if you greet only your own people, what are you doing more than others? Do not even pagans do that?

48 Be perfect, therefore, as your heavenly Father is perfect.

Stay Connected to Christ and Christ will Stay Connect to "YOU"
Read Your Bibles, "DAILY!"

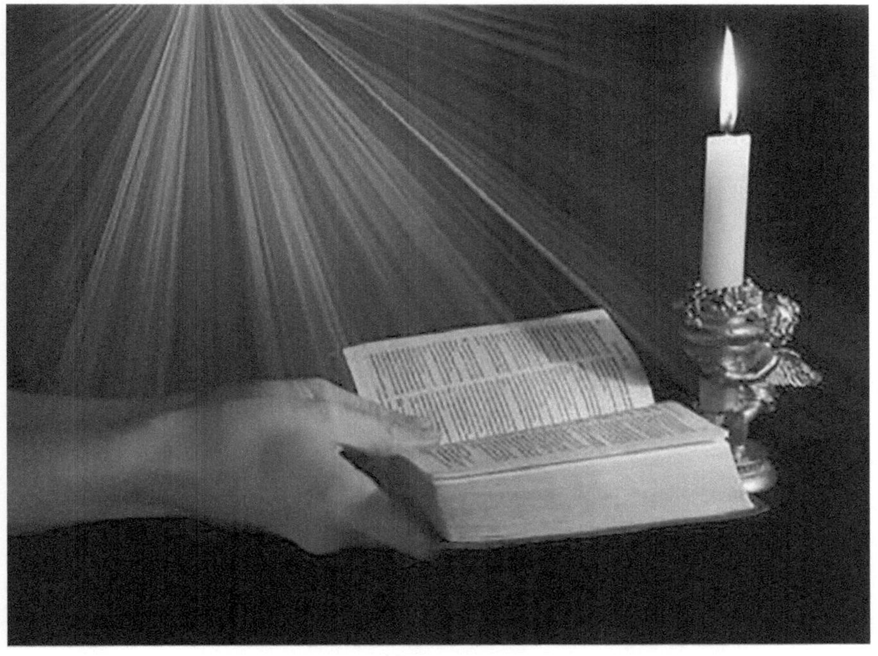

**The teaching of God's word gives light,
so even the simple can understand.** Psalms 119:130

Lord's Prayer

Matthew 6:9-13New International Version
(NIV)
9 "This, then, is how you should pray:
"'Our Father in heaven,
hallowed be your name,
10 your kingdom come,
your will be done,
on earth as it is in heaven.
11 Give us today our daily bread.
12 And forgive us our debts,
as we also have forgiven our debtors.
13 And lead us not into temptation,[a]
but deliver us from the evil one.[b]'

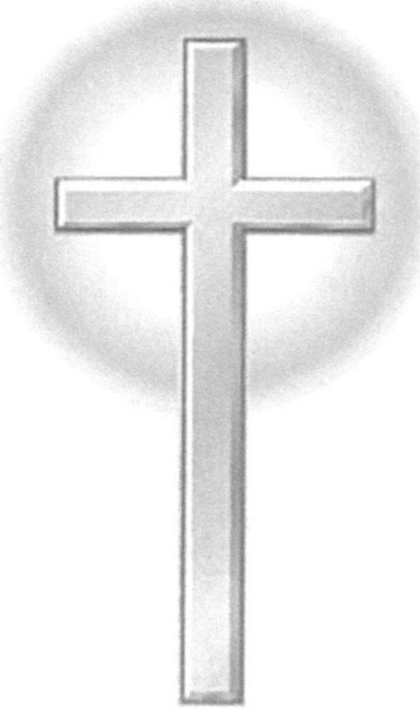

StarN'air's Prayer

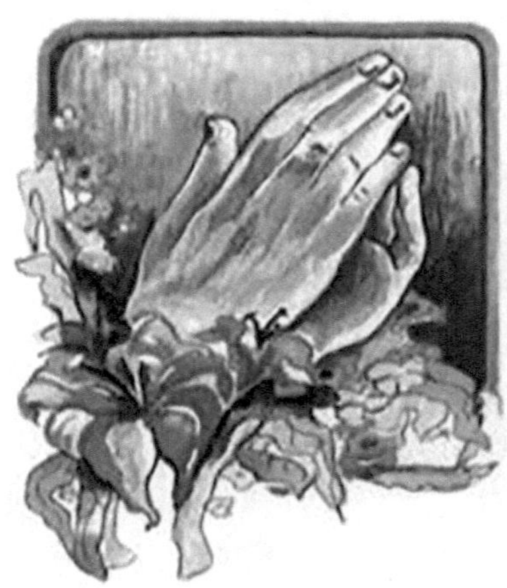

Oh, God, Glorious God of
Abraham, Isaac and Jacob,

I trust you with all my heart,
mind, body and soul

Help me "Move Mountains"

Expand my Horizon, take me places
I've never been use me for Thy
Kingdom

Keep me humble and graceful like you

Let me strive for excellence llow me
good health and prosperity too!

Finally, bring The "Music", The
Symphony of my deepest desire, oh
Lord grant me a song, unlike anything
the world has ever heard. Make it
"Timeless", like you, let me record it,
sing it and deliver it to the universe.

**And God Granted StarN'air's
Request!**

 MISS ASONDRA STARN'AIR

Self

Surrender yourself to God
Eliminate, cast your cares on the **LORD**
Leave your past behind
Focus on the **"Promise Land"**

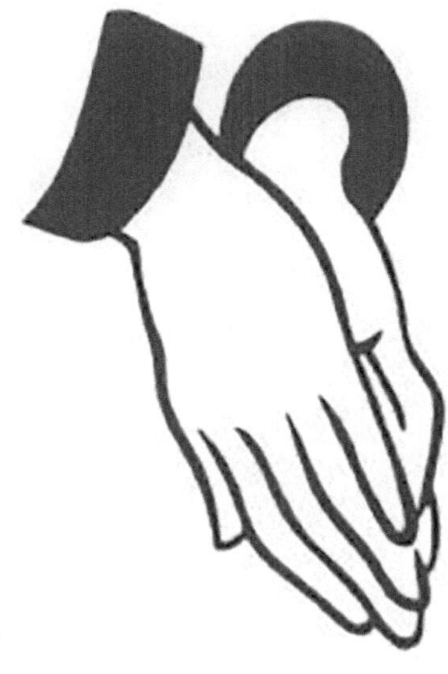

Whatever you ask in prayer you will
receive if you have faith. **Matthew 21:22**

Holy Communion

Holy Communion is open to anyone who's confessed their sins and has decided to make Jesus Lord of their entire lives from this day forward. Children as well. Repentance of sin must be the driving force to become born again, so get born again and when you do, help us win more souls for Christ!

Note: Believers can communion daily! Not limited to one special day.

1 Corinthians 11:23-26 (NIV)

For I received from the Lord what I also passed on to you: The Lord Jesus, on the night he was betrayed, took bread, [24] and when he had given thanks, he broke it and said, "This is my body, which is for you; do this in remembrance of me." [25] In the same way, after supper he took the cup, saying, "This cup is the new covenant in my blood; do this, whenever you drink it, in remembrance of me." For whenever you eat this bread and drink this cup, you proclaim the Lord's death until he comes.

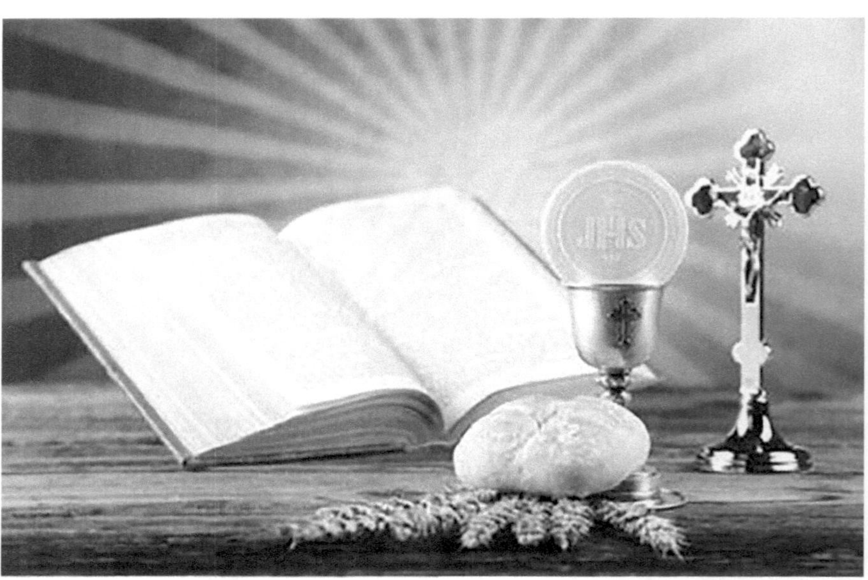

 Miss Asondra StarN'air

For everything there is a season, and a time for every matter under heaven:

a time to be born, and a time to die;
a time to plant, and a time to pluck up what is
planted; a time to kill, and a time to heal;
a time to break down, and a time to build
up; a time to weep, and a time to laugh; a
time to mourn, and a time to dance;
a time to cast away stones, and a time to gather stones
together; a time to embrace, and a time to refrain from
embracing; a time to seek, and a time to lose;
a time to keep, and a time to cast away;
a time to tear, and a time to sew;
a time to keep silence, and a time to
speak; a time to love, and a time to hate;
a time for war, and a time for peace.

For me Miss Asondra StarN'air, it's a time to take back the Promises of God and do something with it! Jesus said I could move mountains, "I shall move them". God promised blessing to me **"I Want Them!"** I know breaking free and taking what God has for me won't be easy. But I've got to fight! Not only for me, but for you too. Caregivers, look, there is nothing in this world we can't achieve, especially if we stay on our knees. Know that, the only one standing in your way is **"YOU"!**

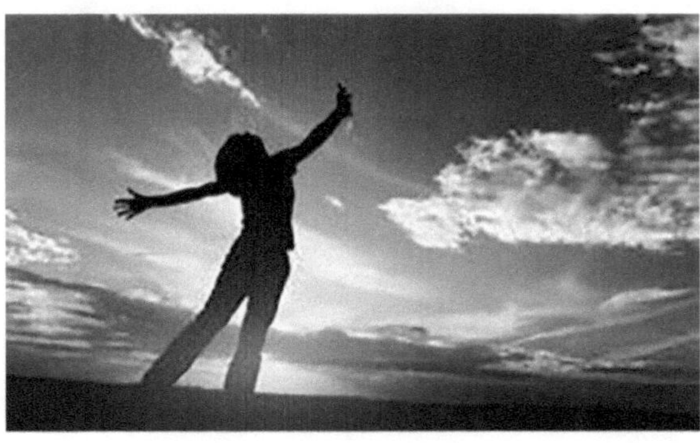

World Hates the Disciples

John 15:18-25

"If the world hates you, keep in mind that it hated me first. If you belonged to the world, it would love you as its own. As it is, you do not belong to the world, but I have chosen you out of the world. That is why the world hates you. Remember what I told you: 'A servant is not greater than his mas-ter.' If they persecuted me, they will persecute you also. If they obeyed my teaching, they will obey yours also. They will treat you this way because of my name, for they do not know the one who sent me. If I had not come and spoken to them, they would not be guilty of sin; but now they have no excuse for their sin. Whoever hates me hates my Father as well. If I had not done among them the works no one else did, they would not be guilty of sin. As it is, they have seen, and yet they have hated both me and my Father. But this is to fulfill what is written in their Law: 'They hated me without reason.

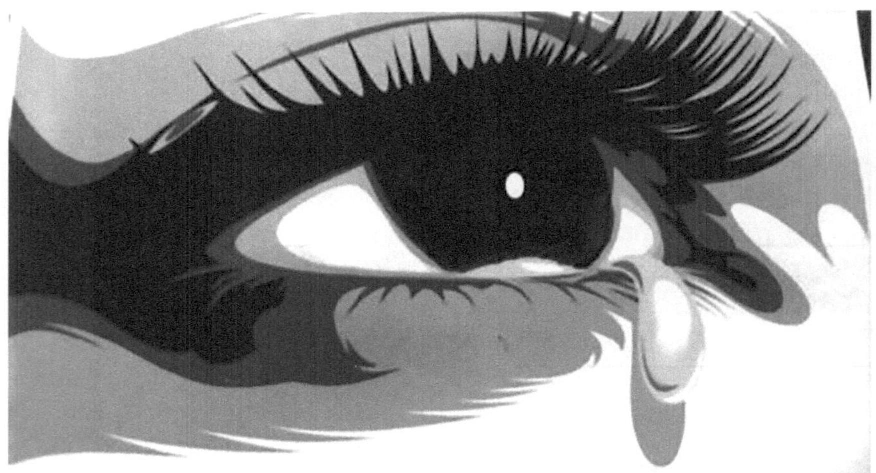

"ME Too!"

The Work of the Holy Spirit

John 15

26 "When the Advocate comes, whom I will send to you from the Father—the Spirit of truth who goes out from the Father—he will testify about me.

27 And you also must testify, for you have been with me from the beginning.

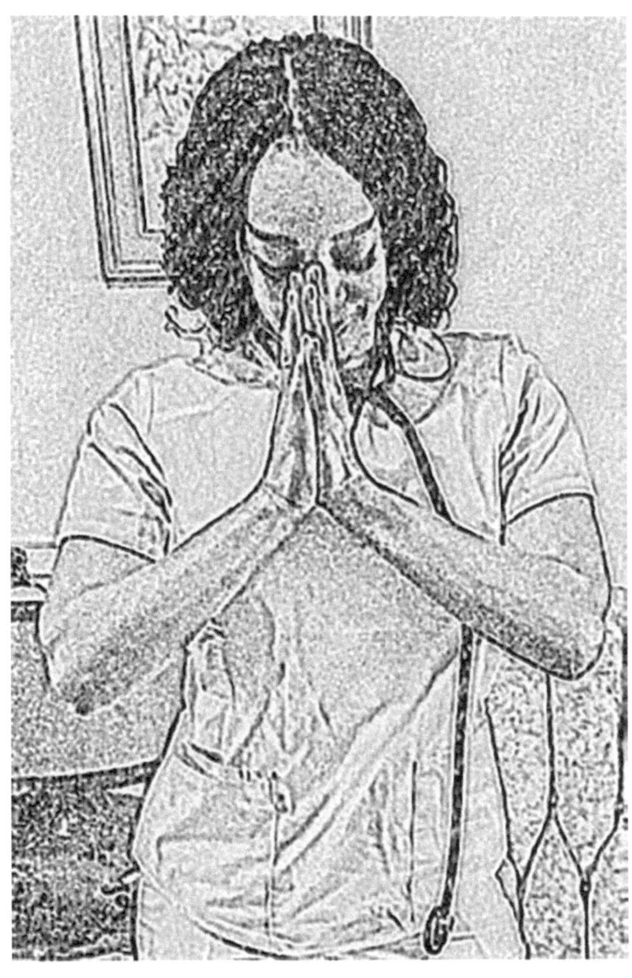

Miss Asondra StarN'air

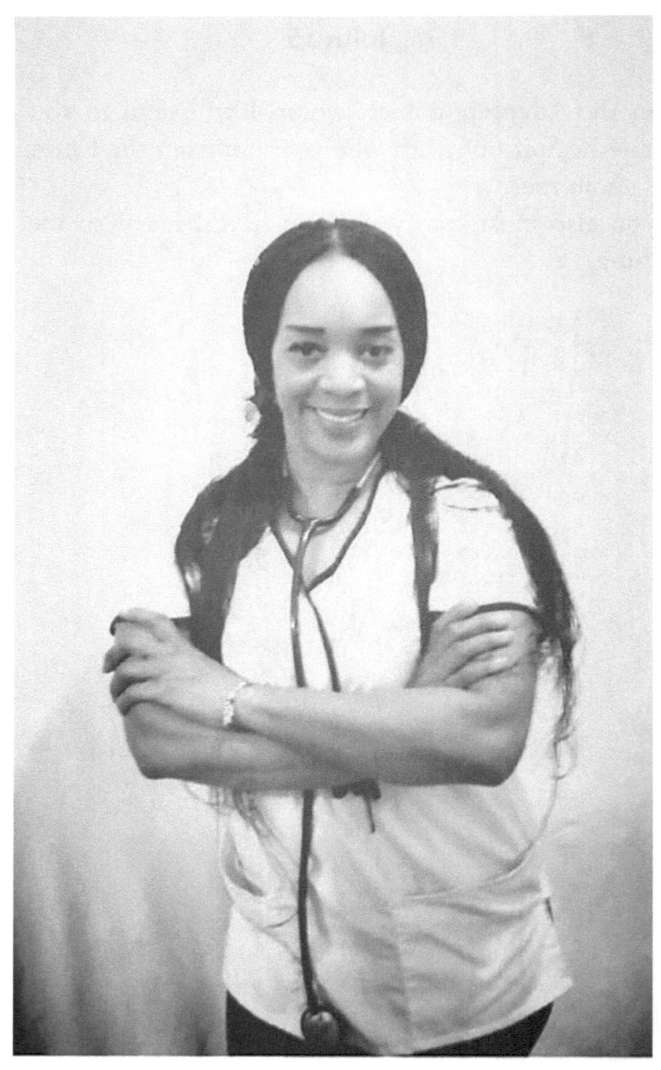

**A Life Without Christ is A Life Wasted!
Make Him Your Everything!
Taste and See that the Lord is Good!**

John 10 New International Version (NIV)
The Good Shepherd and His Sheep

<table>
<tr><td valign="top">

10 "Very truly I tell you Pharisees, anyone who does not enter the sheep pen by the gate, but climbs in by some other way, is a thief and a robber.

2 The one who enters by the gate is the shepherd of the sheep.

3 The gatekeeper opens the gate for him, and the sheep listen to his voice. He calls his own sheep by name and leads them out.

4 When he has brought out all his own, he goes on ahead of them, and his sheep follow him because they know his voice.

5 But they will never follow a stranger; in fact, they will run away from him because they do not recognize a stranger's voice."

6 Jesus used this figure of speech, but the Pharisees did not understand what he was telling them.

7 Therefore Jesus said again, "Very truly I tell you, I am the gate for the sheep.

8 All who have come before me are thieves and robbers, but the sheep have not listened to them.

9 I am the gate; whoever enters through me will be saved.[a] They will come in and go out, and find pasture.

10 The thief comes only to steal and kill and destroy; I have come that they may have life, and have it to the full.

11 "I am the good shepherd. The good shepherd lays down his life for the sheep.

</td><td valign="top">

Caregiver's Call Out!

Here's an Invitation to Christ

Most of your life you've' done what you wanted, still unhappy, struggling can't seem to find consistency in your life, in bondage to things you ought not be doing but can't seem to stop. At the end of the day, you are sad, overworked and feel alone, like nobody cares.

Well you are wrong, remember the Good Shepherd's invitation to you. He's the gate you must walk through, no other way.

He is the good shepherd this world is trying to keep you from and destroying you in the process. Why don't you come, come to Jesus, admit you are a sinner and in need of a savior. Do it today, right now just repeat after me if you can't find the words, to say, say this, Lord, my Father, I want to come home, I am lost without you, and too weak to get out of bondage on my own send the Holy spirit to me now and make me over into the person you want me to be.

In Jesus name, rescue me, set me free!

</td></tr>
</table>

12 The hired hand is not the shepherd and does not own the sheep. So when he sees the wolf coming, he abandons the sheep and runs away. Then the wolf attacks the flock and scatters it.

13 The man runs away because he is a hired hand and cares nothing for the sheep.

14 "I am the good shepherd; I know my sheep and my sheep know me—

15 just as the Father knows me and I know the Father—and I lay down my life for the sheep.

16 I have other sheep that are not of this sheep pen. I must bring them also. They too will listen to my voice, and there shall be one flock and one shepherd.

17 The reason my Father loves me is that I lay down my life—only to take it up again.

18 No one takes it from me, but I lay it down of my own accord. I have authority to lay it down and authority to take it up again. This command I received from my Father."

Help get me away from all those who are stumbling blocks people who just are no good for me to be around anymore, close that door. Lord please give me the strength I need to rebuild my life with you, take away anything that is not honoring or pleasing to you. Take away too my desire to commit sexual sin, help me stop practicing sin on all levels. Give me a brand new life with you Christ.

In Jesus name,

Let the transformation begin

Amen

Everybody, if you prayed that prayer, you just got born again.
Welcome Home!
Read Your Bibles Everyday moving forward! Follow a 'One Year' bible reading plan.

Congratulations!!!!!!!!!!!!!!!!!!!!

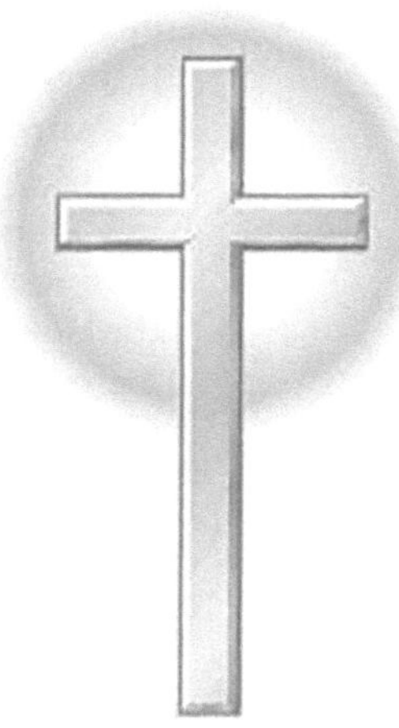

   Miss Asondra StarN'air

SECTION IX

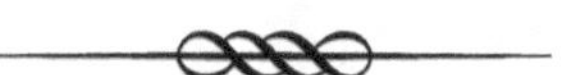

Personal Growth and Development

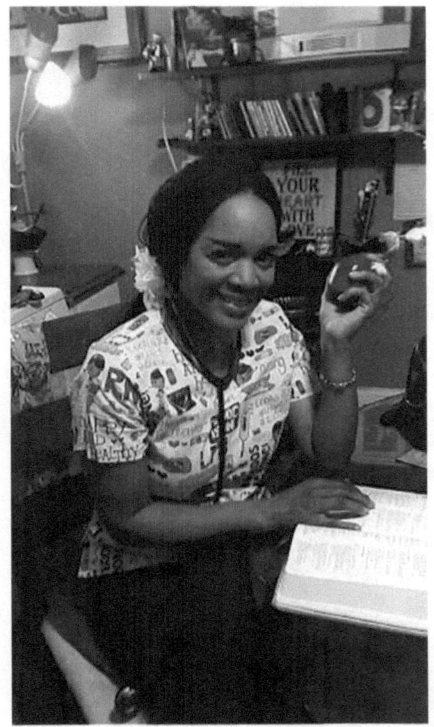

Personal Development In **Christ!**
He must be our role model of Excellence.
Otherwise we will remain out on a limb; lost and
confused and giving into all kinds of pleasures and sin.
Don't go that route, **"Let Jesus In"**!

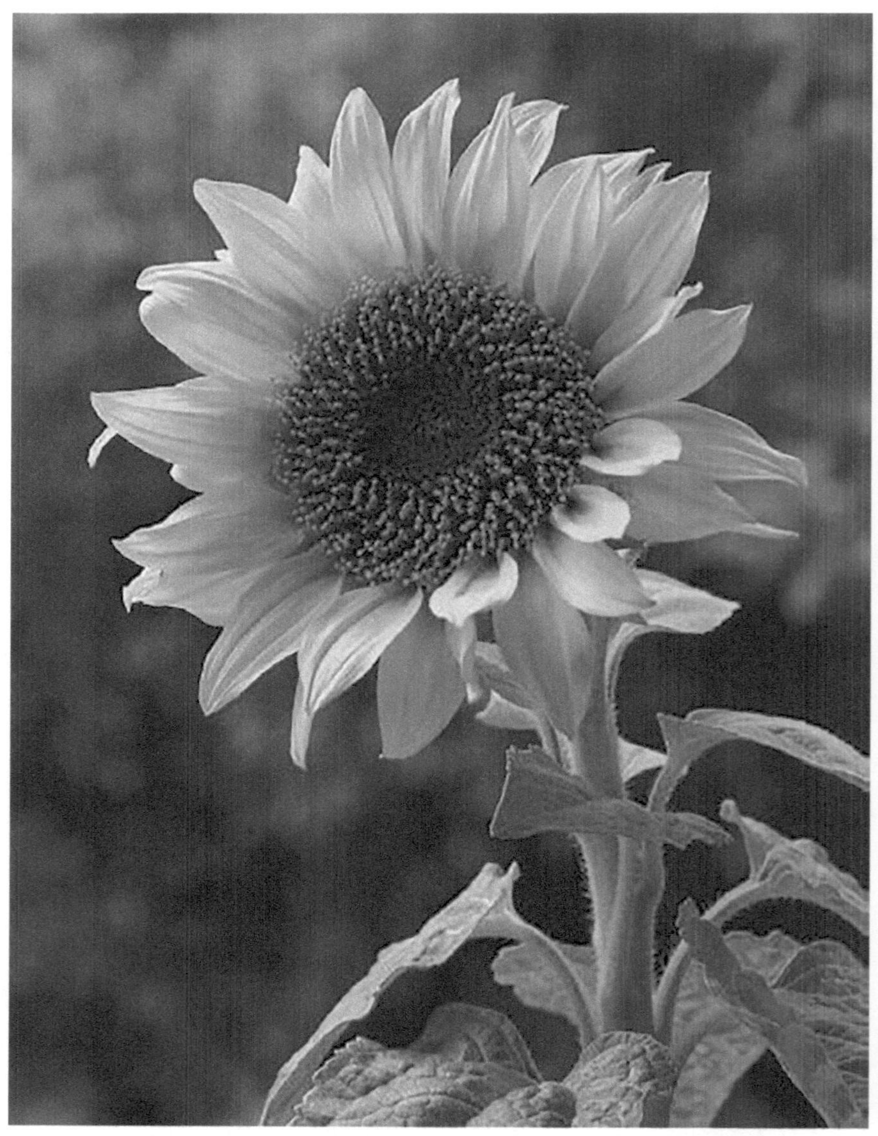

Caregiver's are the Sunflowers of God's heart!

Keep love and service alive in all you do, Jesus loves you and so do I.

 MISS ASONDRA STARN'AIR

Daily Affirmations for CareGivers

I am a professional caregiver.
I am beautiful in every way.
I am successful; I love being a health-care provider.
I am learning new and useful skills.
I am a competent caregiver.
I am supportive of other caregivers.
I am a team player.
I am taking better care of myself.
I am making smarter food choices.
I am exercising more now.
I am starting to drink more water.
I am saying no to junk food.
I am always on time to work.
I am a positive person.
I am done with negativity.
I am minding my own business from now on.
I am done with gossiping.
I am welcoming change, growth, and development in every area of my life now.
I am a child of God, and it shows in my behavior.
I am happy.
I am full of gratitude.
I am starting to rest more. I realize getting a good night's sleep is very important.
I am changing in a great way. I have lots of love and respect for my bosses and coworkers.
I am finding more time to spend with God and his word now.
I am starting to read the Bible a lot more, and I see the difference in my life. I have more peace of mind. I feel like I can do all things in Christ, who strengthens me. **'I Feel Brand New!'**

25 Affirmations for Caregivers

1. I Am an Excellent Caregiver
2. I Am a Professional
3. I Am Smart and Intelligent
4. I Am so blessed
5. I Am doing something about Stress, I'm getting rid of it
6. I Am Patient and Kind
7. I Am Prosperous
8. I Am Faithful to God
9. I Am Sorry for my sin, I shall repent and not do it again
10. I Am A Child Of the most high
11. I Am Developing into what God wants me to be
12. I Am Thankful
13. I Am Learning Something New Everyday
14. I Am becoming a Nicer, More Loving person
15. I Am a Team Player
16. I Am staying away from strife from now on
17. I Am Changing, getting closer and closer to God
18. I Am starting to read my bible everyday now
19. I Am going the extra mile, love does not depend on two hearts, it depend on one(MINE)
20. I love my **"Caregiver Bible to Excellence"** book, I'm telling everyone I know about it
21. I Am an Empathetic, Understanding, Passionate, Reliable, Loving Caregiver
22. I Am ready to do whatever God calls me to do without murmuring or complaining
23. I Am starting to seek God's will and purpose for my life
24. I Am dying to self so Jesus can come and live inside of me
25. I Am giving my life to Christ, I want to follow him now.

 Miss Asondra StarN'air

50 Reasons To Get To Know Jesus

1 - Jesus Was Never Created | Micah 5:2
2 - Jesus Essence Has Never Changed | Hebrews 13:8
3 - Jesus is God | John 1:1
4 - Jesus is The Creator of Everything | Colossians 1:16
5 - Jesus is All-Powerful | Matthew 28:18
6 - Jesus is All-Knowing | Colossians 2:3
7 - Jesus is Ever-Present | Matthew 18:20
8 - Jesus is Holy | Luke 1:35
9 - Jesus is Righteous | Isaiah 53:11
10 - Jesus is Just | Zech 9:9
11 - Jesus Had No Deceit | 1 Peter 2:22
12 - Jesus is Sinless | 2 Corinthians 5:21
13 - Jesus is Spotless | 1 Peter 1:19
14 - Jesus is Innocent | Matthew 27:4
15 - Jesus is Gentle | Matthew 11:29
16 - Jesus is Merciful | Hebrews 2:17
17 - Jesus is Forgiving | Luke 23:34
18 - Jesus Receives Worship by Demons | Mark 5:2,6
19 - Jesus Receives Worship by Men | John 9:38
20 - Jesus Receives Worship by Angels | Hebrews 1:6
21 - Jesus Receives Worship by Disciples | Luke 24:52
22 - Jesus Receives Worship in Heaven | Revelation 7:9-10
23 - Jesus Will Receive Worship from Everyone | Philippians 2:10-11
24 - Jesus Was Human | 1 Timothy 2:5
25 - Jesus Was Conceived by the Holy Spirit | Luke 1:34-35
26 - Jesus Took On Man's Nature | Hebrews 2:9-18
27 - Jesus Humbled Himself | Philippians 2:8
28 - Jesus Was Subject To Human Emotions | Hebrews 5:7
29 - Jesus Raised His Body From The Dead | John 10:18
30 - Jesus Blood Brings Reconciliation With God | Ephesians 2:13-16
31 - Jesus Blood Brings Redemption for Man | Romans 3:24-25
32 - Jesus Blood Allows Man To Be Justified before God | Romans 5:9
33 - Jesus Blood Sanctifies Man | Hebrews 10:29
34 - Jesus Blood Brings Spiritual Victory | Revelation 12:11
35 - Jesus Blood Brings Eternal Life | John 6:53-56
36 - Jesus Came to Save Sinners | Luke 19:10
37 - Jesus Will Bring in Everlasting Righteousness | Daniel 9:24
38 - Jesus Destroyed the Works of Satan | 1 John 3:8
39 - Jesus Fulfilled the Old Testament | Matthew 5:17
40 - Jesus Gives Life Now | John 10:10

41 - **Jesus Is Our Advocate** | <u>1 John 2:1</u>
42 - **Jesus Gives Eternal Life** | <u>John 10:28</u>
43 - **Jesus Is Eternal Life** | <u>1 John 5:20</u>
44 - **Jesus Sends The Holy Spirit To Us** | <u>John 15:26</u>
45 - **Jesus Will Take His People To Heaven** | <u>John 14:3</u>
46 - **Jesus Will Return To The Earth After The Tribulation** | <u>Matthew 24:29</u>
47 - **Jesus Will Return To The Earth In Power & Glory** | <u>Matthew 24:30</u>
48 - **Jesus Completes Revelation** | <u>Hebrews 1:1</u>
49 - **Jesus Will Never Send You Away If You Come To Him** | <u>John 6:37</u>
50 - **Jesus is the Way, the Truth, and the Life** | <u>John 14:6</u>

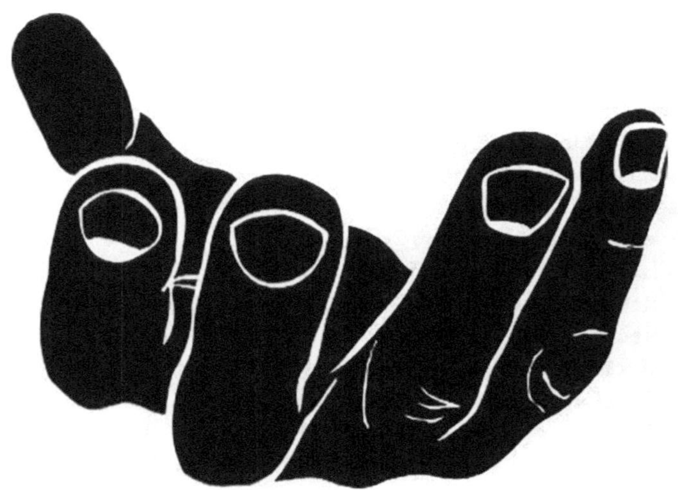

 MISS ASONDRA STARN'AIR

World Out, Jesus In

StarN'air's 'One Year Behavioral Plan'
a plan that will change your life forever!

1. No TV or secular music, only christian programming and spiritual/gospel hymns, melody in your heart to the Lord.
2. No profanity or lewd jokes or negative conversations.
3. Restrain from sex outside of marriage/and intimacy, no romantic relationship, just you and Jesus for one whole year.
4. Remove yourself from those buddies or so called friends that are not taking this one year plan with you. You become what you hang out with, troublemakers, fools, nonbelievers and hypocrites, don't even eat with them anymore. Oh my, there goes 90 percent of your life.
5. This may also include family members who have not committed their lives to Christ. Jesus said in **Matthew 10:23**, *"Do not think I came to bring peace on earth; I did not come to bring peace but a sword."* He goes on to say "He who loves his mother or father more than me is not worthy of me." And he also says a person's enemies will be a member of his own household. I'm just sayin'!
6. Do my one-year weight loss and management boot camp for caregivers. It is written that our bodies are not our own, it was bought with a price, **"JESUS"**! Therefore, it's time to get in the best shape ever and stay that way because we have a lot of ground breaking to do.
7. Bond with someone you hurt or mistreated, especially if that person was an innocent co-worker. If you are not guilty of this, then choose someone else you've been cruel or unfair to and heal that relationship. One full year—put them on your **"Christlike Love List"**.
8. No more **"Gossiping"**, or hanging out with **"Gossipers"** people who badmouth others. Too, God hates haughty eyes and lying tongues!!! Gossips many times turns into hearts that devise wicked plans. Again, boycott, no gossip of any kind. This includes TV shows and magazines.
9. Along with your bible, if there's time, read *'A Caregiver's Bible to Excellence'*, regularly, to help keep you on top of your game. Plus, you'll find Christ all through this book, so get hooked!
10. **Tithe**, give to God what belongs to him.

Wow, We're Halfway Through!

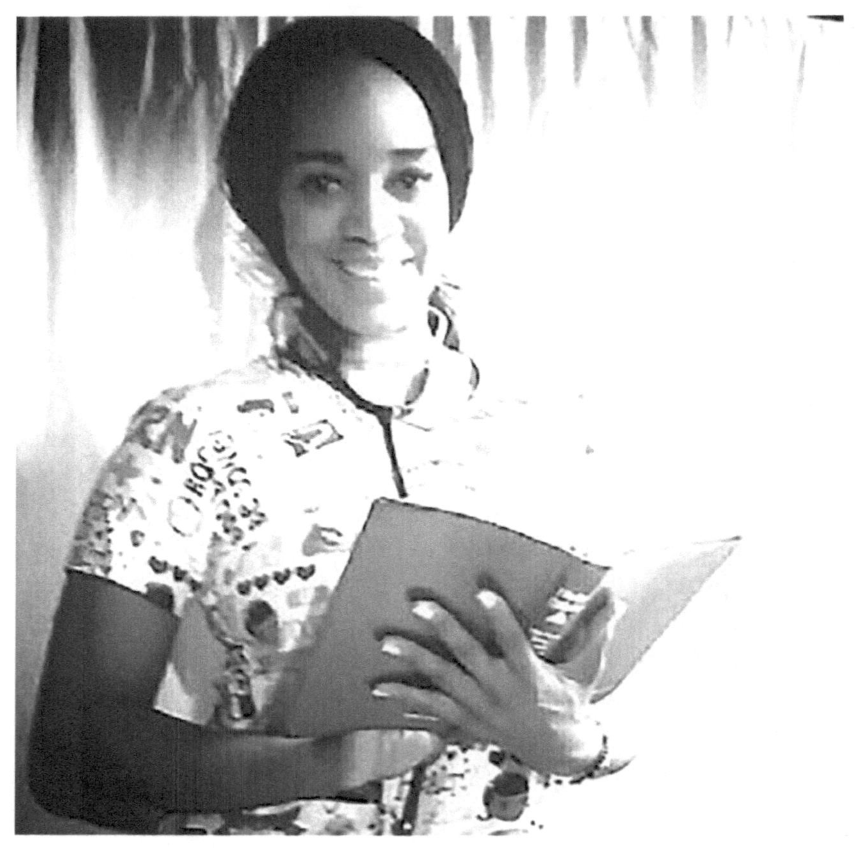

Wow, I'm Lovin' This Crew!

"Commercial Brake"

Have a heart, help others, give more this year,
more than you've ever given before.

Giving is Living, Try it You'll See

Giving Will Set You Free!

Scriptures Of Love

1 Corinthians 13:4-8 - Charity suffereth long, [and] is kind; charity envieth not; charity vaunteth not itself, is not puffed up,

1 Corinthians 16:14 - Let all your things be done with charity.

John 13:34-35 - A new commandment I give unto you, That ye love one another; as I have loved you, that ye also love one another.

1 John 4:8 - He that loveth not knoweth not God; for God is love.

Colossians 3:14 - And above all these things [put on] charity, which is the bond of perfectness.

John 15:13 - Greater love hath no man than this, that a man lay down his life for his friends.

1 John 4:7 - Beloved, let us love one another: for love is of God; and every one that loveth is born of God, and knoweth God.

1 John 4:19 - We love him, because he first loved us.

1 Peter 4:8 - And above all things have fervent charity among yourselves: for charity shall cover the multitude of sins.

John 3:16 - For God so loved the world, that he gave his only begotten Son, that whosoever believeth in him should not perish, but have everlasting life.

1 Corinthians 13:1-13 - Though I speak with the tongues of men and of angels, and have not charity, I am become [as] sounding brass, or a tinkling cymbal.

1 John 4:18 - There is no fear in love; but perfect love casteth out fear: because fear hath torment. He that feareth is not made perfect in love.

Mark 12:31 - And the second [is] like, [namely] this, Thou shalt love thy neighbour as thyself. There is none other commandment greater than these.

Luke 6:35 - But love ye your enemies, and do good, and lend, hoping for nothing again; and your reward shall be great, and ye shall be the children of the Highest: for he is kind unto the unthankful and [to] the evil.

Ephesians 5:25 - Husbands, love your wives, even as Christ also loved the church, and gave himself for it;

> **No matter what life throws at you, never leave the love position!**
> **Love's A Home Run!**

Ephesians 4:15
Instead, speaking the truth in love, we will grow to become in every respect the mature body of him who is the head, that is, Christ.

1 Thessalonians 3:12
May the Lord make your love increase and overflow for each other and for everyone else, just as ours does for you.

Proverbs 21:21
Whoever pursues righteousness and love finds life, prosperity and honor.

Romans 8:38-39
For I am convinced that neither death nor life, neither angels nor demons, neither the present nor the future, nor any powers, neither height nor depth, nor anything else in all creation, will be able to separate us from the love of God that is in Christ Jesus our Lord.

Proverbs 10:12
Hatred stirs up conflict,
but love covers over all wrongs.

1 Corinthians 13:1
If I speak in the tongues of men or of angels, but do not have love, I am only a resounding gong or a clanging cymbal.

Mark 12:31
The second is this: 'Love your neighbor as yourself.' There is no commandment greater than these.

Psalm 116:1-2
I love the Lord, for he heard my
voice; he heard my cry for mercy.
Because he turned his ear to me,
I will call on him as long as I live.

Mark 12:30
Love the Lord your God with all your heart and with all your soul and with all your mind and with all your strength.

Psalm 30:5
For his anger lasts only a moment,
but his favor lasts a lifetime;
weeping may stay for the night, but
rejoicing comes in the morning.

1 Peter 3:10-11
For, Whoever would love life
and see good days
must keep their tongue from evil and
their lips from deceitful speech. They
must turn from evil and do good; they
must seek peace and pursue it.

Leviticus 19:17-18
Do not hate a fellow Israelite in your heart. Rebuke your neighbor frankly so you will not share in their guilt. Do not seek revenge or bear a grudge against anyone among your people, but love your neighbor as yourself. I am the Lord.

1 Corinthians 10:24

No one should seek their own good, but the good of others.

2 Timothy 1:7

For the Spirit God gave us does not make us timid, but gives us power, love and self-discipline.

Psalm 103:8

The Lord is compassionate and gracious,
slow to anger, abounding in love.

1 Timothy 4:12

Don't let anyone look down on you because you are young, but set an example for the believers in speech, in conduct, in love, in faith and in purity.

1 John 4:10

This is love: not that we loved God, but that he loved us and sent his Son as an atoning sacrifice for our sins.

Romans 8:35

Who shall separate us from the love of Christ? Shall trouble or hardship or persecution or famine or nakedness or danger or sword?

Psalm 42:8

By day the Lord directs his love,
at night his song is with me—
a prayer to the God of my life.

1 John 4:8

Whoever does not love does not know God, because God is love.

Matthew 5:44

But I tell you, love your enemies and pray for those who persecute you.

Ephesians 5:2

And walk in the way of love, just as Christ loved us and gave himself up for us as a fragrant offering and sacrifice to God.

1 Timothy 6:11

But you, man of God, flee from all this, and pursue righteousness, godliness, faith, love, endurance and gentleness.

1 Corinthians 13:3

If I give all I possess to the poor and give over my body to hardship that I may boast, but do not have love, I gain nothing.

Romans 13:10

Love does no harm to a neighbor. Therefore love is the fulfillment of the law.

Luke 10:27

He answered, "'Love the Lord your God with all your heart and with all your soul and with all your strength and with all your mind'; and, 'Love your neighbor as yourself.'"

John 14:21

Whoever has my commands and keeps them is the one who loves me. The one who loves me will be loved by my Father, and I too will love them and show myself to them.

Psalm 94:18

When I said, "My foot is slipping," your unfailing love, Lord, supported me.

1 John 3:11

For this is the message you heard from the beginning: We should love one another.

1 John 4:11

Dear friends, since God so loved us, we also ought to love one another.

1 John 4:9

This is how God showed his love among us: He sent his one and only Son into the world that we might live through him.

Hebrews 13:1-2

Keep on loving one another as brothers and sisters. Do not forget to show hospitality to strangers, for by so doing some people have shown hospitality to angels without knowing it.

Jude 1:2

Mercy, peace and love be yours in abundance.

Lamentations 3:22-23

Because of the Lord's great love we are not
consumed, for his compassions never fail. They are
new every morning;
great is your faithfulness.

John 13:34

A new command I give you: Love one another. As I have loved you, so you must love one another.

1 John 2:15

Do not love the world or anything in the world. If anyone loves the world, love for the Father is not in them.

Psalm 86:5

You, Lord, are forgiving and good, abounding in love to all who call to you.

Revelation 3:19

Those whom I love I rebuke and discipline. So be earnest and repent.

Psalm 103:13

As a father has compassion on his children,

so the Lord has compassion on those who fear him.

John 13:35

"By this everyone will know that you are my disciples, if you love one another."

Romans 13:9

The commandments, "You shall not commit adultery," "You shall not murder," "You shall not steal," "You shall not covet," and whatever other command there may be, are summed up in this one command: "Love your neighbor as yourself."

John 14:15

If you love me, keep my commands.

Romans 8:28

And we know that in all things God works for the good of those who love him, who have been called according to his purpose.

Galatians 5:14

For the entire law is fulfilled in keeping this one command: "Love your neighbor as yourself."

Deuteronomy 6:4-5

Hear, O Israel: The Lord our God, the Lord is one. Love the Lord your God with all your heart and with all your soul and with all your strength.

Ephesians 2:4-5

But because of his great love for us, God, who is rich in mercy, made us alive with Christ even when we were dead in transgressions—it is by grace you have been saved.

Galatians 5:13

You, my brothers and sisters, were called to be free. But do not use your freedom to indulge the flesh; rather, serve one another humbly in love.

2 Thessalonians 1:3

We ought always to thank God for you, brothers and sisters, and rightly so, because your faith is growing more and more, and the love all of you have for one another is increasing.

Psalm 33:5 | NIV

The Lord loves righteousness and justice; the earth is full of his unfailing love.

Luke 10:27

He answered, "'Love the Lord your God with all your heart and with all your soul and with all your strength and with all your mind'; and, 'Love your neighbor as yourself.'"

John 14:21

Whoever has my commands and keeps them is the one who loves me. The one who loves me will be loved by my Father, and I too will love them and show myself to them.

Psalm 94:18

When I said, "My foot is slipping," your unfailing love, Lord, supported me.

1 John 3:11

For this is the message you heard from the beginning: We should love one another.

1 John 4:11

Dear friends, since God so loved us, we also ought to love one another.

1 John 4:9

This is how God showed his love among us: He sent his one and only Son into the world that we might live through him.

Hebrews 13:1-2

Keep on loving one another as brothers and sisters. Do not forget to show hospitality to strangers, for by so doing some people have shown hospitality to angels without knowing it.

Jude 1:2

Mercy, peace and love be yours in abundance.

Lamentations 3:22-23
Because of the Lord's great love we are not
consumed, for his compassions never fail. They are
new every morning;
great is your faithfulness.

John 13:34
A new command I give you: Love one another. As I have loved you, so
you must love one another.

1 John 2:15
Do not love the world or anything in the world. If anyone loves the
world, love for the Father is not in them.

Psalm 86:5
You, Lord, are forgiving and good, abounding in love to all who call
to you.

Revelation 3:19
Those whom I love I rebuke and discipline. So be earnest and repent.

Psalm 103:13
As a father has compassion on his children,
so the Lord has compassion on those who fear him.

John 13:35
"By this everyone will know that you are my disciples, if you love one
another."

Romans 13:9
The commandments, "You shall not commit adultery," "You shall not
murder," "You shall not steal," "You shall not covet," and whatever other
command there may be, are summed up in this one command: "Love
your neighbor as yourself."

John 14:15
If you love me, keep my commands.

 Miss Asondra StarN'air

Romans 8:28

And we know that in all things God works for the good of those who love him, who have been called according to his purpose.

Galatians 5:14

For the entire law is fulfilled in keeping this one command: "Love your neighbor as yourself."

Hear, O Israel: The Lord our God, the Lord is one. Love the Lord your God with all your heart and with all your soul and with all your strength.

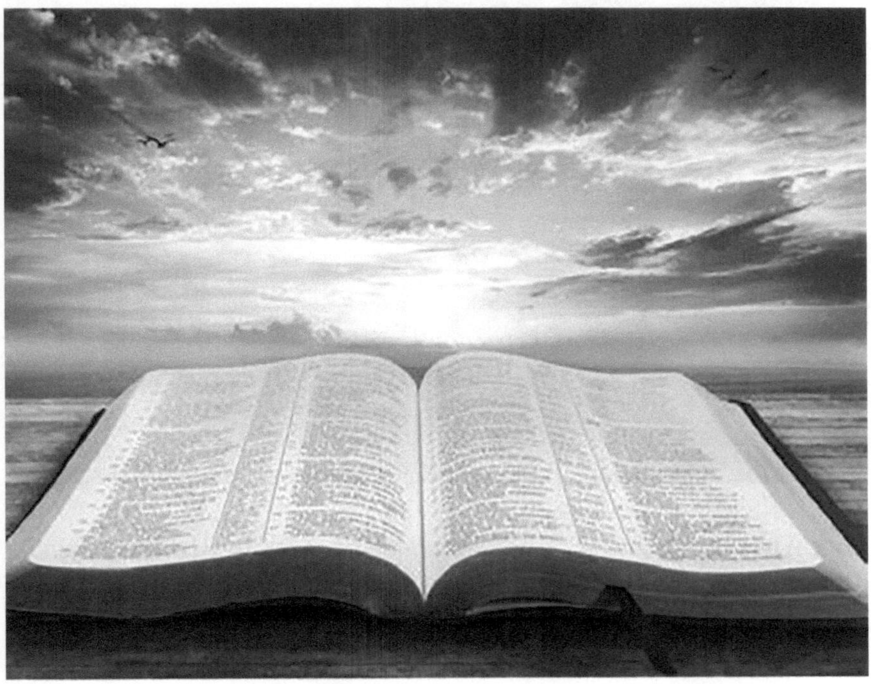

The Message, "LOVE"!

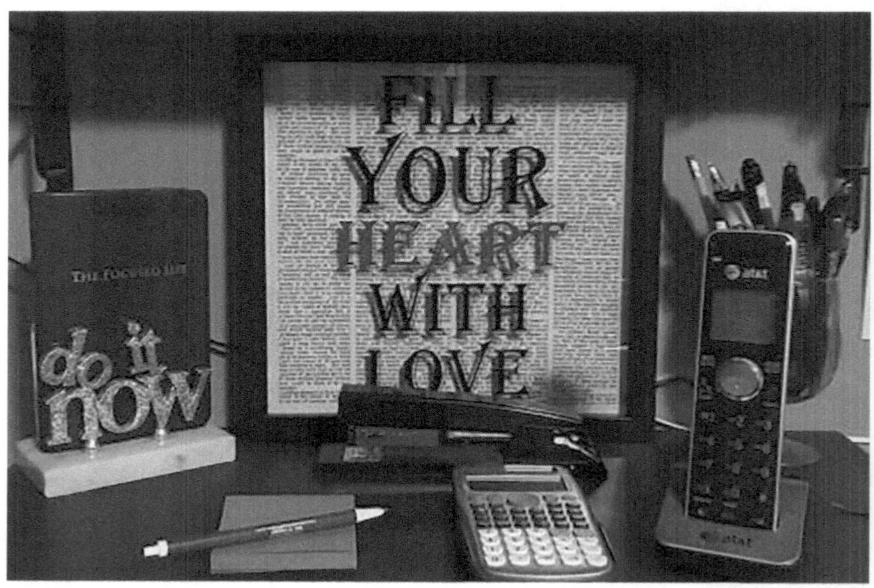

Love Always, not just at church or among your family and close friends, fill your heart with love, for **"Everybody, Everywhere"**! Treat your co-workers and bosses well too. Put into practice **'A Focus Life'** do everything it takes to live right!

Do It Now!

Mind Body & Soul

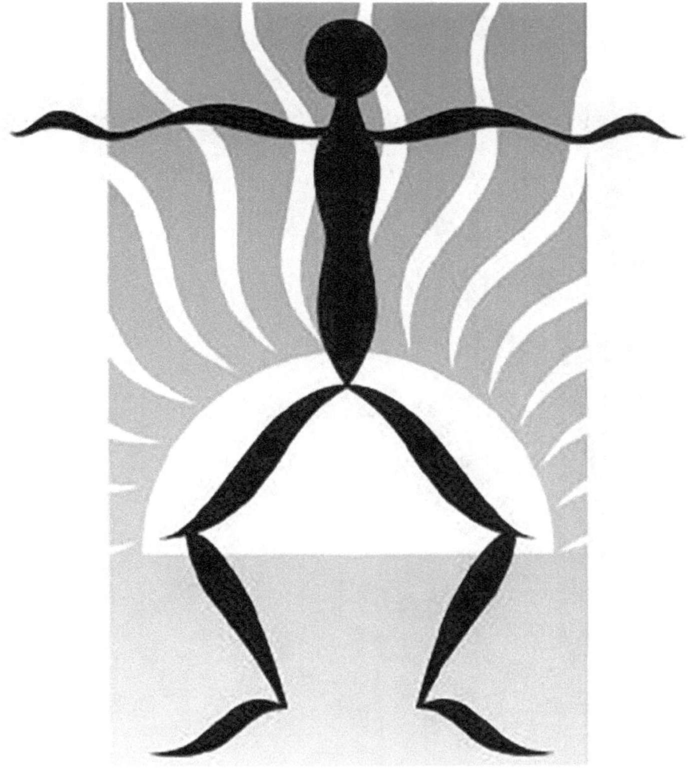

Meditate On God's Word, "Read"!

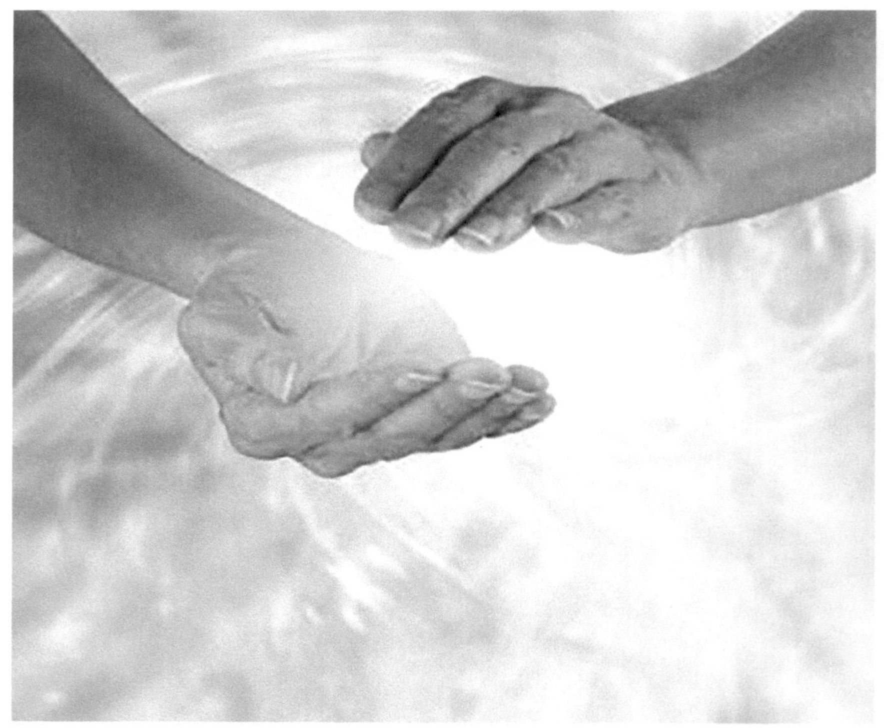

Stay Focus, "Breathe"!

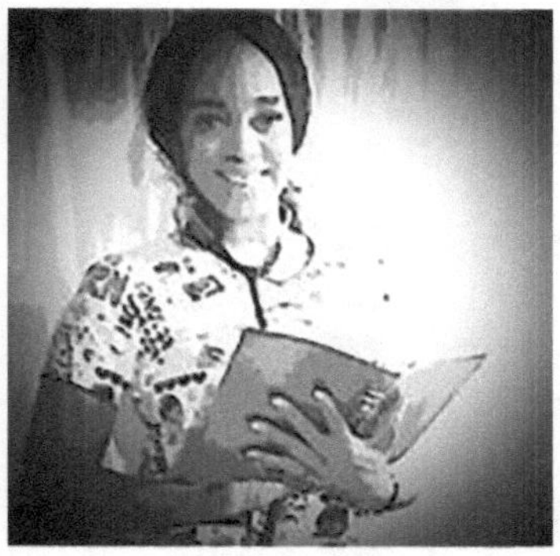

In order to be and live the kind of life God has for us, Caregivers, we must get in shape, and get healthy. There is just no getting around that, all of us **"Think Health"**! Join me with that mindset, **"THINK HEALTH"** Let us make that our daily practice.

- We are what we eat!
- We need plenty of sleep!
- Let our **LORD** lead!
- Lastly, pull out your bibles, **READ!**

THINK HAPPY

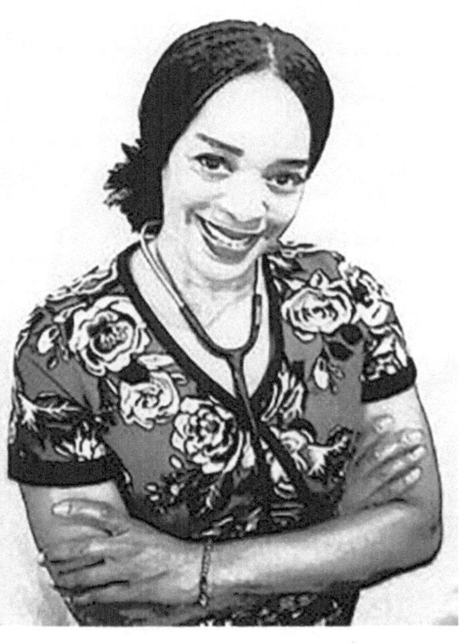

BE HAPPY TOO!

THINK HEALTH, LIVE WELL, LIVE DAILY

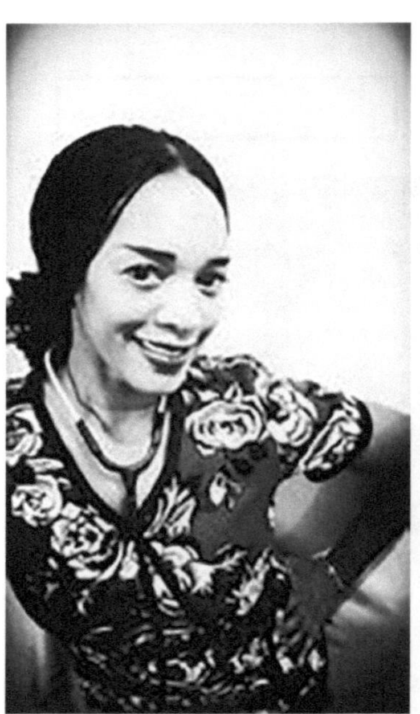

- Exercise
- Sleep
- Read
- Smile though your heart is breaking.
- Love your enemies
- Develop a prayer life
- Forgiver all who have hurt you.
- Laugh at your hater, love them anyway, always stay in the love position.
- Remove gossip out of your life
- Get out of abusive relationships
- Realize that sex is not worth dying for, reframe from sex outside of marriage.
- Turn TV off and Jesus on!
- Reduce alcohol by 90% or more, yes it's true Jesus drank wine but he did not become a drunken fool.
- Learn to have a Jesus kinda life, it will take you places you never dreamed of.

"LIFE"

A Life Review

A life Review, is a progressive return to consciousness of memories and unresolved pass conflicts for re-evaluation and resolution.

A Life Reimagined

A life Reimagined, means we can start all over again, we can win. We can change, we can leave all our mistakes and bad stuff behind, We can learn to be more gentle and kind, and guess what? We can find love again too!

A New Calling

A New Calling yes, there's a new calling on your life, time to change directions, time to give more love and affection.

A Change Maker

A Change Maker is Jesus and those who follow him, for it is written in John 14:12, Verily, verily, I say unto you, the person that believeth on me, the work that I do shall they do also and greater than these shall they do; because I go unto my father. **It's Our Turn Now, "Yours and Mine".**

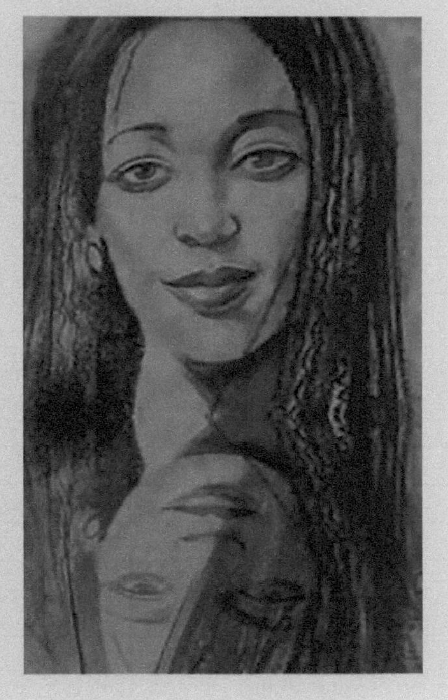

Meditate, Talk To God!

Who I Use To Be

Who I Am Now

My Goals In Life

My Dreams and Desires

My Legacy

SECTION X

Scriptures to Walk by, Talk by, Live by

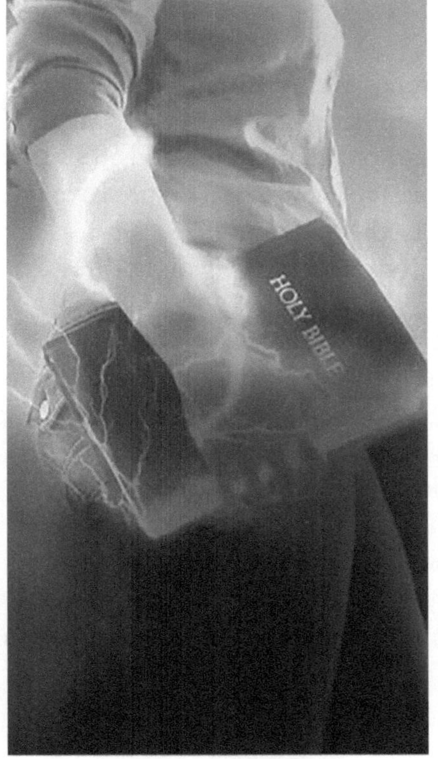

Scriptures On the Go!

Today, I'll have some scriptures for lunch instead of gossip, instead of strife, or conflict, mightiest well throw in some *Jesus Water* in on the side.

LOVE

No matter what we accomplish in Life If we have not Loved, none of it will matter in the end!

1 Corinthians 13:1–3

"If I speak in the tongues of men or of angels, but do not have love, I am only a resounding gong or a clanging cymbal. If I have the gift of prophecy and can fathom all mysteries and all knowledge, and if I have a faith that can move mountains, but do not have love, I am nothing. If I give all I possess to the poor and give over my body to hardship that I may boast but do not have love, I gain nothing."

That's right, you gain nothing! You end up with you in the end, and life is not about you, never has been and never will be. No matter what your title, financial status, or popularity—if you are stuck up, full of pride, self-indulged, mega-star, athlete, even president. Again, if you have not loved, all the work you have done is for nothing.

And, caregivers, we have no excuse because we are supposed to be the Florence Nightingales of this world. If "WE" don't show love, the world is in trouble, because we are the chosen ones to be a light of love in a world that is crying out for help. We **MUST**, show love, We **MUST** give love, and We **MUST** be love!

Spiritual Gifts for all of God's Caregivers

1 Corinthians 12:12

Spiritual Gifts

Now, dear brothers and sisters, regarding your question about the special abilities the Spirit gives us. I don't want you to misunderstand this. You know that when you were still pagans, you were led astray and swept along in worshiping speechless idols. So I want you to know that no one speaking by the Spirit of God will curse Jesus, and no one can say Jesus is Lord, except by the Holy Spirit.

There are different kinds of spiritual gifts, but the same Spirit is the source of them all. There are different kinds of service, but we serve the same Lord. God works in different ways, but it is the same God who does the work in all of us.

A spiritual gift is given to each of us so we can help each other. To one person the Spirit gives the ability to give wise advice; to another the same Spirit gives a message of special knowledge. The same Spirit gives great faith to another, and to someone else the one Spirit gives the gift of healing. He gives one person the power to perform miracles, and another the ability to prophesy. He gives someone else the ability to discern whether a message is from the Spirit of God or from another spirit. Still another person is given the ability to speak in unknown languages, while another is given the ability to interpret what is being said. It is the one and only Spirit who distributes all these gifts. He alone decides which gift each person should have.

Everybody's Got a Gift, If You Look Inside You'll Find It!

Jesus Is Our Healer!

1. (Exodus 15:26 NKJV) and said, "If you diligently heed the voice of the LORD your God and do what is right in His sight, give ear to His commandments and keep all His statutes, I will put none of the diseases on you which I have brought on the Egyptians. For I am the LORD who heals you."

2. (Deuteronomy 32:39 NKJV) 'Now see that I, even I, am He, And there is no God besides Me; I kill and I make alive; I wound and I heal; Nor is there any who can deliver from My hand.

3. (2 Chronicles 7:14 NKJV) "If My people who are called by My name will humble themselves, and pray and seek My face, and turn from their wicked ways, then I will hear from heaven, and will forgive their sin and heal their land.

4. (Psalms 30:2 NKJV) O LORD my God, I cried out to You, And You healed me.

5. (Psalms 6:2 NKJV) Have mercy on me, O LORD, for I am weak; O LORD, heal me, for my bones are troubled.

6. (Psalms 103:1-4 NKJV) Bless the LORD, O my soul; And all that is within me, bless His holy name! {2} Bless the LORD, O my soul, And forget not all His benefits: {3} Who forgives all your iniquities, Who heals all your diseases, {4} Who redeems your life from destruction, Who crowns you with loving, kindness and tender mercies,

7. (Psalms 107:20 NKJV) He sent His word and healed them, And delivered them from their destructions.

8. (Psalms 147:3 NKJV) He heals the brokenhearted And binds up their wounds.

9. (Proverbs 3:7-8 NKJV) Do not be wise in your own eyes; Fear the LORD and depart from evil. {8} It will be health to your flesh, And strength to your bones.

10. (Proverbs 4:20-22 NKJV) My son, give attention to my words; Incline your ear to my sayings. {21} Do not let them depart from your eyes; Keep them in the midst of your heart; {22} For they are life to those who find them, And health to all their flesh.

11. (Isaiah 53:5 NKJV) But He was wounded for our transgressions, He was bruised for our iniquities; The chastisement for our peace was upon Him, And by His stripes we are healed.

12. (Isaiah 58:8 NKJV) Then your light shall break forth like the morning, Your healing shall spring forth speedily, And your righteousness shall go before you; The glory of the LORD shall be your rear guard.

13. (Isaiah 61:1 NKJV) "The Spirit of the Lord GOD is upon Me, Because the LORD has anointed Me To preach good tidings to the poor; He has sent Me to heal the brokenhearted, To proclaim liberty to the captives, And the opening of the prison to those who are bound;

14. (Jeremiah 3:22 NKJV) "Return, you backsliding children, And I will heal your backslidings." "Indeed we do come to You, For You are the LORD our God.

15. (Jeremiah 17:14 NKJV) Heal me, O LORD, and I shall be healed; Save me, and I shall be saved, For You are my praise.

16. (Jeremiah 30:17 NKJV) For I will restore health to you And heal you of your wounds,' says the LORD, 'Because they called you an outcast saying: "This is Zion; No one seeks her."'

17. (Jeremiah 33:6 NKJV) 'Behold, I will bring it health and healing; I will heal them and reveal to them the abundance of peace and truth.

18. (Hosea 6:1 NKJV) Come, and let us return to the LORD; For He has torn, but He will heal us; He has stricken, but He will bind us up.

19. (Hosea 14:4 NKJV) "I will heal their backsliding, I will love them freely, For My anger has turned away from him.

20. (Malachi 4:2 NKJV) But to you who fear My name The Sun of Righteousness shall arise With healing in His wings; And you shall go out And grow fat like stall-fed calves.

21. (Matthew 4:23 NKJV) And Jesus went about all Galilee, teaching in their synagogues, preaching the gospel of the kingdom, and healing all kinds of sickness and all kinds of disease among the people.

22. (Matthew 8:13 NKJV) Then Jesus said to the centurion, "Go your way; and as you have believed, so let it be done for you." And his servant was healed that same hour.

23. (Matthew 8:16 NKJV) When evening had come, they brought to Him many who were demon-possessed. And He cast out the spirits with a word, and healed all who were sick,

24. (Matthew 9:35 NKJV) Then Jesus went about all the cities and villages, teaching in their synagogues, preaching the gospel of the kingdom, and healing every sickness and every disease among the people.

25. (Matthew 10:1 NKJV) And when He had called His twelve disciples to Him, He gave them power over unclean spirits, to cast them out, and to heal all kinds of sickness and all kinds of disease.

26. (Matthew 10:8 NKJV) "Heal the sick, cleanse the lepers, raise the dead, cast out demons. Freely you have received, freely give.

27. (Matthew 12:22 NKJV) Then one was brought to Him who was demon-possessed, blind and mute; and He healed him, so that the blind and mute man both spoke and saw.

28. (Matthew 14:14 NKJV) And when Jesus went out He saw a great multitude; and He was moved with compassion for them, and healed their sick.

29. (Luke 6:19 NKJV) And the whole multitude sought to touch Him, for power went out from Him and healed them all.

30. (Luke 9:6 NKJV) So they departed and went through the towns, preaching the gospel and healing everywhere.(The twelve are sent out)

31. (Luke 10:8-9 NKJV) "Whatever city you enter, and they receive you, eat such things as are set before you. {9} "And heal the sick there, and say to them, 'The kingdom of God has come near to you.'(The seventy are sent out)

32. (Luke 17:15 NKJV) And one of them, when he saw that he was healed, returned, and with a loud voice glorified God,(The story of the ten lepers)

33. (Acts 3:12 NKJV) So when Peter saw it, he responded to the people: "Men of Israel, why do you marvel at this? Or why look so intently at us, as though by our own power or godliness we had made this man walk?

34. (Healing of the lame man at the Gate Beautiful) (Acts 4:29-31 NKJV) "Now, Lord, look on their threats, and grant to Your servants that with all boldness they may speak Your word, {30} "by

 Miss Asondra StarN'air

stretching out Your hand to heal, and that signs and wonders may be done through the name of Your holy Servant Jesus." {31} And when they had prayed, the place where they were assembled together was shaken; and they were all filled with the Holy Spirit, and they spoke the word of God with boldness.

35. (1 Corinthians 12:9 NKJV) to another faith by the same Spirit, to another gifts of healings by the same Spirit,

36. (James 5:14-16 NKJV) Is anyone among you sick? Let him call for the elders of the church, and let them pray over him, anointing him with oil in the name of the Lord. {15} And the prayer of faith will save the sick, and the Lord will raise him up. And if he has committed sins, he will be forgiven. {16} Confess your trespasses to one another, and pray for one another, that you may be healed. The effective, fervent prayer of a righteous man avails much.

37. (Revelation 22:2 NKJV) In the middle of its street, and on either side of the river, was the tree of life, which bore twelve fruits, each tree yielding its fruit every month. The leaves of the tree were for the healing of the nations.

38. (Luke 8:47 NKJV) Now when the woman saw that she was not hidden, she came trembling; and falling down before Him, she declared to Him in the presence of all the people the reason she had touched Him and how she was healed immediately.

39. (Luke 8:48 NKJV) And He said to her, "Daughter, be of good cheer; your faith has made you well. Go in peace."

40. (Luke 5:17 NKJV) Now it happened on a certain day, as He was teaching, that there were Pharisees and teachers of the law sitting by, who had come out of every town of Galilee, Judea, and Jerusalem. And the power of the Lord was present to heal them.

Salt and Light

13 "You are the salt of the earth. But if the salt loses its saltiness, how can it be made salty again? It is no longer good for anything, except to be thrown out and trampled underfoot.

14 "You are the light of the world. A town built on a hill cannot be hidden. 15 Neither do people light a lamp and put it under a bowl. Instead they put it on its stand, and it gives light to everyone in the house. 16 In the same way, let your light shine before others, that they may see your good deeds and glorify your Father in heaven.

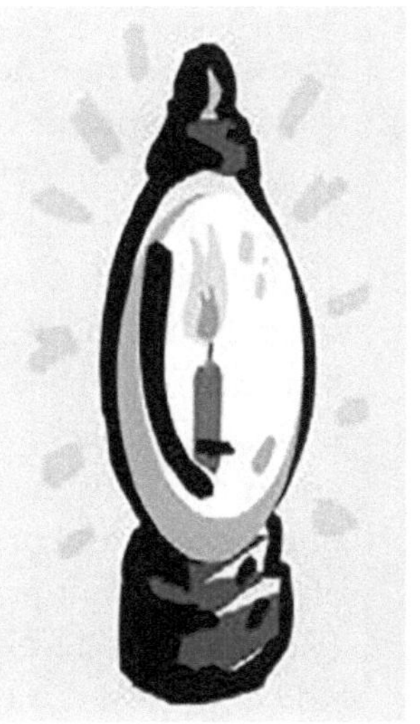

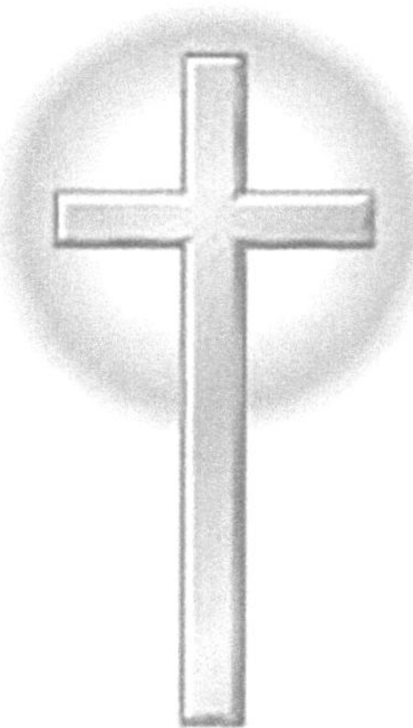

The **8** Beatitudes' of Jesus

"Blessed are the poor in spirit,
for theirs is the kingdom of heaven.

Blessed are they who mourn,
for they shall be comforted.

Blessed are the meek,
for they shall inherit the earth.

Blessed are they who hunger and thirst for righteousness,
for they shall be satisfied.

Blessed are the merciful,
for they shall obtain mercy.

Blessed are the pure of heart,
for they shall see God.

Blessed are the peacemakers,
for they shall be called children of God.

Blessed are they who are persecuted for the sake of
righteousness, for theirs is the kingdom of heaven."

Gospel of St. Matthew 5:3-10

You Got to have Faith

Mark 9:42—But whoever causes one of these little ones who **believe** in Me to stumble, it would be better for him if a millstone were hung around his neck, and he were thrown into the sea.

Luke 8:12—Those by the wayside are the ones who hear; then the devil comes and takes away the word out of their hearts, lest they should **believe** and be saved.

John 1:12—But as many as received Him, to them He gave the right to become children of God, to those who **believe** in His name.

John 2:23—Now when He was in Jerusalem at the Passover, during the feast, many **believed** in His name when they saw the signs which He did.

John 3:14-18—And as Moses lifted up the serpent in the wilderness, even so must the Son of Man be lifted up, that whoever **believes** in Him should not perish but have eternal life. For God so loved the world that He gave His only begotten Son, that whoever **believes** in Him should not perish but have everlasting life. For God did not send His Son into the world to condemn the world, but that the world through Him might be saved. He who **believes** in Him is not condemned; but he who does not **believe** is condemned already, because he has not **believed** in the name of the only begotten Son of God.

John 3:36—He who **believes** in the Son has everlasting life; and he who does not **believe** the Son shall not see life, but the wrath of God abides on him.

John 6:29—Jesus answered and said to them, "This is the work of God, that you **believe** in Him whom He sent."

John 6:35—And Jesus said to them, "I am the bread of life. He who comes [by faith] to Me shall <u>never hunger</u>, and he who **believes** <u>in Me</u> shall <u>never thirst</u>."

John 6:40—And this is the will of Him who sent Me, that everyone who sees the Son and **believes** <u>in Him</u> may have <u>everlasting life</u>; and <u>I will raise him up at the last day</u>.

John 6:47—Most assuredly, I say to you, he who **believes** <u>in Me</u> has <u>everlasting life</u>.

John 6:59—Also we have come to **believe** and know <u>that You are the Christ, the Son of the living God</u>.

John 7:38—He who **believes** <u>in Me</u>, as the Scripture has said, <u>out of his heart will flow rivers of living water</u>.

John 8:24, 58—Therefore I said to you that you will die in your sins; for if you do not **believe** that <u>I am He</u>, you will die in your sins . . . Jesus said to them, "Most assuredly, I say to you, before Abraham was, I AM."

John 9:35-38—Jesus heard that they had cast him out; and when He had found him, He said to him, "Do you **believe** <u>in the Son of God</u>?" He answered and said, "Who is He, Lord, that I may believe in Him?" And Jesus said to him, "You have both seen Him and it is He who is talking with you." Then he said, "Lord, I believe!" And he worshiped Him.

John 10:38—but if I do, though you do not believe Me, believe the works, that you may know and **believe** that <u>the Father is in Me, and I in Him</u>.

John 11:25-27—Jesus said to her, "I am the resurrection and the life. He who **believes** <u>in Me</u>, though he may die, he <u>shall live</u>. And whoever lives and **believes** <u>in Me</u> shall <u>never die</u>. Do you believe this?" She said to Him, "Yes, Lord, I **believe** that <u>You are the Christ, the Son of God</u>, who is to come into the world."

John 12:44, 45—Then Jesus cried out and said, "He who **believes** *in Me*, believes not in Me but in Him who sent Me. And he who sees Me sees Him who sent Me.

John 14:11—**Believe** Me that I am in the Father and the Father in Me, or else believe Me for the sake of the works themselves.

John 20:31—But these are written that you may **believe** that Jesus is the Christ, the Son of God, and that believing you may have life in His name.

Acts 8:37—Then Philip said, "If you **believe** with all your heart, you may." And he answered and said, "I **believe** that Jesus Christ is the Son of God."

Acts 10:43—To Him all the prophets witness that, through His name, whoever **believes** in Him will receive remission of sins.

Acts 11:17—If therefore God gave them the same gift as He gave us when we **believed** on the Lord Jesus Christ, who was I that I could withstand God?

Acts 14:23—So when they had appointed elders in every church, and prayed with fasting, they commended them to the Lord in whom they had **believed**.

Acts 15:9—And made no distinction between us and them, purifying their hearts **by faith**.

Acts 16:31, 34—So they said, "**Believe** on the Lord Jesus Christ, and you will be saved, you and your household." . . . Now when he had brought them into his house, he set food before them; and he rejoiced, having **believed** in God [confirmation of Christ's deity) with all his household.

 MISS ASONDRA StarN'air

Acts 18:8—Then Crispus, the ruler of the synagogue, **believed** on the Lord with all his household. And many of the Corinthians, hearing, believed and were baptized.

Acts 19:4—Then Paul said, "John indeed baptized with a baptism of repentance, saying to the people that they should **believe** on Him who would come after him, that is, on Christ Jesus."

Acts 20:21—Testifying to Jews, and also to Greeks, repentance toward God and [by] **faith** toward our Lord Jesus Christ.

Acts 26:18—To open their eyes, in order to turn them from darkness to light, and from the power of Satan to God, that they may receive forgiveness of sins and an inheritance among those who are sanctified **by faith** in Me.

Romans 1:17—For in it the righteousness of God is revealed from faith to faith [an expression meaning completely, from first to last]; as it is written, "The just shall live **by faith**." (See **Habakkuk 2:4; Romans 2:20; Galatians 3:11; Hebrews 10:38**)

Romans 3:21, 22—But now the righteousness of God apart from the law is revealed, being witnessed by the Law and the Prophets, even the righteousness of God, **through faith** in Jesus Christ, to all and on all who believe. (cf. **21-30**)

Romans 4:3—For what does the Scripture say? "Abraham **believed** God, and it was accounted to him for righteousness." (See **Romans 4:9, 11; Galatians 3:6; James 2:23**)

Romans 4:5—But to him who does not work but **believes** on Him who justifies the ungodly, his **faith** is accounted for righteousness.

Romans 5:1, 2—Therefore, having been justified **by faith**, we have peace with God through our Lord Jesus Christ, through whom also we have access **by faith** into this grace in which we stand, and rejoice in hope of the glory of God.

Romans 9:30—What shall we say then? That Gentiles, who did not pursue righteousness, have attained to righteousness, even the <u>righteousness</u> **of faith**.

Romans 10:8-11—But what does it say? "The word is near you, in your mouth and in your heart" (that is, the word of faith which we preach): that if you **confess** with your mouth [an expression confirming genuineness of action] <u>the Lord Jesus</u> and **believe** <u>in your heart</u> [reinforcing the fact that faith must be genuine] that <u>God has raised Him from the dead</u>, you will be saved. For with the heart one **believes** <u>unto righteousness</u>, and with the mouth confession is made unto salvation [the natural outgrowth of an inward imputation of righteousness, which is solely by faith]. For the Scripture says, "Whoever **believes** <u>on Him</u> will not be put to shame."

1 Corinthians 1:21—For since, in the wisdom of God, the world through wisdom did not know God, it pleased God through the foolishness of the message preached to <u>save</u> those who **believe**.

Galatians 2:16—Knowing that a man is not <u>justified</u> by the works of the law but **by faith** <u>in Jesus Christ</u>, even we have **believed** <u>in Christ Jesus</u>, that we might be <u>justified</u> **by faith** <u>in Christ</u> and not by the works of the law; for by the works of the law no flesh shall be justified.

Galatians 2:20—I have been crucified with Christ; it is no longer I who live, but Christ lives in me; and the life which I now live in the flesh I <u>live</u> **by faith** <u>in the Son of God</u>, who loved me and gave Himself for me. (See **Habakkuk 2:4; Romans 1:17; Galatians 3:11; Hebrews 10:38**)

Galatians 3:22—But the Scripture has confined all under sin, that the promise **by faith** <u>in Jesus Christ</u> might be given to those who **believe**.

Galatians 3:24— Therefore the law was our tutor to bring us to Christ, that we might be <u>justified</u> **by faith**.

Ephesians 1:13—<u>In Him</u> you also <u>trusted</u>, after you heard the word of truth, the gospel of your salvation; <u>in whom</u> also, having **believed**, you were <u>sealed with the Holy Spirit</u> of promise.

Ephesians 2:8, 9— For by grace you have been <u>saved</u> **through faith**, and that not of yourselves; it is the gift of God, not of works, lest anyone should boast.

Philippians 3:9— And be found in Him, not having my own <u>righteousness</u>, which is from the law, but that which is **through faith in Christ**, the <u>righteousness</u> which is <u>from God</u> **by faith**.

1 Timothy 1:16—However, for this reason I obtained mercy, that in me first Jesus Christ might show all longsuffering, as a pattern to those who are going to **believe** <u>on Him</u> for <u>everlasting life</u>.

1 Timothy 3:16—And without controversy great is the mystery of godliness: <u>God was manifested in the flesh</u> [confirmation of Christ's deity], justified in the Spirit, seen by angels, preached among the Gentiles, **believed** <u>on</u> in the world, received up in glory.

1 Timothy 4:10—For to this end we both labor and suffer reproach, because we **trust in** the <u>living God</u>, who is the <u>Savior</u> of all men, especially of those who **believe**.

1 Peter 1:3-5— Blessed be the God and Father of our Lord Jesus Christ, who according to His abundant mercy has <u>begotten us again</u> to a <u>living hope</u> through the resurrection of Jesus Christ from the dead, to an <u>inheritance incorruptible and undefiled</u> and that <u>does not fade away</u>, <u>reserved in heaven</u> for you, who are <u>kept by the power of God</u> **through faith** for <u>salvation</u> ready to be revealed in the last time.

1 Peter 2:6—Therefore it is also contained in the Scripture, "Behold, I lay in Zion A chief cornerstone, elect, precious, and he who **believes** <u>on Him</u> will by no means be put to shame."

1 John 3:23—And this is His commandment: that we should **believe** <u>on the name of His Son Jesus Christ</u> and love one another, as He gave us commandment.

1 John 5:1, 5—Whoever **believes** that <u>Jesus is the Christ</u> is born of God, and everyone who loves Him who begot also loves him who is begotten of Him . . . Who is he who overcomes the world, but he who **believes** that <u>Jesus is the Son of God</u>?

1 John 5:13—These things I have written to you who **believe** <u>in the name of the Son of God</u>, that you may <u>know that you have eternal life</u>, and that you may continue to **believe** <u>in the name of the Son of God</u>.

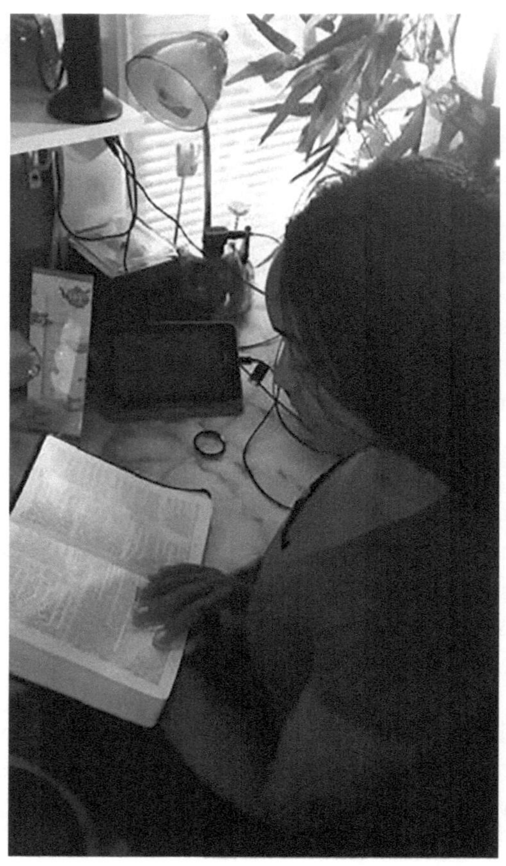

 Miss Asondra StarN'air

You Got To Have Faith

My story, when God, when? I'm sure you too have asked that question. I know I have many times. It's going on two decades, and God still has not given me the desires of my heart. But I still trust him, I have faith God knows what he's doing in my life. Patience is a virtue, not meant to deny or hurt you! Wait on God! In the meantime, I keep loving and serving him.

And if for some reason, God does not give me what I ask for, so what! I'm still going to love and serve him for the rest of my days. Sometimes our desire can conflict with God's plan for our lives. I wanted to be a global recording artist make hit records, but as you can see God had other plans. And I like it! I like that I get a chance to minister to others by writing books. I would have never thought God would take me this route but he did, He said to me "write my book and call it *"A Caregiver's Bible To Excellence!"* I answered the call, and with faith we'll show them all, I am what God says I am! And so are you, stay true to you, no matter what your circumstances, hold on to God. Hold on to his promises, hold on to your goals and dreams don't ever give up. Keep Jesus in your cup! Dear love ones, **"YOU GOT TO HAVE FAITH"** that God is going to work everything out in your favor. But also true too, you got to do what He ask you to do, faith without works on your part is dead. You must do some work too, to help **"YOU"** because God is not going to do all the work. I know sometimes life hurts. But we must be strong and press on. 'Everybody, Everywhere' know pain. There are two types of pains, one that hurts you and one that changes you. And that's what this book is all about, changing hearts one Caregiver at a time.

I encourage all of you to find out God's will for your life and have faith that he will get you to where you need to be. All your hard work, pain, and suffering—don't let it be for nothing. Keep pressing on, keep believing, keep loving and forgiving. And remember, faith without works is dead. Press on my brothers and sister out there, Keep the faith and faith will keep you moving forward to your destine, look at me, today I'm exactly where I'm supposed to be **"FREE!"**

You Got To Have Faith!

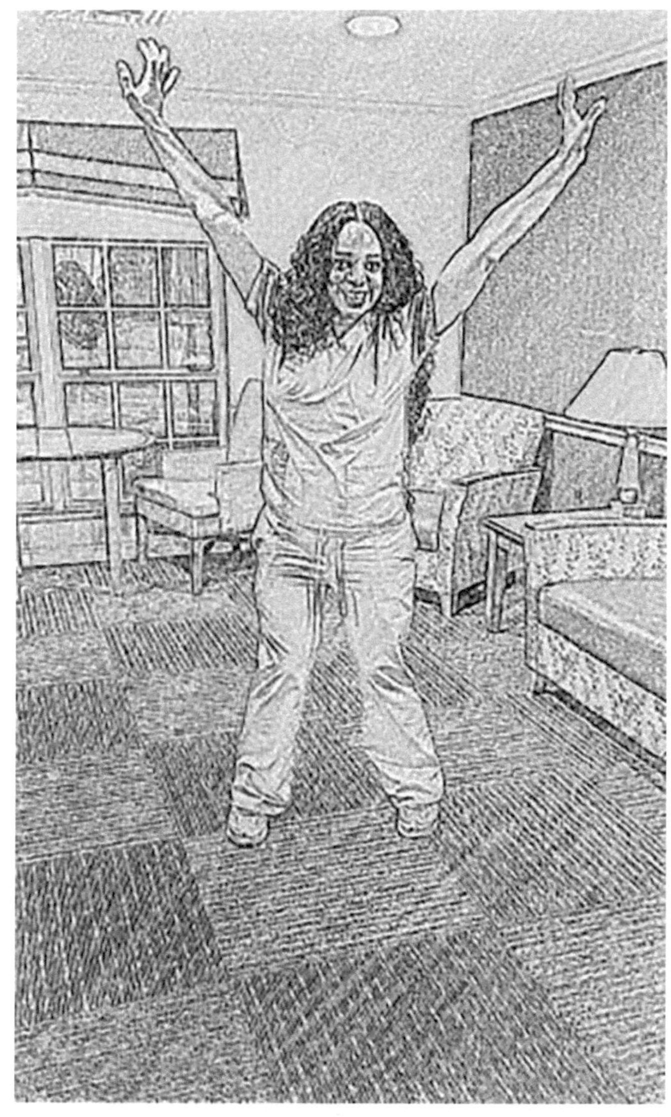

I Did It!

 Miss Asondra StarN'air

The Scriptures

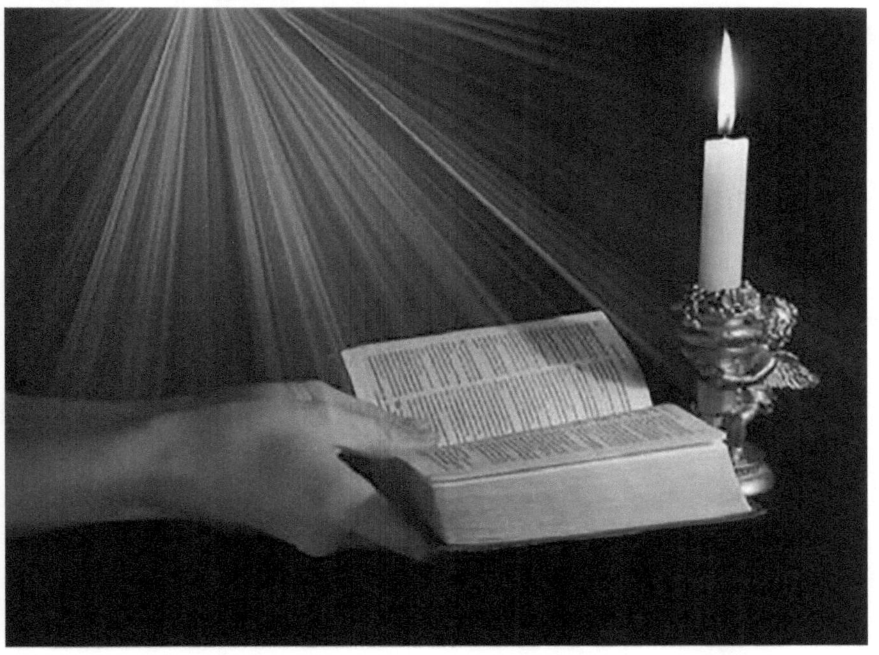

Caregivers, listen, Thy word is a lamp unto our feet, a light that will protect and guide us, **"In God We Trust"** Psalms 119:105
Never Ever Give Up!

My Favorite Scriptures!

Found in the book of ______________ The Scripture _______________________
Notes: ____
Found in the book of ______________ The Scripture _______________________
Notes: ____
Found in the book of ______________ The Scripture _______________________
Notes: ____
Found in the book of ______________ The Scripture _______________________
Notes: ____
Found in the book of ______________ The Scripture _______________________
Notes: ____
Found in the book of ______________ The Scripture _______________________
Notes: ____
Found in the book of ______________ The Scripture _______________________
Notes: ____
Found in the book of ______________ The Scripture _______________________
Notes: ____
Found in the book of ______________ The Scripture _______________________
Notes: ____
Found in the book of ______________ The Scripture _______________________
Notes: ____
Found in the book of ______________ The Scripture _______________________
Notes: ____
Found in the book of ______________ The Scripture _______________________
Notes: ____
Found in the book of ______________ The Scripture _______________________

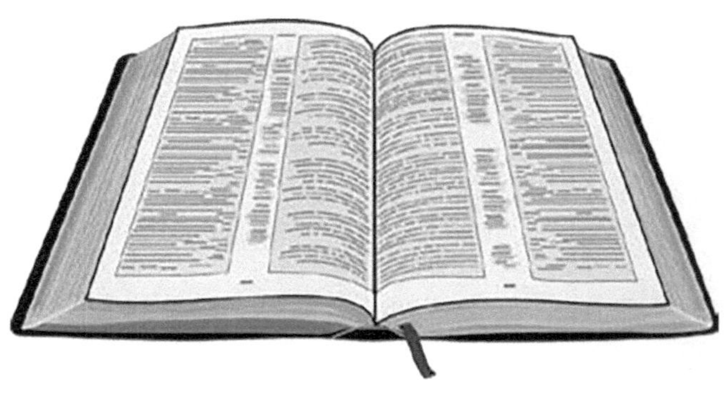

 Miss Asondra StarN'air

My Favorite Scriptures!

Found in the book of _______________   The Scripture _________________________

Notes: ____

Found in the book of _______________   The Scripture _________________________

Notes: ____

Found in the book of _______________   The Scripture _________________________

Notes: ____

Found in the book of _______________   The Scripture _________________________

Notes: ____

Found in the book of _______________   The Scripture _________________________

Notes: ____

Found in the book of _______________   The Scripture _________________________

Notes: ____

Found in the book of _______________   The Scripture _________________________

Notes: ____

Found in the book of _______________   The Scripture _________________________

Notes: ____

Found in the book of _______________   The Scripture _________________________

Notes: ____

Found in the book of _______________   The Scripture _________________________

Notes: ____

Found in the book of _______________   The Scripture _________________________

Notes: ____

Found in the book of _______________   The Scripture _________________________

Notes: ____

Found in the book of _______________   The Scripture _________________________

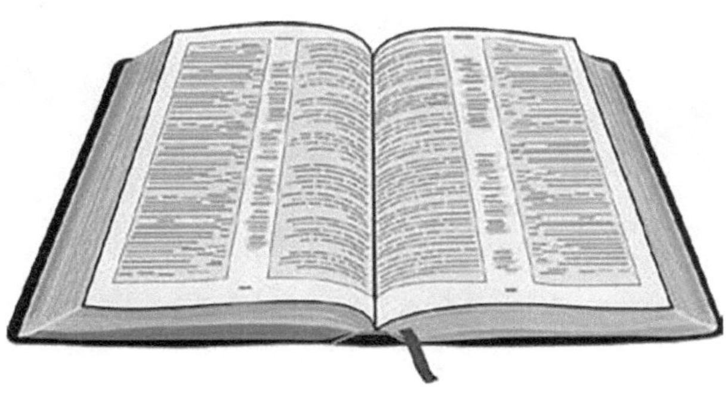

GOD is with YOU!

Your name ____

The Lord is my shepherd; I shall not want.

He maketh me to lie down in green pastures; He leadeth me beside the still waters. He restoreth my soul; He leadeth me in the paths of righteousness for His name's sake. Yea, though I walk through the valley of the shadow of death, I will fear no evil; for Thou art with me; Thy rod and Thy staff, they comfort me. Thou preparest a table before me in the presence of mine enemies; Thou anointest my head with oil; my cup runneth over. Surely goodness and mercy shall follow me all the days of my life; and I will dwell in the house of the Lord forever.

Amen

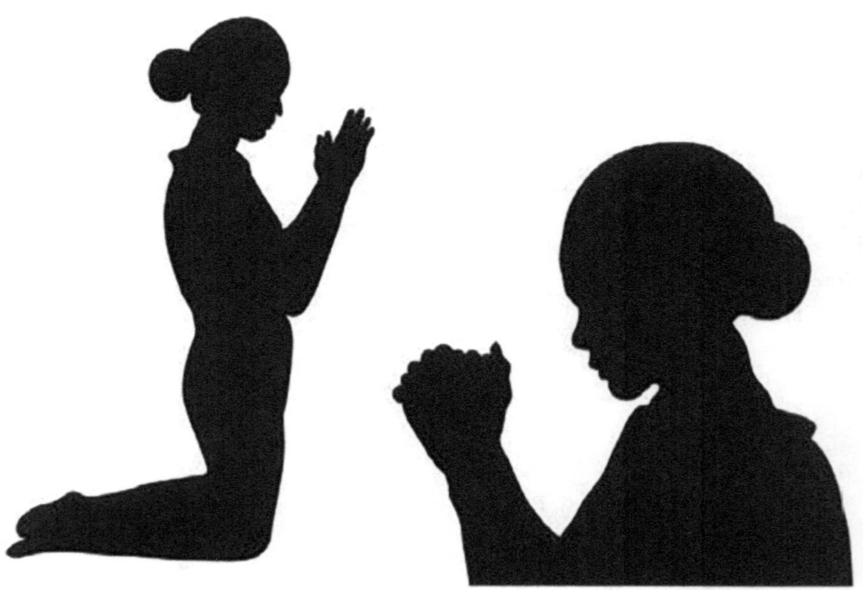

   MISS ASONDRA STARN'AIR

SECTION XI

Life Coach, Therapy Session

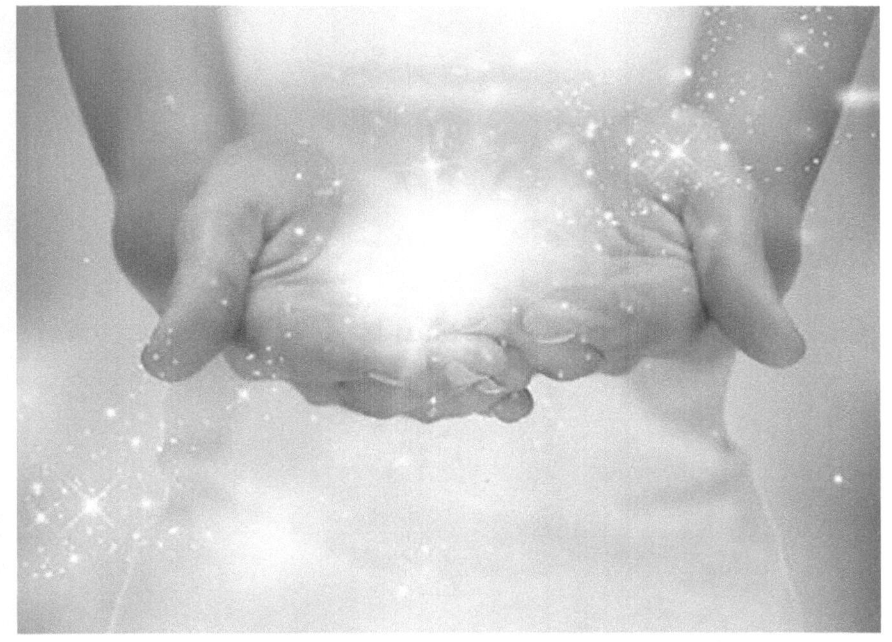

S.O.A.P

Serve Those in Need

Obey God's Word

Apply What You Read

Pray for Understanding

Once we do all that, "Our Hands" will really be clean!

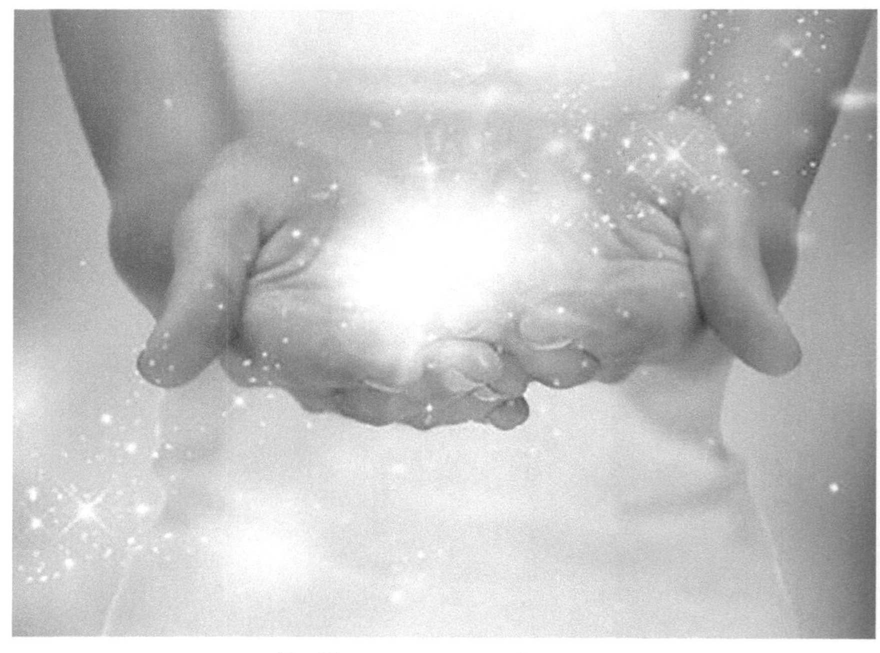

In Jesus name, Amen!

Hello

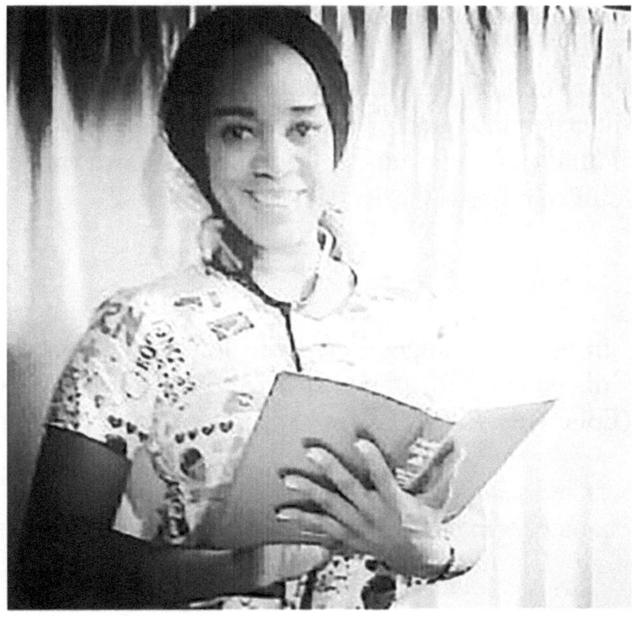

How are we doing so far, I know we have covered a lot, well it is a Caregiver's Bible, I just wanted to make sure you have everything you need to be great, **"Excellent!"** We are **'The New Day Caregivers',** we are not aides anymore, God's opening up new doors. With that being said, we still must deal with everyday life so I have come to you as a oracle of the Lord to encourage **"All Of Humanity"** especially the caregiver to read God's word daily. God gave humans life, but also, He felt it wise to leave behind a manual too, **B**asic **I**nstructions **B**efore **L**eaving **E**arth book. **"The Bible"** was left behind for believers, god's children, you and me, sisters and brothers, black and white and all in-between, in it, it is written that in this world, we are going to have trials and tribulations, no getting around it; but like superman, "to the recuse" God's word is here to help pull us through those troubling and tough times! I have provided some life coaching scriptures that's sure to have you up and running, strong and feeling divine in no time!

Enjoy!

Anxiety

Don't worry about anything; instead, pray about everything.

Tell God what you need, and thank him for all he has done. If you do this, you will experience God's peace, which is far more wonderful than the human mind can understand. His peace will guard your hearts and minds as you live in Jesus Christ. (Philippians 4:6–7)

Anger

And don't sin by letting anger gain control over you; don't let the sun go down while you are still angry, for anger gives a mighty foothold to the devil. (Ephesians 4:26–27)

Dear brothers and sisters, be quick to listen, slow to speak, and to anger. Your anger can never make things right in God's sight. (James 1:19–20)

Bravery

Be strong and courageous, do not be afraid or tremble at them, for the Lord your God is the one who goes with you. He will not fail you or forsake you. (Deuteronomy 31:6–7)

Brokenheartedness

The Lord is close to the brokenhearted. (Psalm 43:18)

Trust in the Lord with all your heart and do not lean on your own understanding. In all your ways acknowledge him, and he will make straight your paths. (Proverbs 3:5–6)

Depression

The Lord hears his people when they call to him for help. He rescues them from all their troubles . . . The righteous face many troubles, but the Lord rescues them from each and every one. (Psalm 34:17, 19)

 MISS ASONDRA STARN'AIR

Death

And, now sisters and brothers, I want you to know what happens to the Christians who have died so you will not be full of sorrow like people who have no hope. For since we believe that Jesus died and was raised to life again, we also believe that when Jesus comes, God will bring back with Jesus all the Christians who died. (Thessalonians 4:13–14)

Eternality

Jesus told her, "I am the resurrection and the life. Those who believe in me, even though they die like everyone else, will live again. They are given eternal life for believing in me and will never perish. (John 11:25–26)

Fear

Don't be afraid, for I am with you. Do not be dismayed, for I am your God. I will strengthen you, I will help you. I will uphold you with my victorious right hand. (Isaiah 41:10)

THEY do not fear bad news; they confidently trust the LORD to care for them, They are confident and fearless and can face their foes triumphantly. (Psalm 112:7–8)

For YOU are my hiding place; you protect me from trouble. You surround me with songs of victory. (Psalm 32:7)

Frustration

Patient endurance is what you need now, so you will continue to do God's will. Then you will receive all that he promised. (Hebrews 10:36)

Guilt

"Come now and let us argue this out," says the LORD. "No matter how deep the stain of your sin, I can remove it, I can make you as clean as freshly fallen snow. Even if you are stained as red as crimson, I can make you as white as wool." (Isaiah 1:18)

And I will forgive their wrongdoings, and I will never again remember their sins. (Hebrews 8:12)

Healing

In one of the villages, Jesus met a man with an advanced case of leprosy. When the man saw Jesus, he fell to the ground, face down in the dust, begging to be healed, Lord "he said "if you want to, you can make me well again."

Jesus reached out and touched the man." I want to." he said "Be healed!" And instantly the leprosy disappeared. (Luke 5:12–13)

Confess your sin to each other and pray for each other so that you may be healed; the earnest prayer of a righteous person has great power and wonderful results. (James 5:13–16)

Impatience

BE STILL in the presence of the LORD, and wait patiently for him to act. Don't worry about evil people who prosper or fret about their wicked schemes. (Psalm 37:7)

Insecurity

I am holding you by your right hand—I the LORD your God. And I say to you "Do not be afraid, I am here to help you." (Isaiah 41:13)

What can we say about such wonderful things as these? If God is for us who can be against us? Since God did not spare even his Son but gave him up for all, won't God, who gave up Christ, also give us everything else? (Romans 8:31–32)

Insult

God bless those who are persecuted because they live for God, for the Kingdom of Heaven is theirs.

God blesses you when you are mocked and persecuted and lied about because you are my followers. Be happy about it! Be very glad! For a great reward awaits you in heaven, And remember, the ancient prophets were persecuted too . . .

But I say, love your enemies! Pray for those who persecute you! In that way, you will be acting as true children of your Father in heaven. For he gives his sunlight to both evil and the good, and he sends rain on the just and on the unjust too. (Matthew 5:10–12, 44–55)

Jealousy

But if you are bitterly jealous and there is selfish ambition in your heart, don't brag about being wise, that is the worst kind if lie. For jealousy and selfishness are not God's kind of wisdom. Such things are earthly, unspiritual and motivated by the Devil. For wherever there is jealousy and selfish ambition m there you will find disorder and ever kind of evil. (James 3:14–16)

So don't be dismayed when the wicked grow rich, and their homes become splendid. For when they die, they carry nothing with them. their wealth will not follow them into the grave. (Psalm 49:16–17)

Loneliness

"For the mountains may depart and the hills disappear, but even then I will remain loyal to you. My covenant of blessing will never be broken," says the LORD, who has mercy on you. (Isaiah 54:10)

No I will not abandon you as orphans—I will come to you. (John 14:18)

Low Self–Esteem

As God's messenger, I give each of you this warning. Be honest in your estimate of yourself, measuring your value by how much faith God has given you. Just as our bodies have many parts and each part has a special function, so it is with Christ's body. We are all parts of his own body, and each of us has different work to do. And since we are all one body of Christ, we belong to each other, and each of us needs all the others. (Romans 12:3–5)

Pain

For our present troubles are quite small and won't last long. Yet they produce for us an immeasurably great glory that will last forever! . . .

I have received wonderful revelations from God. But to keep me from getting puffed up, I was given a thorn in my flesh, a messenger from satin to torment me and keep me from getting proud. Three different times I begged the Lord to take it away, each time he said, "My gracious favor is all you need. My power works best in your weakness, So no I am glad to boast about my weaknesses, so that the power of Christ may work through me, since I know it is all for Christ's good. I am quite content with my weaknesses and with insults, hardships, persecutions, and calamities. For when I am weak, then I am strong. (2 Corinthians 4:17; 12:7–10)

Sickness

The Lord nurses them when they are sick and eases their pain and discomfort. (Psalm 41:3)

You must serve only the Lord your God. if you do, I will bless you with food and water, and I will keep you healthy. There will be no miscarriages or infidelity (sex outside of marriage) among your people, and I will give you long and full lives. (Exodus 23:25–26)

Temptation

God *blesses* the people who patiently endure testing. Afterward, they will receive the crown of life that God has promised to those who love him. And remember, no one who wants to do wrong should ever say, "God is tempting me." God is never tempted to do wrong, and he never tempts anyone either . . . so humble yourself before God. Resist the devil and he will flee from you. (James 1:12–13; 4:7)

But REMEMBER that the temptations that come into your life are no different from what other experience. And God is faithful. He will keep the temptation from becoming so strong that you can't stand up against it. When you are tempted, he will show you a way out so that you will not give in to it. (1 Corinthians 10:13)

Weariness

Then Jesus said, "come to me all of you who are weary and carry heavy burdens, and I will give you rest. Take my yoke upon you. Let me teach you, because I am humbled and gentle, and you will find rest for your souls. For my yoke fits perfectly, and my burden I give you is light. (Matthew 11:28–30)

But those who wait on the Lord will find new strengths. They will fly high on wings like eagles. They will run and not grow weary. They will walk and not faint. (Isaiah 40:31)

Worry

You will keep in perfect peace all who trust in you, whose thoughts are fixed on you! Trust in the LORD always, for the LORD GOD is the "Eternal Rock." (Isaiah 26:3–4)

Give all your worries and cares to God, for he cares about what happens to you. (1 Peter 5:7)

Then turning to his disciples, Jesus said, "So I tell you, don't worry about everyday life—whether you have enough food to eat or clothes to wear. For life consists of far more than food or clothing. Look at the ravens. They don't need to plant or harvest or put food in barns because God feeds them. And you are far more valuable to him than any birds! Can all your worry add a single moment to your life? Of course not! And if worry can't do little things like that, what's the use in worrying over bigger things? Look at the lilies and how they grow. They don't work or make their clothing, yet Solomon in all his glory was not dressed as beautiful as they are. And if god cares so wonderfully for flowers that are here today and gone tomorrow, won't he more surely care for you? You have so little faith!" (Luke 12:22–28)

Wait, There's More!

Friendship

Whoever walk with the wise will become wise; whoever walks with the fools will suffer harm.

DON'T be selfish; don't live to make a good impression on others. Be humble, thinking of others as better than yourself. Don't think only about your affairs, but be interested in others, too, and what they are doing. (Philippians 2:3–4)

Injustice

In his Kingdom God called you to his eternal glory by means of Jesus Christ. After you have suffered as little while, he will restore, support, and strengthen you. and he will place you on a firm foundation. All power is his forever and ever. Amen. (1 Peter 5:10–11)

Love

I have love you even as the Father has loved me. Remain in my love. When you obey me, you remain in my love, just as I obey my Father and remain in his love. I have told you this so you will be filled with my joy. Yes, your joy will overflow! I command you to love each other in the same way that I love you. And here is how to measure it —the greatest love is shown when people lay down their lives for their friends. You are my friends if you obey me. I no longer call you servants, because a master doesn't confide in servants. Now you are my friend since I told you everything the master has told me. You did not choose me. I chose you. I appointed you to go produce fruit that will last, so that the Father will give you whatever you ask, using my name. (John 15:9–16)

Marriage

And further, you will submit to one another out of reverence for Christ. You wives will submit to your husbands as you do to the Lord . . . and you husbands must love your wives with the same love Christ shows the church. (Ephesians 5:21, 25)

Parents

And now a word to the fathers, don't make your children angry by the way you treat them. Rather, bring them up with the discipline and instructions approved by the Lord. (Ephesians 1:4)

Children

CHILDREN, obey your parents because you belong to the Lord, for this is the right thing to do. "Honor your father and mother." This is the first of the Ten Commandments that ends with a promise. And this is the promise: If you honor your mother and father, "you will live a long life, full of blessing." (Ephesians 1:1–3)

Money Management

Those who love money will never have enough. How absurd to think that wealth brings true happiness! (Ecclesiastes 5:10)

And the same God who takes care of me will supply all your needs from his glorious riches, which have been given us in Christ Jesus. (Philippians 4:19)

Owe nothing to anyone except love one another, for he who loves his neighbor has fulfilled the law. (Romans 13:8)

Just as the rich rule the poor, so the borrower is servant to the lender. (Proverbs 22:7)

For where your treasure is, there your heart will be also. (Matthew 6:21)

Bring the whole tithe into the storehouse, that there may be food in my house. Test me in this says the LORD Almighty, "and see if I will not throw open the floodgates of heaven and pour out so much blessing that there will not be room enough to store it. (Matthew 3:10)

Debt

Keep out of debt and owe no man anything, except to love one another; for he who loves his neighbor [who practices loving others] has fulfilled the Law [relating to one's fellowmen, meeting all its requirements]. (Romans 13:8)

When the Lord your God blesses you as He promised you, then you shall lend to many nations, but you shall not borrow; and you shall rule over many nations, but they shall not rule over you. (Deuteronomy 1:6)

But don't begin until you count the cost. For who would begin construction of a building without first getting estimates and then checking to see if there is enough money to pay the bills? (Luke 14:28)

Trust

Trust in the lord with all your heart; do not depend on your own understanding. Seek his will in all that you do, and he will direct your path. (Proverbs 3:5–6)

     Miss Asondra StarN'air

Faith

So then Faith come by hearing and hearing by the word of God. Roman 10:17

Simply put, read your bibles daily, get in a good Bible-living and teaching church.

Truly I tell you if you had faith as small as a mustard seed, you can say to this mountain, move from here to there and it will move. (Matthew 17:19)

Born Again

Jesus replied. "I assure you, unless you are born again, you can never see the Kingdom of God . . .

Those who have been born into God's family do not sin, because God's life is in them. So they can't keep on sinning, because they have been born of God. (1 John 3:9)

Finding God

His purpose in all of this was that the nations should seek him after God and perhaps feel their way toward him and find him—though he is not far from anyone of us. For in him we live and move and exist. As one of your own poets says, "We are his offspring." (Acts 17:27–28)

"For I know the plans I have for you," says the LORD, "they are plans for good and not for disaster, to give you a future and a hope. In those days when you pray, I will listen. If you look for me in earnest, you will find me when you seek me." (Jeremiah 29:11–13)

Knowing God

However at that time, when you did not know God, you were slaves to those which by nature are no gods. But now that you have come to know God, or rather to be known by God, how is it that you turn back again to the weak and worthless elemental things, to which you desire to be enslaved all over again? (Galatians 4:8–9)

And this I pray, that your love may abound still more and more in real knowledge and all discernment, so that you may approve the things that are excellent, in order to be sincere and blameless until the day of Christ; having been filled with the fruit of righteousness which comes through Jesus Christ, to the glory and praise of God. (Philippians 1:9–11)

By this the children of God and the children of the devil are obvious: anyone who does not practice righteousness is not of God, nor the one who does not love his brother 1 john 3:10.

Knowing Jesus Christ

But seek first His kingdom and His righteousness, and all these things will be added to you. (Matthew 6:33)

Many will say to Me on that day, "Lord, Lord, did we not prophesy in Your name, and in Your name cast out demons, and in Your name perform many miracles?" And then I will declare to them, "I never knew you; depart from me, you who practice lawlessness." (Matthew 7:22–23)

For the Lord is a great God and a great King above all gods. (Psalm 95:3)

Prayer

But you, when you pray, go into your inner room, close your door and pray to your Father who is in secret, and your Father, who sees what is done in secret, will reward you. And when you are praying, do not use meaningless repetition as the Gentiles do, for they suppose that they will be heard for their many words. So do not be like them; for your Father knows what you need before you ask Him. (Matthew 6:6–9)

If my people, who are called by my name, will humble themselves and pray and seek my face and turn from their wicked ways, then I will hear from heaven, and I will forgive their sin and will heal their land. (2 Chronicles 7:14)

Therefore I tell you, whatever you ask for in prayer, believe that you have received it, and it will be yours. (Mark 11:24)

God's Word Matters!

The name of the Lord is a strong tower; the righteous run into it and are safe. **Proverbs 18:10**

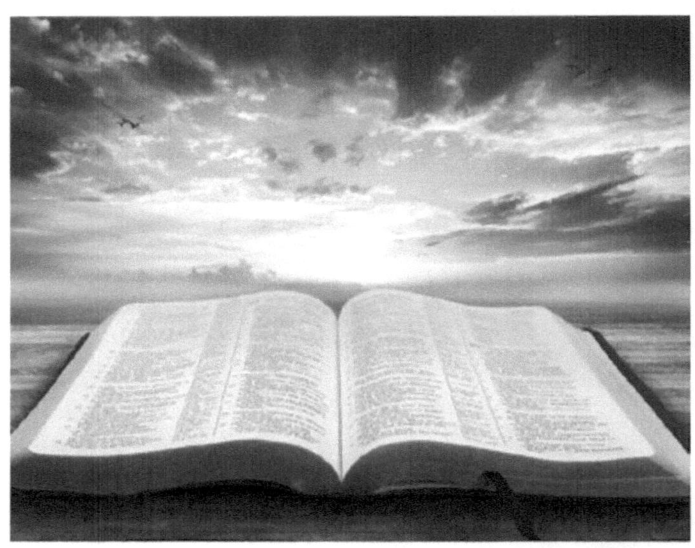

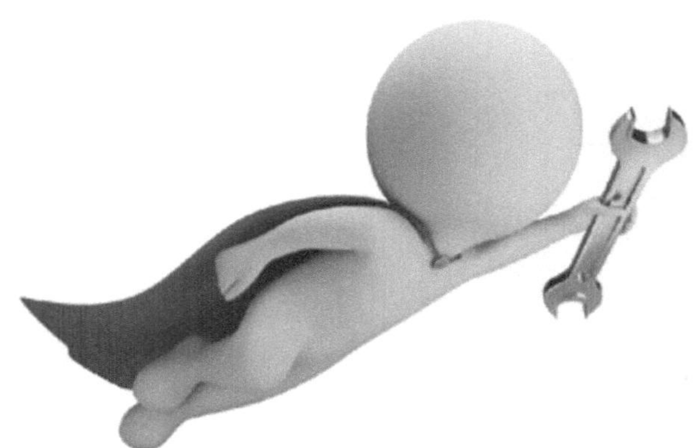

There is Nothing in Your Life God Can't Fix Always Remember This! "NOTHING".

SECTION XII

First Time Moms

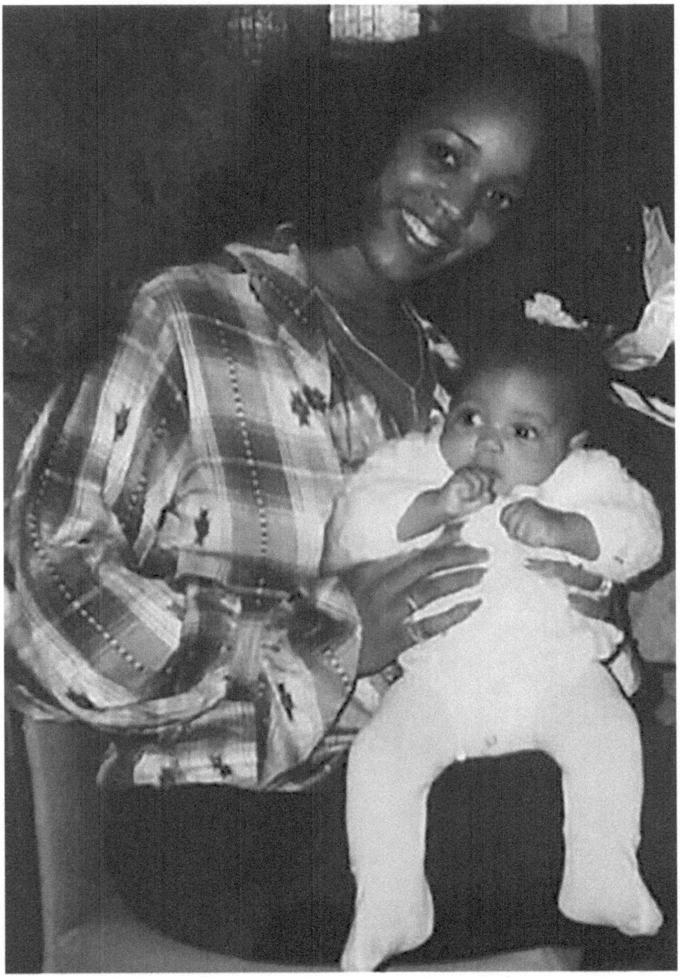

And Dad's

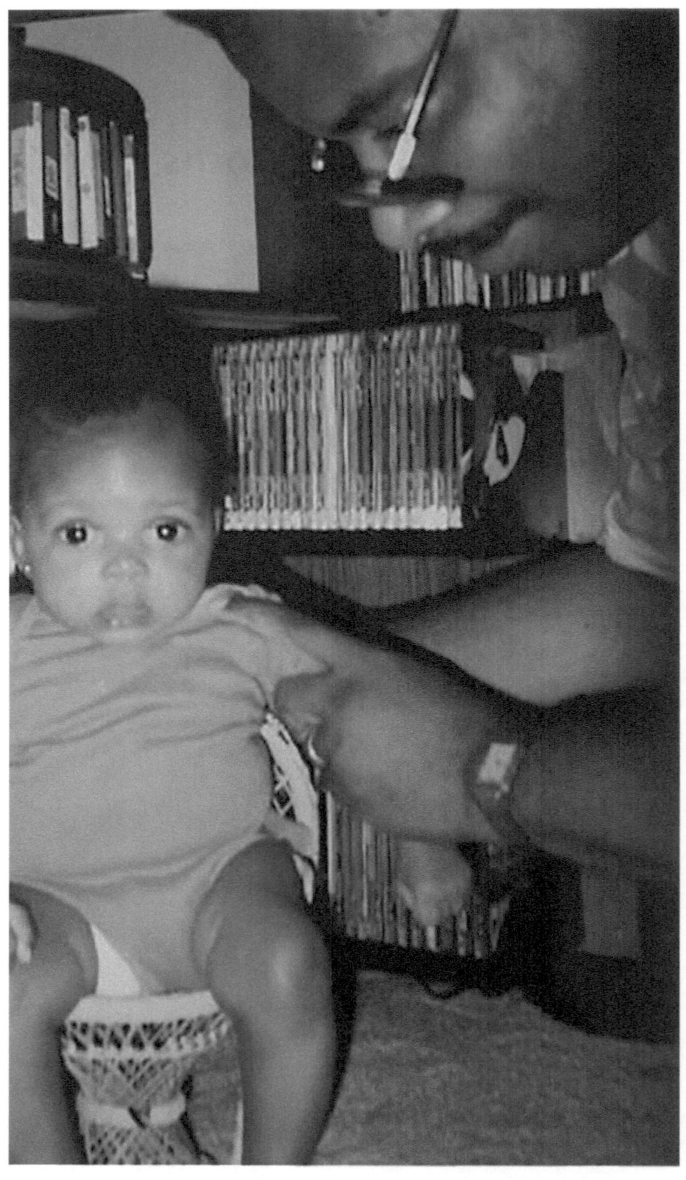

 Miss Asondra StarN'air

Moms To Be

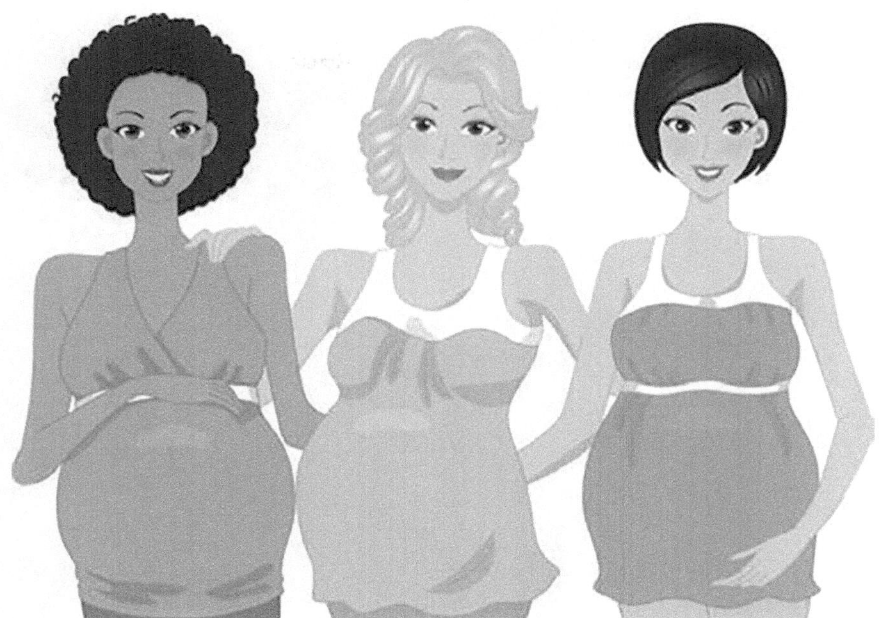

Choose **Life!**

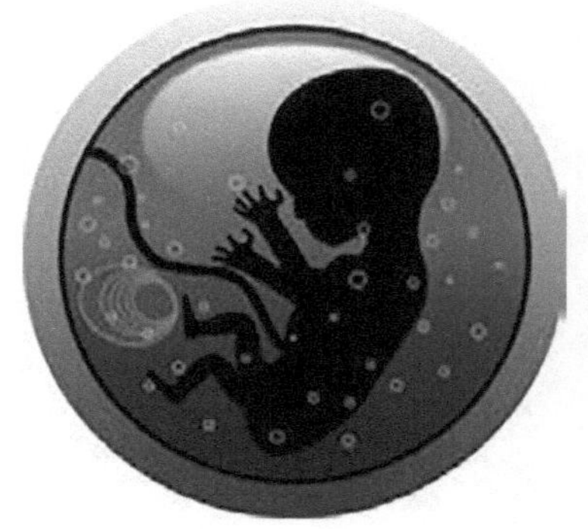

L_{et}

I_{nfants come down}

F_{ull term to}

E_{arth}

 Miss Asondra StarN'air

First-Time Moms and Dads

Welcome, welcome, welcome to the world of caregiving!

If you are a mom or dad, you are a caregiver too I want to welcome you. This book is packed with a lot of information. Just take want you need and leave the rest until you are ready to explore other areas of caregiving. Being a first-time parent, you are about to embark on a lifetime journey that's not only rewarding but fun too.

It is my hope that you educate yourself on the stages of development, also known as life span. It's an in-depth study on the entire life span of an individual, starting from birth to death. It also helps caregivers deal and understand various illnesses and options.

It is also very important, parents, that you understand, **"YOU"** have a child now, and things are going to be different. So make all the necessary adjustments as soon as possible.

If you are married—and I hope you are—help each other.

- Make sure there is a balance there because it's going to take both of you.

- Eat smart, give up on junk food.

- Moms get plenty of rest, when the baby rest, **'YOU REST'**!

- If you are a single mom, **"You Can Do It!"** God will help you!

- Each day pray for guidance.

- Make it your goal to be excellent at what you do. Again, parents welcome to the world of care giving!

First-Time Mom

Becoming a first-time mom can be exciting as well as overwhelming.

You are about to be a caregiver too. This baby will rely on **YOU** to provide for all its needs. But relax and rest assured you are not alone. This section of the book was created just for you. Inside it ladies you will find so many wonderful things to help make becoming a first time new mom, a lot easier. Congratulations on your new baby!

Enjoy Your Little Ones!

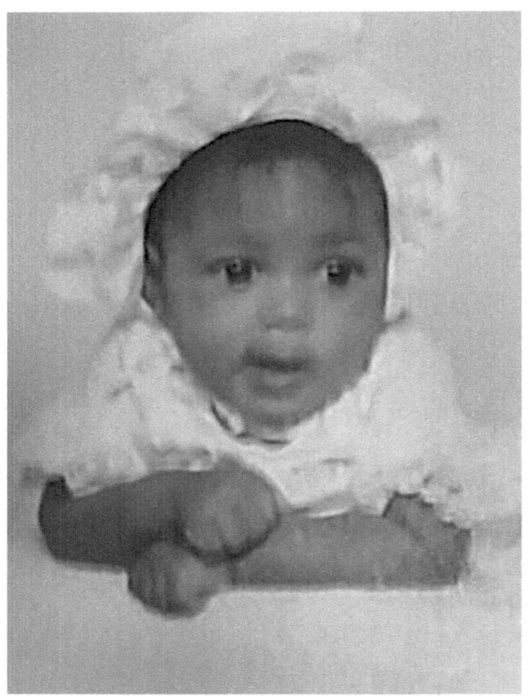

 Miss Asondra StarN'air

Circle: Is it a Boy or Girl?

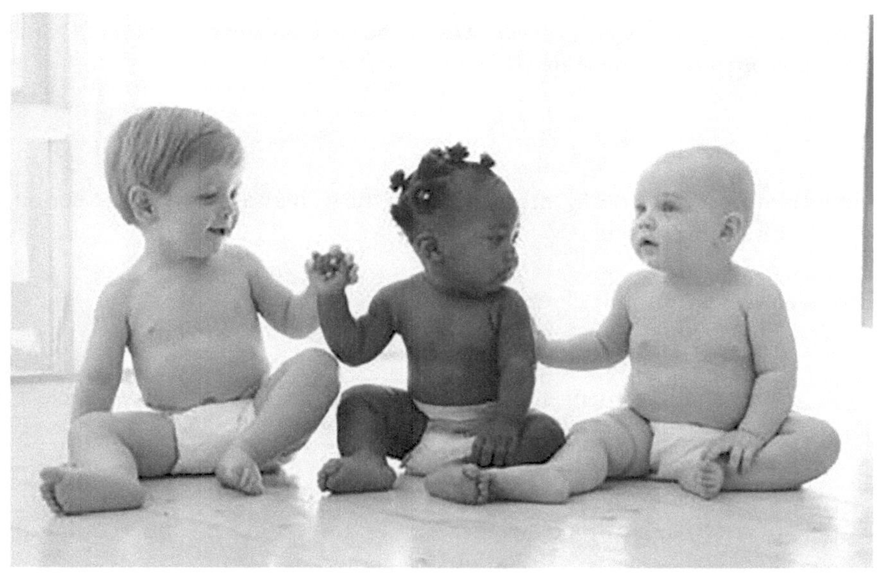

The Stages OF Pregnancy

The typical pregnancy last 40 weeks from the first day of your last menstrual period to birth of the neonate (Baby)

It is divided into 3 stages called Trimesters

First Trimester - 12th week, early changes in the woman's body. Missed period along with other changes.

Physical and emotional changes

- Extreme fatigue
- Breast enlargement, tender, nipples may protrude,
- Nausea, morning sickness, throwing up.
- weight gain, or loss
- unusual craving, increased or decreased appetites
- Mood swings, mood swings, mood swings, did I say mood swings!
- Headaches, heartburn, heaviness, happiness

In just 4 weeks your baby is developing

- The Nervous system (brain and spinal cord)
- The heart is forming
- Arms and leg bud are growing
- Your little one is now an embryo and 1/25 of an inch long, it's a baby! pick a name, Life has truly begun. "Let the little baby live, don't abort your unborn child. Just be strong and courageous and place all your love, faith and trust in the Lord, He will work everything out. He does it each and every time, you and your child will be fine. Better Than Fine!

By the end of the 12 weeks, your baby is fully developing, external sex organs shows girl or boy.

Second Trimester – 13 to 28 weeks this trimester you will find easier than the first trimester. Your morning sickness, and fatigue may lessen or completely go away, but remember, it is still very important that you rest. In this trimester you will get what we call "A baby bump," you will start to show a little. You may notice other body changes too.

   Miss Asondra StarN'air

Body Changes Due to Pregnancy

- Aches and Pains
- darkening around the skin of your nipples
- Itching on the abdomen, palms and sole of feet.
- patches of darker skin, usually over the cheeks, forehead, nose or upper lip.
- Stretch marks on your breast, buttocks or thighs.
- Longer and thicker hair or the opposite, lose hair.
- Longer and stronger nails
- Become tired easily **(REST)**
- More weight gain. Alert! If you are gaining or losing weight rapidly call your doctor immediately, this could be a sign of something more serious going on.

At 16 weeks your little one is still developing and getting stronger!

- The Musculoskeletal system continues to form.
- Your baby begins sucking
- Its skin is forming and is nearly translucent
- Your baby's meconium develops in his or her intestinal tract. This will be your baby's first bowel movement.

Now your baby is 4 to 5 inches long and still growing it weighs almost 3 ounce.

At 20 weeks baby is still growing, eyelashes, hair, fingernails, are visible they can hear and swallow too now.

By the end of this second trimester, just about everything's in place, including its personality.

Third Trimester—Week 29 until birth.

This is the final stage of pregnancy. In this stage, you may continue to get aches and pains plus some new ones. This is because as the baby grows, more pressure is on your internal organs, which means you may have some difficulty breathing from time to time or find yourself having to urinate more often than usual, I did but this is normal. Once you have the baby, these problems should go away. Hang in there pregnant mom, you're almost there, no worries, no fears, don't be scared, God is with you, *He's* there.

Some More Discomforts and Changes:

- Swelling in face, fingers, ankles.
- Hemorrhoids.
- Breasts may be very tender and may leak a watery pre-milk called colostrum.
- Protruding belly.
- The baby is moving lower in your abdomen, known as "dropping."
- Contractions, which can be real or false labor.
- Heartburn.
- Shortness of breath (SOB) and difficulty sleeping.

Other Changes as the Due Date Approaches (DDA)

Your cervix becomes thinner and softer in a process called effacement, which helps the cervix open during childbirth.

At thirty-two weeks, your baby is still not done growing. God is making sure all the organs and vital minerals, such as iron and calcium, are being distributed.

- Bones are still growing; they are soft but fully formed.
- Eyes can now open and close; sleeping pattern is established too.
- Your baby is gaining about ½ pound a week and is about 15 to 17 inches long.
- More things are happening too. Lungs are still developing, and fine hair is falling off.

Hang in there! Eight more weeks to go . . .

Finally, you are approaching your due date and are now between thirty-seven and forty weeks. By the end of week 37, your baby is considered full-term:

- Your baby's organs are capable of functioning on their own.
- Your baby may now turn into a head position, ready to be born.

- Average birth weight is 6 pounds, 2 ounces to 9 pounds, 2 ounces.
- Average length 19 to 21 inches. But "healthy babies" come in many weights and sizes, so don't be alarmed if they are not in the normal range.

Congratulations!

You are a brand-new mom and dad! Enjoy your new bundle of joy!
Welcome to the world of caregiving.
Let Jesus lead the way!

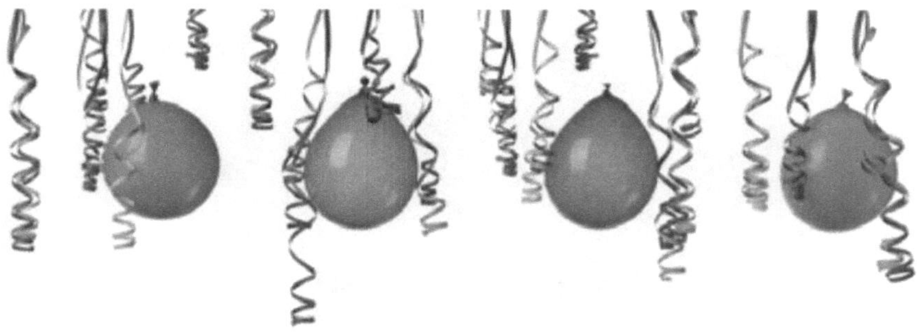

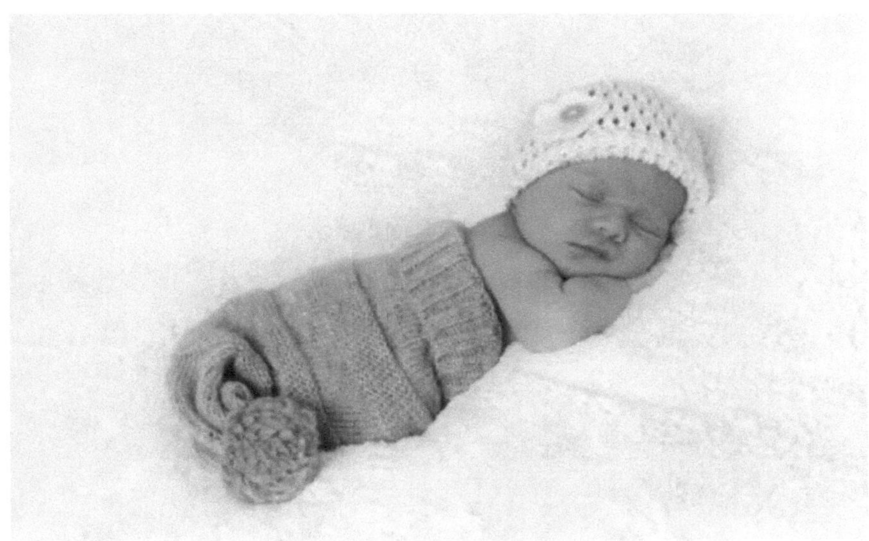

New Mom, New Baby, Both Adjusting!

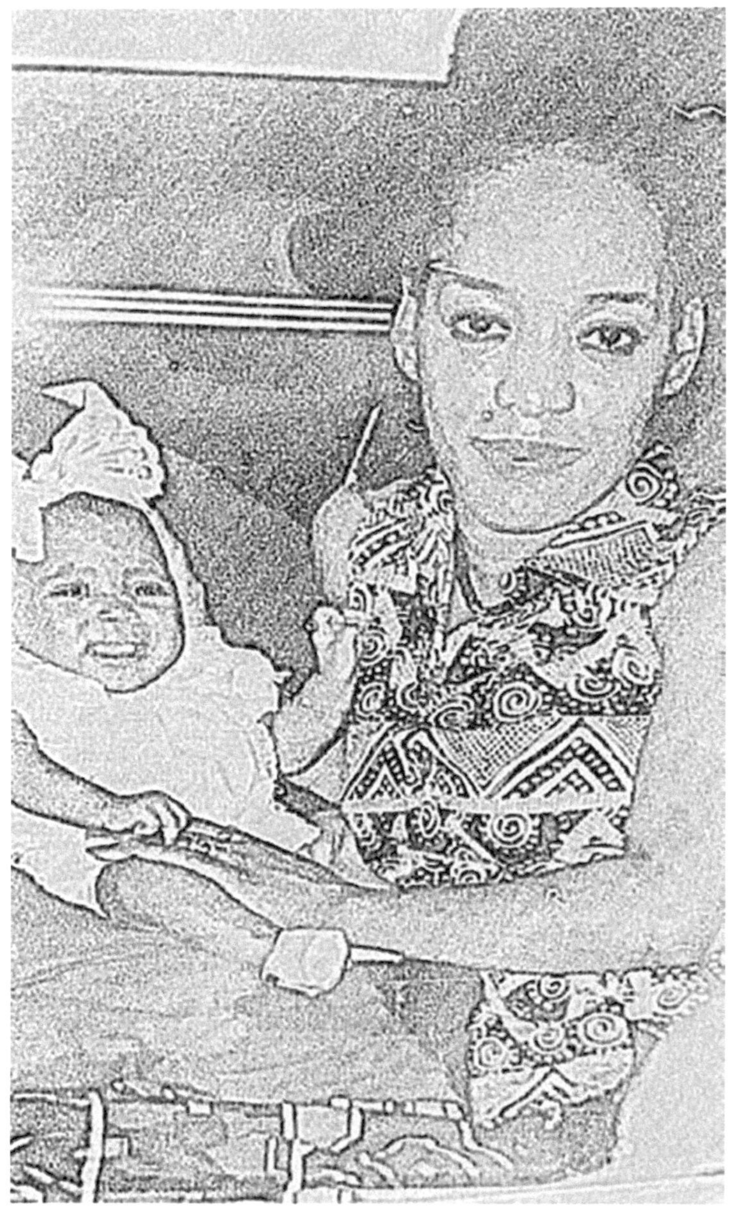

 Miss Asondra StarN'air

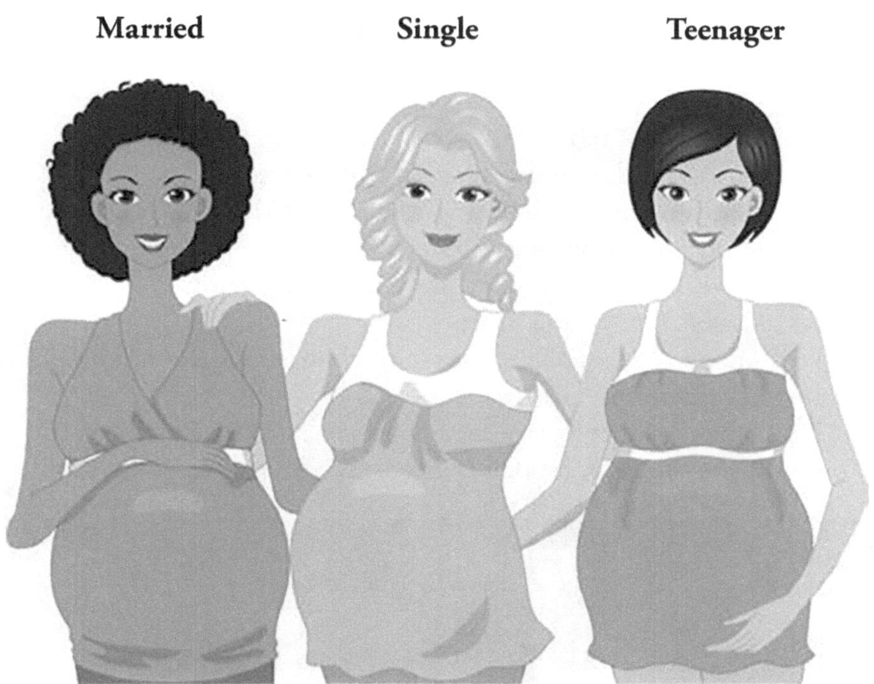

Affirmations for First-Time Moms

"I Will" Affirmations for New Moms

1. I will be the best mom ever.
2. I will do all it takes to ensure a good life for my child.
3. I will use biblical principles and discipline with my child.
4. I will find a good Bible-teaching family-church home.
5. I will make being an excellent mom my first priority.
6. I will invest in my child's future.
7. I will choose a respectable name for my child, strong and meaningful.
8. I will keep my child clean and safe.
9. I will open a savings account now for my child's education.
10. I will be a good role model. In my home, we will serve the Lord!

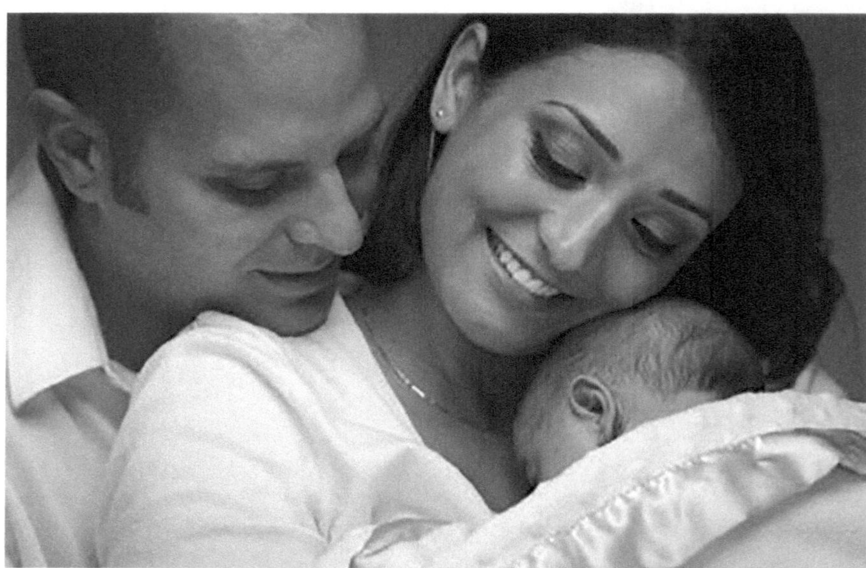

 Miss Asondra StarN'air

Affirmation for Teenage Moms or under 21

1. I will get my priorities straight, I will become a great parent.
2. I will not take advantage of my parents. I will learn to care and raise my child myself. I made the child, I take care of the child.
3. I will not feel like a failure, I will use this unplanned pregnancy as an opportunity to turn my life around and be the best mom ever.
4. I will still get my education and go to college if I so choose, I still have a great future and so does my child.
5. I will change my priorities now, I will no long hand out in the streets, I will commit to raising child whole heartedly.
6. I will reframe from having sex outside of marriage from now on, I will wait until I'm married.
7. I will now look to God to guide me and my child.
8. I will put away childish ways, grow up and start making smarter decision moving forward.
9. I will not hang out with anyone who does not want to live for God anymore.
10. Today I will cut some people out of my life, but wish them well, so that I can be all God has called me to be.

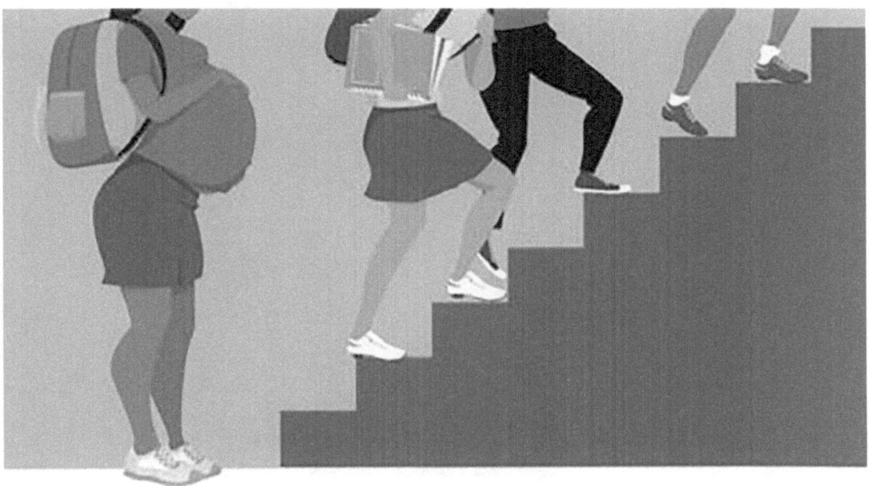

Affirmations for Single Moms

1. I will raise my child with the help of the Almighty.
2. I will look to Jesus to be the missing parent.
3. I will reframe from sex outside of marriage.
4. I will forgive those who hurt or abandoned me.
5. I will raise my child using biblical principles along with discipline.
6. I will rearrange my life in a way that makes it smarter and easier on both me and my child.
7. I will bless the Lord at all times His praise shall continually be in my mouth.
8. I will not allow worldly men to come in on me and my child. As for me and my house, we shall serve the Lord.
9. I will choose a job/career that has benefits and flexibility.
10. I will not give up on excellence. My family's future looks bright. With God on our side, who can be against us? ***"Nobody"!***

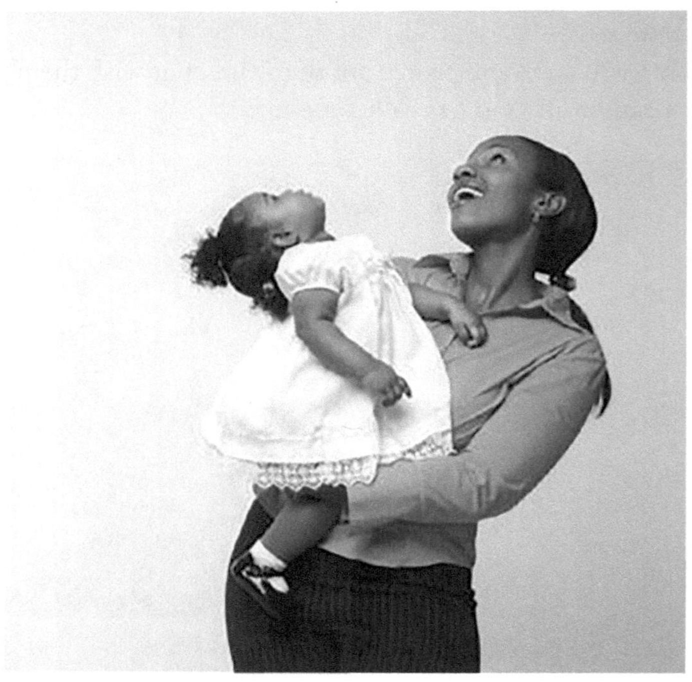

 MISS ASONDRA STARN'AIR

Tips on choosing a baby name

- Make sure it means some-thing positive.
- Make it sing, a powerful note.
- Simplify the spelling, but make it original too.
- Keep with powerful tradition.
- Look at the initials; create a smooth blend.
- Ask yourself if your child would be proud of the name.
- Can your child build upon that name? Is it powerful and inspiring?
- Is it a name of respect?
- Does it sound great coming off your tongue?
- Does the name make you and others smile or proud?
- Try it out on your friends and family; see and hear their response.
- Select ten names and pray on them. Ask God to help pick the perfect name for your child.
- Consider your baby's daddy; you both decide. Don't leave him out. It's his child too.
- Write it down; see how it looks on paper.
- Choose one you love.
- Finally, make your choice!

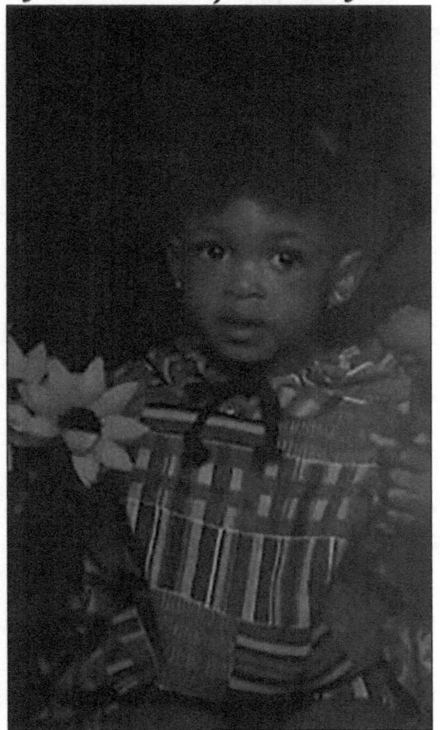

My Jazzy Jazz!

Jazz Adonna Njeri' Akili Jones

My daughter at age 2

What Every Child Needs to Thrive

- God fearing parents
- Good nutritious food
- Positive environments/ shelter
- Adequate sleep
- Exercise/playtime
- Immunizations
- Godly righteous leadership in the home
- Safe and secure surrounding
- Love, love, and more love
- Activities and social stimulations
- Supportive teachers and caregivers
- Education and opportunities to thrive/achieve
- Attention and companionship
- Appropriate guidance and discipline
- Good role models, **"Family Matters"**
- Taught about God/Jesus
- The consequence of deception and thievery
- Room to grow and develop
- Respect
- To be listened and talked to
- Understanding and Guidance
- Healthy "Nourished" good growth and development
- Respect the word **"NO"**
- Respect and honor parents and authority
- "You" the parent/caretaker
- To know they are loved!

Three Infant Temperaments

1. **Easy Babies:** Positive disposition
2. **Difficult Babies:** Negative moods, slow to adapt to new situation
3. **Slow to Warm Babies:** inactive, calm reaction to environment, negative moods and they withdraw from situations.

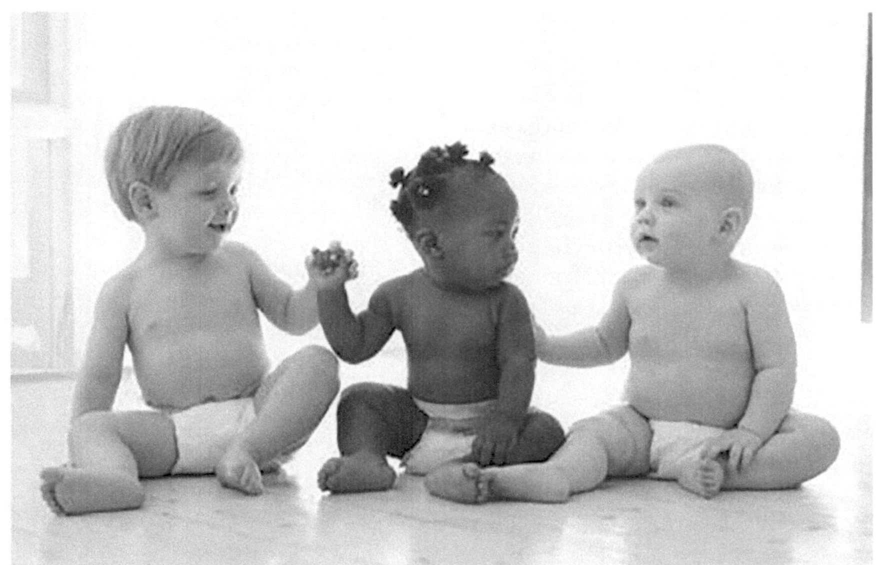

CPR for Infants and Children

If you are alone with the unconscious infant give 2 minutes of **CPR** before calling 911.

Time is of the essence when dealing with **CPR** especially for infants, permanent brain damage or death can occur within minutes if a baby's blood flow stops. So no time to be scared to do **CPR**, you MUST do **CPR**! Many times the need for **CPR** happens after drowning, suffocation, Chocking, and in children it may be due to some other injuries.

CPR involves Rescue Breathing, which provides oxygen to the lungs and Chest compressions, that helps keep the blood flowing.

Anyone working with children should be certified, anyone who is a parent too, should be certified. And anyone who is neither should be certified!

CPR saves lives, we never know in life what we may be faced with, mightiest well be prepared to help The **Zero** and be a **Hero**!

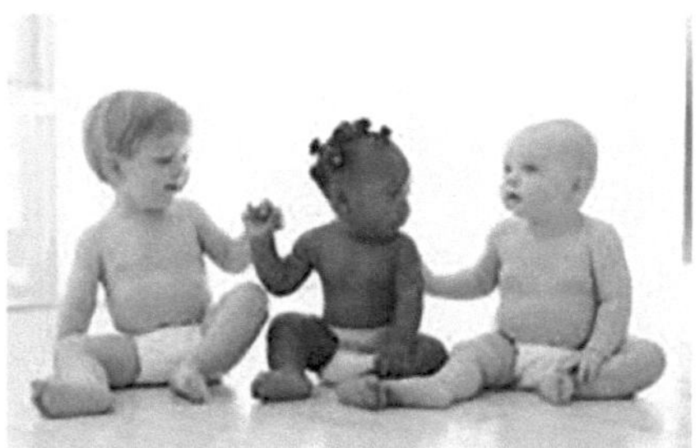

You can do it CPR

First do the **3 C's** Check the scene
Check the victim
Call for help

Second if the child is not responding Put phone on speaker mode **LISTEN** to disputer, Start **CPR**

If you do not have a phone, here's what you do.

1. **Shout and tap** if the child does not respond, isn't breathing or is breathing but not normal. position the baby on its back and start **CPR**
2. Give 30 gentle chest compressions at a rate of 100 to -120 / minutes. Use two of three fingers, place those fingers directly in the center of the child's chest just below the nipples. Now press down about one – third the depth of the chest, which is about 1 and a half inches.
3. Open the air way by tilting the head back, lift the chin up. Gently do not tilt the child head back too far.
4. If the chest doesn't rise, open airway again and repeat all **CPR** steps until help arrives. We are caregivers we **MUST** help save lives.
5. Just remember to stay:
Calm, Cool and Collected
"You Got This!"

You Can Do It!

Things for First Time Mom!

FIRST TIME MOM'S CHECKLIST

Infant Care

Nursing/Feeding
- Bottles (5-8)
- Bottle Warmer
- Bottle Brush
- Dishwasher Caddy
- Extra Nipples
- Bottle Sterilizer
- Bottle Drying Rack
- Insulated Tote
- Breast Pump
- Nursing Accessories (Pads, Storage Bags)
- Nursing Pillow or Boppy
- Burp Cloths (8-12)
- Bibs (8-12)
- Pacifiers (3-5)

Baby/Care
- Parenting Books
- Rattles
- Teethers
- Grooming Kit (Nail Clippers, Brush, Comb)
- Thermometer
- First Aid Kit
- Humidifier/Vaporizer
- Diaper Pail
- Monitor

Bath
- Infant Bathtub
- Hooded Bath Towels (2-4)
- Washcloths (2-4)
- Bath Toys

Diapering Accessories
- Wipes Warmer
- Diaper Bag
- Baby Changing Mat

Baby Gear

Safety
- Cabinet and Door Latches
- Safety Gates
- Outlet Covers
- Car Travel Mirror

Car Seats
- Infant or Convertible Car Seat
- Strap Covers
- Head Support
- Car Seat Toys
- Car Seat Undermat
- Car Sunshade

Strollers
- Stroller or Travel System
- Umbrella Stroller

Entertainers/Swings/Play Yards
- Full-size Swing or Travel Swing
- Jumper
- Stationary Entertainer
- Bouncer/Rocker
- Baby Carrier
- Play Yard
- Play Yard Sheets (2-3)

High Chairs
- High Chair
- Booster Seat
- High Chair Accessories (Splat Mat, Chair Cover)

Nursery

Cradles/Bassinets
- Cradle, Bassinet or Portable Crib
- Cradle, Bassinet or Portable Crib Bedding Set
- Cradle, Bassinet or Portable Crib Sheets (2-3)

Nursery Furniture
- Crib
- Changing Table
- Armoire/Dresser/Chest
- Glider or Rocker
- Ottoman
- Crib Mattress

Bedding/Room Décor
- Crib Bedding Set
- Mattress Pads (2-3)
- Waterproof Crib Pad
- Fitted Crib Sheets (3-5)
- Blankets (3-6)
- Changing Table Pad
- Changing Table Pad Covers (2-4)
- Baskets/Storage Bins (2-4)
- Crib Mobile
- Lamp
- Rug
- Hamper
- Sleep Positioner
- Diaper Stacker
- Hangers

Toys/Gifts

Toys, Books & Music
- Crib Toys
- Playmat
- Books
- DVDs
- CDs
- Activity Toys

Keepsakes
- Baby Book/Photo Album
- Picture Frames

Clothing

(Various Sizes)
- Homecoming Outfit
- Bodysuits (8-10)
- Cap and Bootie Sets (2-4)
- Gowns (3-5)
- Socks
- Baby Mittens
- Sleep 'n Plays (3-6)
- Seasonal Outerwear

Baby **Shower** Invitation

Baby Shower **S**implified! Ask everyone to include a package of diapers and baby wipes with their gifts. You are going to need these more than anything else for the next twelve months.

Load up on these two items—fifty people, fifty packages of diapers and wipes. This will save you hundreds of dollars the first year of your baby's life. Here's a sample title and invite.

> **Diapers, Wipes, and Gift for Baby Shower Celebration!**
> **For:** _________________________
> **Please include these two items with your gift.**
> **Thank you. See you there!**

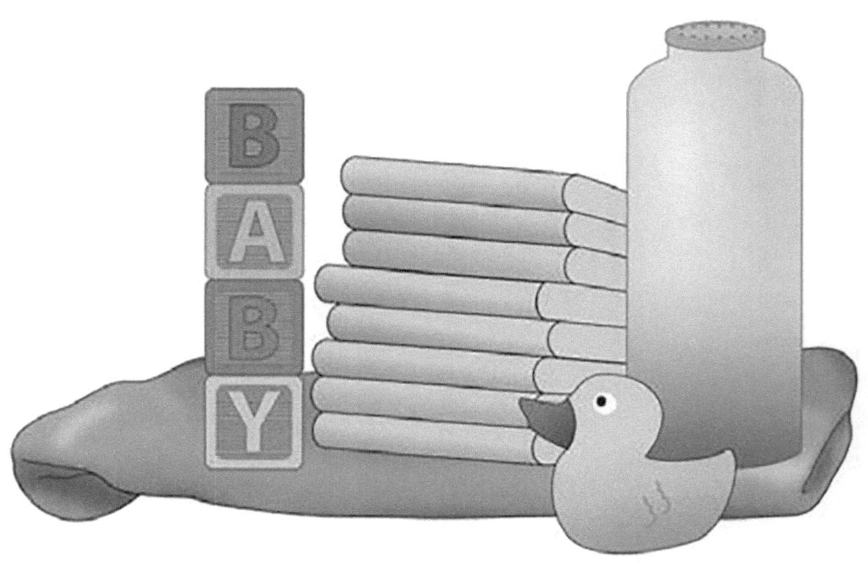

Wish List

Menu

Meats	Vegetables	Fruits
____________	____________	____________
____________	____________	____________
____________	____________	____________
____________	____________	____________

Beverages	Breads	Side Dishes
____________	____________	____________
____________	____________	____________
____________	____________	____________
____________	____________	____________

Host ____

Time and Place ________________________________

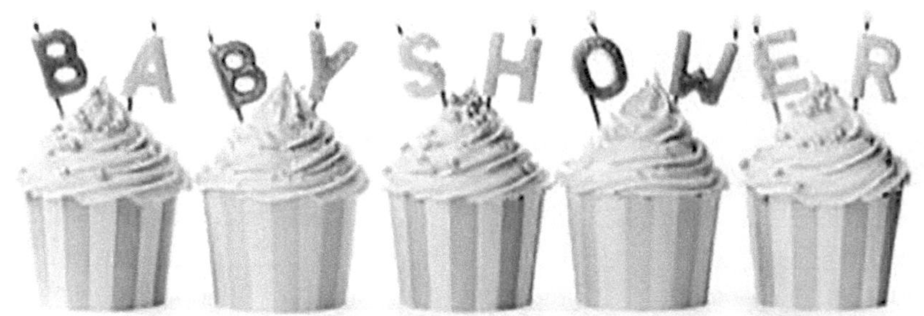

 Miss Asondra StarN'air

Thank-You Gift List

Name	Gift

Spare the Rod, Spoil the Child!

Whoever spares the rod hates their children, but the one who loves their children is careful to discipline them. **Proverbs 13:24**

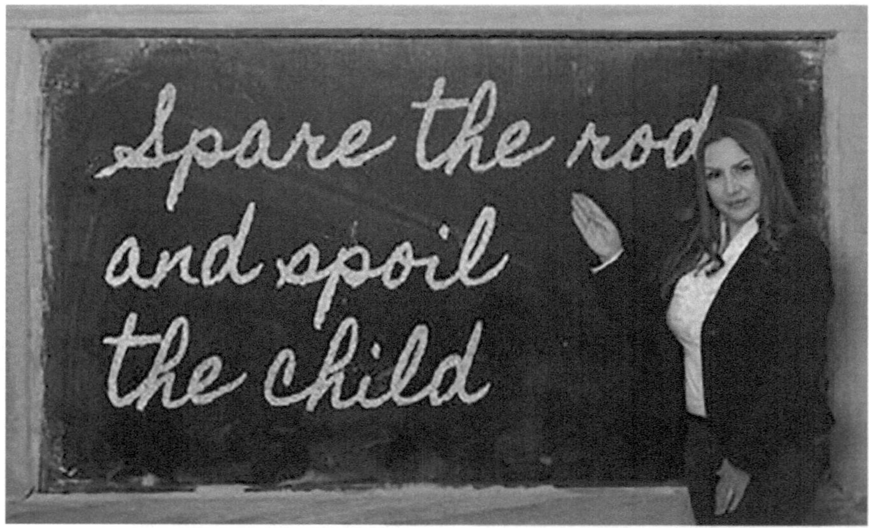

 MISS ASONDRA STARN'AIR

Raising Children God's Way!

Proverbs 13:24
Whoever spares the rod hates his son, but he who loves him is diligent to discipline him.

Colossians 3:21
Fathers, do not provoke your children, lest they become discouraged.

Proverbs 29:17
Discipline your son, and he will give you rest; he will give delight to your heart.

Psalm 127:3–5
Behold, children are a heritage from the Lord, the fruit of the womb a reward. Like arrows in the hand of a warrior are the children of one's youth. Blessed is the man who fills his quiver with them! He shall not be put to shame when he speaks with his enemies in the gate.

Proverbs 22:15
Folly is bound up in the heart of a child, but the rod of discipline drives it far from him.

Psalm 127:3
Behold, children are a heritage from the Lord, the fruit of the womb a reward.

2 Timothy 3:16
All Scripture is breathed out by God and profitable for teaching, for reproof, for correction, and for training in righteousness,

Proverbs 19:18
Discipline your son, for there is hope; do not set your heart on putting him to death.

Proverbs 15:5
A fool despises his father's instruction, but whoever heeds reproof is prudent.

2 Timothy 3:14–17

But as for you, continue in what you have learned and have firmly believed, knowing from whom you learned it and how from childhood you have been acquainted with the sacred writings, which are able to make you wise for salvation through faith in Christ Jesus. All Scripture is breathed out by God and profitable for teaching, for reproof, for correction, and for training in righteousness, that the man of God may be competent, equipped for every good work.

Matthew 19:14

But Jesus said, "Let the little children come to me and do not hinder them, for to such belongs the kingdom of heaven."

1 Timothy 5:8

But if anyone does not provide for his relatives, and especially for members of his household, he has denied the faith and is worse than an unbeliever.

1 Samuel 1:27–28

For this child I prayed, and the Lord has granted me my petition that I made to him. Therefore I have lent him to the Lord. As long as he lives, he is lent to the Lord." And he worshiped the Lord there.

Proverbs 20:11 even a child can makes himself known by his acts, by whether his conduct is pure and upright.

Leviticus 19:29

"Do not profane your daughter by making her a prostitute, lest the land fall into prostitution and the land become full of depravity.

Romans 8:28

And we know that for those who love God all things work together for good, for those who are called according to his purpose.

Isaiah 54:13

All your children shall be taught by the Lord, and great shall be the peace of your children.

3 John 1:4

I have no greater joy than to hear that my children are walking in the truth.

2 Timothy 3:17

That the man of God may be competent, equipped for every good work.

1 Peter 2:20

For what credit is it if, when you sin and are beaten for it, you endure? But if when you do good and suffer for it you endure, this is a gracious thing in the sight of God.

Proverbs 31:27–28

She looks well to the ways of her household and does not eat the bread of idleness. Her children rise up and call her blessed; her husband also, and he praises her:

Matthew 12:33

"Either make the tree good and its fruit good, or make the tree bad and its fruit bad, for the tree is known by its fruit.

Psalm 127:4–5

Like arrows in the hand of a warrior are the children of one's youth. Blessed is the man who fills his quiver with them! He shall not be put to shame when he speaks with his enemies in the gate.

Deuteronomy 21:18–21

"If a man has a stubborn and rebellious son who will not obey the voice of his father or the voice of his mother, and, though they discipline him, will not listen to them, then his father and his mother shall take hold of him and bring him out to the elders of his city at the gate of the place where he lives, and they shall say to the elders of his city, 'This our son is stubborn and rebellious; he will not obey our voice; he is a glutton and a drunkard.' Then all the men of the city shall stone him to death with stones. So you shall purge the evil from your midst, and all Israel shall hear, and fear.

Ephesians 5:1

Therefore be imitators of God, as beloved children.

Jeremiah 29:11

For I know the plans I have for you, declares the Lord, plans for welfare and not for evil, to give you a future and a hope.

Lamentations 2:19

"Arise, cry out in the night, at the beginning of the night watches! Pour out your heart like water before the presence of the Lord! Lift your hands to him for the lives of your children, who faint for hunger at the head of every street."

Luke 2:52

And Jesus increased in wisdom and in stature and in favor with God and man.

Proverbs 23:14

If you strike him with the rod, you will save his soul from Sheol.

1 Samuel 2:26

Now the young man Samuel continued to grow both in stature and in favor with the Lord and also with man.

Malachi 2:15

Did he not make them one, with a portion of the Spirit in their union? And what was the one God seeking? Godly offspring. So guard your-selves in your spirit, and let none of you be faithless to the wife of your youth

Matthew 18:10

"See that you do not despise one of these little ones. For I tell you that in heaven their angels always see the face of my Father who is in heaven.

Deuteronomy 28:32

Your sons and your daughters shall be given to another people, while your eyes look on and fail with longing for them all day long, but you shall be helpless.

Acts 2:17

"'And in the last days it shall be, God declares, that I will pour out my Spirit on all flesh, and your sons and your daughters shall prophesy, and your young men shall see visions, and your old men shall dream dreams;

Isaiah 59:20–21

"And a Redeemer will come to Zion, to those in Jacob who turn from transgression," declares the Lord. "And as for me, this is my covenant with them," says the Lord: "My Spirit that is upon you, and my words that I have put in your mouth, shall not depart out of your mouth, or out of the mouth of your offspring, or out of the mouth of your children's offspring," says the Lord, "from this time forth and forevermore."

Psalm 145:4

One generation shall commend your works to another, and shall declare your mighty acts.

1 Thessalonians 4:1–13

Finally, then, brothers, we ask and urge you in the Lord Jesus, that as you received from us how you ought to walk and to please God, just as you are doing, that you do so more and more. For you know what instructions we gave you through the Lord Jesus. For this is the will of God, your sanctification: that you abstain from sexual immorality; that each one of you know how to control his own body in holiness and honor, not in the passion of lust like the Gentiles who do not know God;...

Psalm 92:1–15

A Psalm. A Song for the Sabbath. It is good to give thanks to the Lord, to sing praises to your name, O Most High; to declare your steadfast love in the morning, and your faithfulness by night, to the music of the lute and the harp, to the melody of the lyre. For you, O Lord, have made me glad by your work; at the works of your hands I sing for joy. How great are your works, O Lord! Your thoughts are very deep!

BABY JOURNAL

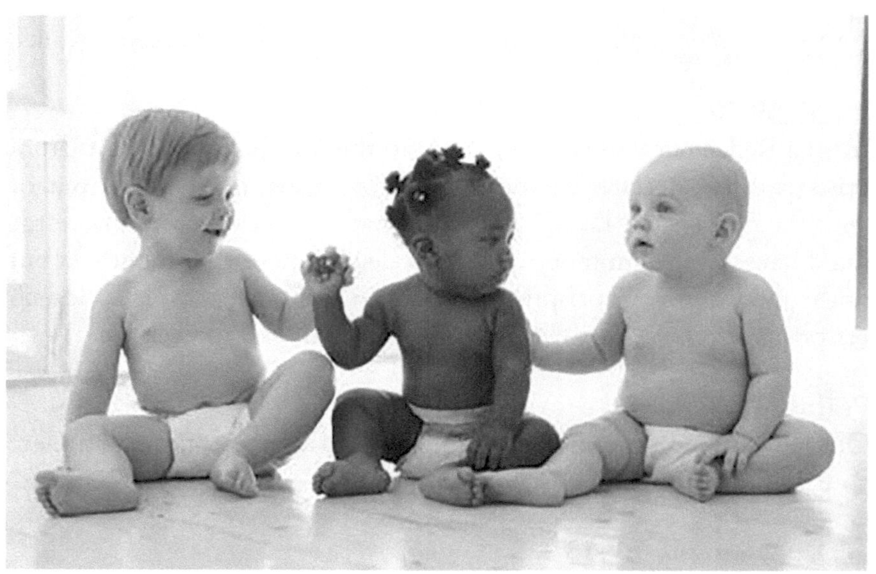

 Miss Asondra StarN'air

Your Child's Body Parts

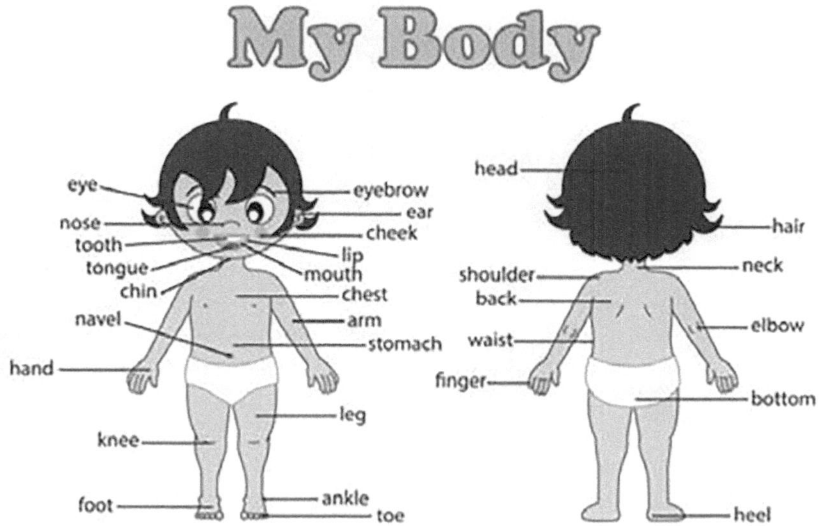

Is Healthy and Strong!

Baby Journal One

Baby's full name ________________ Came to this world on _______________

Born at __________________ Hospital/Other _________________________

United States/Other ____

Weight __________ Ounces __________ Height _________ Eye Color ________

Parents: Mother ___________________ Father _______________________

Godparents are/is____

Morals and values instilled in this child will be ___________________________

____

____

____

____

____

____

____

____

____

____

My role as a parent will be to ______________________________________

____

____

____

____

____

____

____

I vow to make sure ____

____

____

____

____

____

____

The scripture I will use to help me become a Christian caregiver to this child
of God is

____

     Miss Asondra StarN'air

<h3 align="center">Mom's Childbearing Labor Experience Baby One</h3>

How much weight did you gain from this pregnancy? _______________

What was this experience for you like with baby _______________

____

____

____

____

____

____

____

____

____

____

<h3 align="center">Infant Temperament (Circle one)</h3>

Easy Babies 40%	Difficult Babies 10%	Slow to Warm Babies 15%
Positive disposition	Negative moods, slow to adapt to new situations	Inactive, calm reaction to environment, negative moods withdraw from new situations

How long did it take for the neonate (infant) to adjust to a more positive temperament? Circle one.

3 Months   6 Months   One Year /Other

Finally, how long did it take for you to get back in shape? _______________

What did you do to get the weight off? _______________

What do you love about being a mom/caregiver/parent? _______________

____

____

____

Scripture you used to regain your confidence and discipline to get back in shape

____

____

Things Parents Should Know About His or Her Child's Early Years

First smile ____
Favorite foods ____
Favorite toys ____
Cartoons ____
First word ____
First time called Mommy, or Daddy ____
First tooth date ____
First attempt to form words and sentences _______________________________________
First crawl ____
First step ____
First time slept whole night ____
First time used sippy cup ____
First time feeding themselves ____
Age when they potty-trained _____________ and how long it took _____________
First birthday party ___________________________ Christening __________________________
First day of school/day care ____
First time you had to discipline ____
First time you read to them and introduced them to Jesus ___________________________
First restaurant you took them to ____
First behavior report ____
First report card ____
First school picture taken ____
First Christmas and what they received ____
First time they said "I love you" ____
First fall/cut/accident ____
First fight ____
Health-care issues and allergies ____
Personality type ____

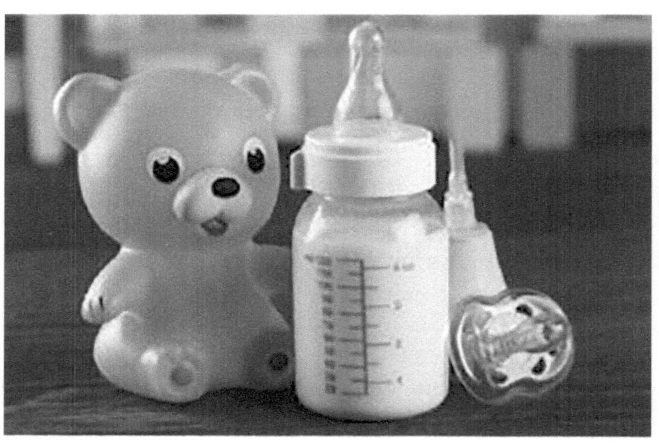

 Miss Asondra StarN'air

Baby Journal Two

Baby's full name ________________________Came to this world on ________________

Born at ____________________ Hospital/Other____________________________________

United States/Other ____

Weight __________ Ounces ___________Height __________ Eye Color _________

Parents: Mother ____________________Father ________________________________

Godparents are/is____

Morals and values instilled in this child will be ________________________________

____

____

____

____

____

____

____

____

____

My role as a parent will be to ____

____

____

____

____

____

____

____

I vow to make sure ____

____

____

____

____

____

____

The scripture I will use to help me become a Christian caregiver to this child
of God is

____

Mom's Childbearing Labor Experience Baby Two

How much weight did you gain from this pregnancy? _______________________

What was this experience for you like with baby _______________________

____

____

____

____

____

____

____

____

____

____

Infant Temperament (Circle one)

Easy Babies 40%	Difficult Babies 10%	Slow to Warm Babies 15%
Positive disposition	Negative moods, slow to adapt to new situations	Inactive, calm reaction to environment, negative moods withdraw from new situations

How long did it take for the neonate (infant) to adjust to a more positive temperament? Circle one.

3 Months   6 Months   One Year /Other

Finally, how long did it take for you to get back in shape? _______________

What did you do to get the weight off? _______________________

What do you love about being a mom/caregiver/parent? _______________

____

____

____

Scripture you used to regain your confidence and discipline to get back in shape

____

____

Things Parents Should Know About His or Her Child's Early Years

First smile ____
Favorite foods ____
Favorite toys ____
Cartoons ____
First word ____
First time called Mommy, or Daddy ____________________________________
First tooth date ____
First attempt to form words and sentences _____________________________
First crawl ____
First step ____
First time slept whole night ____
First time used sippy cup ____
First time feeding themselves ____
Age when they potty-trained ____________ and how long it took ___________
First birthday party _________________ Christening ____________________
First day of school/day care ____
First time you had to discipline _______________________________________
First time you read to them and introduced them to Jesus _______________
First restaurant you took them to ______________________________________
First behavior report ____
First report card ____
First school picture taken ____

First Christmas and what they received _________________________________
First time they said "I love you" _______________________________________
First fall/cut/accident ____
First fight ____
Health-care issues and allergies _______________________________________
Personality type ____

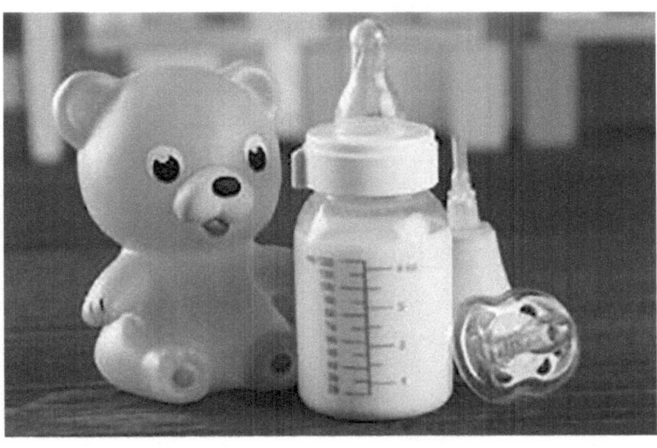

Baby Journal Three

Baby's full name _________________Came to this world on _______________

Born at _________________ Hospital/Other_______________________________

United States/Other ____

Weight __________ Ounces ___________Height _________ Eye Color ________

Parents: Mother _________________Father ______________________________

Godparents are/is____

Morals and values instilled in this child will be ________________________

____

____

____

____

____

____

____

____

____

My role as a parent will be to ____

____

____

____

____

____

____

____

I vow to make sure ____

____

____

____

____

____

____

The scripture I will use to help me become a Christian caregiver to this child
of God is

____

 MISS ASONDRA STARN'AIR

How much weight did you gain from this pregnancy? ________________________

What was this experience for you like with baby _________________________

____

____

____

____

____

____

____

____

____

____

Infant Temperament (Circle one)

Easy Babies 40%	Difficult Babies 10%	Slow to Warm Babies 15%
Positive disposition	Negative moods, slow to adapt to new situations	Inactive, calm reaction to environment, negative moods withdraw from new situations

How long did it take for the neonate (infant) to adjust to a more positive temperament? Circle one.

3 Months   6 Months   One Year /Other

Finally, how long did it take for you to get back in shape? ________________

What did you do to get the weight off? _________________________________

What do you love about being a mom/caregiver/parent? ___________________

____

____

____

Scripture you used to regain your confidence and discipline to get back in shape

____

____

Things Parents Should Know About His or Her Child's Early Years

First smile ____
Favorite foods ____
Favorite toys ____
Cartoons ____
First word ____
First time called Mommy, or Daddy __________________________
First tooth date ____
First attempt to form words and sentences _________________
First crawl ____
First step ____
First time slept whole night ______________________________
First time used sippy cup _________________________________
First time feeding themselves _____________________________
Age when they potty-trained ___________ and how long it took ___________
First birthday party _________________ Christening ________________
First day of school/day care ______________________________
First time you had to discipline __________________________
First time you read to them and introduced them to Jesus ___________
First restaurant you took them to _________________________
First behavior report _____________________________________
First report card ____
First school picture taken ________________________________
First Christmas and what they received ____________________
First time they said "I love you" _________________________
First fall/cut/accident ___________________________________
First fight ____
Health-care issues and allergies __________________________
Personality type ____

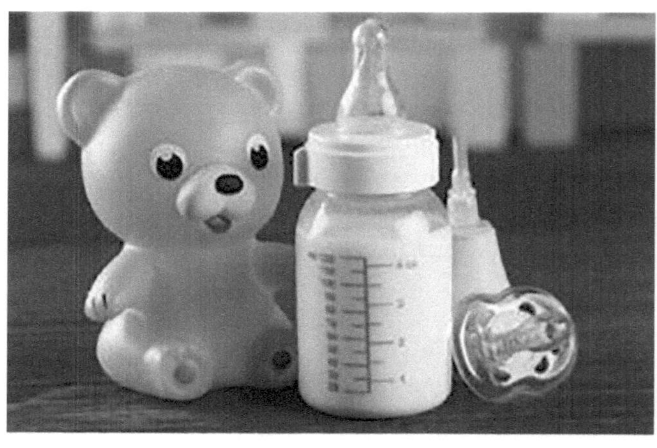

   Miss Asondra StarN'air

Baby Journal Four

Baby's full name _______________________Came to this world on _______________

Born at ___________________ Hospital/Other_________________________________

United States/Other ____

Weight __________ Ounces ___________Height __________ Eye Color _________

Parents: Mother ____________________Father _________________________________

Godparents are/is____

Morals and values instilled in this child will be ___________________________________

____

____

____

____

____

____

____

____

____

____

My role as a parent will be to ____

____

____

____

____

____

____

____

____

I vow to make sure ____

____

____

____

____

____

____

____

The scripture I will use to help me become a Christian caregiver to this child
of God is

____

<h3 style="text-align:center">Mom's Childbearing Labor Experience Baby Four</h3>

How much weight did you gain from this pregnancy? _______________________

What was this experience for you like with baby ______________________

____

____

____

____

____

____

____

____

____

____

Infant Temperament (Circle one)

Easy Babies 40%	Difficult Babies 10%	Slow to Warm Babies 15%
Positive disposition	Negative moods, slow to adapt to new situations	Inactive, calm reaction to environment, negative moods withdraw from new situations

How long did it take for the neonate (infant) to adjust to a more positive temperament? Circle one.

3 Months   6 Months   One Year /Other

Finally, how long did it take for you to get back in shape? _______________

What did you do to get the weight off? _______________________

What do you love about being a mom/caregiver/parent? _______________

____

____

____

Scripture you used to regain your confidence and discipline to get back in shape

____

____

Things Parents Should Know About His or Her Child's Early Years

First smile ____

Favorite foods ____

Favorite toys ____

Cartoons ____

First word ____

First time called Mommy, or Daddy ____

First tooth date ____

First attempt to form words and sentences ________________________________

First crawl ____

First step ____

First time slept whole night ____

First time used sippy cup ____

First time feeding themselves ____

Age when they potty-trained ____________ and how long it took ____________

First birthday party ____________________ Christening ___________________

First day of school/day care ____

First time you had to discipline ____

First time you read to them and introduced them to Jesus _________________

First restaurant you took them to ____

First behavior report ____

First report card ____

First school picture taken ____

First Christmas and what they received ___________________________________

First time they said "I love you" ____

First fall/cut/accident ____

First fight ____

Health-care issues and allergies ____

Personality type ____

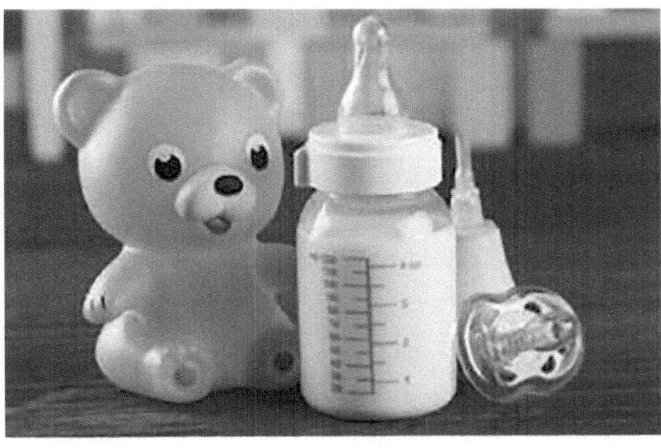

Baby Journal Five

Baby's full name ___________________Came to this world on ______________

Born at ___________________ Hospital/Other_________________________________

United States/Other ____

Weight __________ Ounces ___________Height __________ Eye Color _________

Parents: Mother _____________________Father _______________________________

Godparents are/is____

Morals and values instilled in this child will be ______________________________

____

____

____

____

____

____

____

____

____

My role as a parent will be to ____

____

____

____

____

____

____

____

I vow to make sure ____

____

____

____

____

____

____

____

The scripture I will use to help me become a Christian caregiver to this child
of God is

____

 MISS ASONDRA StarN'air

Mom's Childbearing Labor Experience Baby Five

How much weight did you gain from this pregnancy? _______________________

What was this experience for you like with baby _______________________

____

____

____

____

____

____

____

____

____

____

Infant Temperament (Circle one)

Easy Babies 40%	Difficult Babies 10%	Slow to Warm Babies 15%
Positive disposition	Negative moods, slow to adapt to new situations	Inactive, calm reaction to environment, negative moods withdraw from new situations

How long did it take for the neonate (infant) to adjust to a more positive temperament? Circle one.

3 Months   6 Months   One Year /Other

Finally, how long did it take for you to get back in shape? _______________

What did you do to get the weight off? _______________________________

What do you love about being a mom/caregiver/parent? _______________

____

____

____

Scripture you used to regain your confidence and discipline to get back in shape

____

____

Things Parents Should Know About His or Her Child's Early Years

First smile ____
Favorite foods ____
Favorite toys ____
Cartoons ____
First word ____
First time called Mommy, or Daddy _____________________________
First tooth date ____
First attempt to form words and sentences _______________________
First crawl ____
First step ____
First time slept whole night ___________________________________
First time used sippy cup _____________________________________
First time feeding themselves __________________________________
Age when they potty-trained ____________ and how long it took __________
First birthday party ____________________ Christening _____________
First day of school/day care ___________________________________
First time you had to discipline ________________________________
First time you read to them and introduced them to Jesus __________
First restaurant you took them to ______________________________
First behavior report ____
First report card ____
First school picture taken _____________________________________
First Christmas and what they received __________________________
First time they said "I love you" _______________________________
First fall/cut/accident ____
First fight ____
Health-care issues and allergies ________________________________
Personality type ____

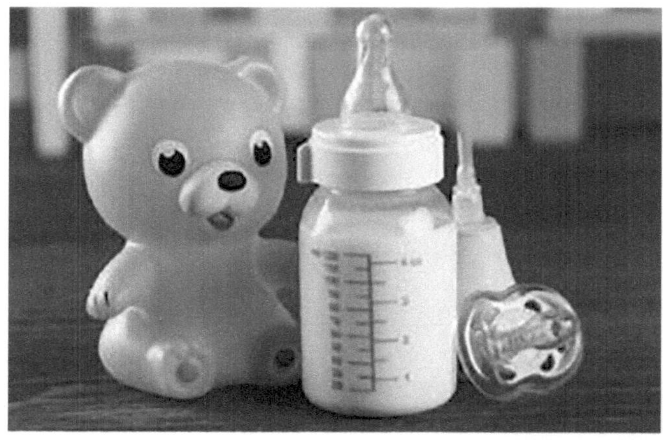

  Miss Asondra StarN'air

Postpartum Depression

What is postpartum Depression? A severe form of depression occurring after childbirth and pregnancy. One study found that out of ten thousand participants one out of every seven mothers with newborns experience postpartum depression.

Postpartum depression is unique to every pregnancy and may affect both experienced and first–time moms alike.

If you have just had a baby and are now feeling sad and blue, it may very well be postpartum depression.

Call on the name of Jesus, he will help you, or contact your doctor, do not try to go this alone.

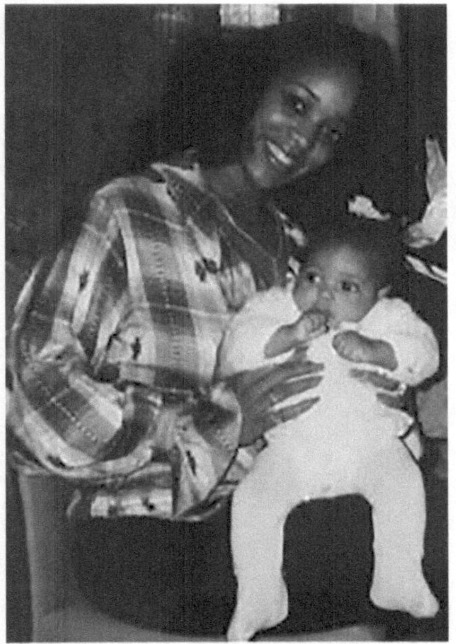

Trust in God, Let "Him" heal you.
Just take it one day at a time!

Signs of Postpartum

- Severe mood swings
- Sad feeling
- Change in Appetite
- Intense Anger
- Irritability
- Insomnia or fatigue
- Feel like a failure
- Fear and worry
- Un-motivated
- Worthlessness
- Problems thinking clearly
- Feel loss and unsure
- Not good enough
- Feel fat, ugly, unattractive
- Insecure about baby's daddy and the relationship
- Issues of trust
- Job issues
- Feel lost and alone

Help Tips

- Pray to God.
- Read Scriptures.
- Watch Comedy.
- Get up and get dress, do your hair.
- Talk with other moms.
- Know that this too shall pass.
- Play with your new beautiful baby.
- Focus on God, not on you. Be full of gratitude!

Tips on How to Lose the Baby Weight!

1. Exercise four days a week.
2. Drinks six to 8 glass of water daily.
3. Eat whatever you want on a smaller plate, do not go back for seconds.
4. Breast feed as long as you can, it gets the weight off much faster. However, if you can't breast feed because of work or just don't want to, that's not a problem, choose well balance snacks in between meals.
5. **Rest, Rest, Rest!** Sleep does the body good! It gives you the energy to want to work out, do not under-estimate the power of sleep. Rest and good sleep gets you up and on your feet, so put some music on, move, dance to the beat! Move for one hour, shed those pounds and keep watching how much you eat.
6. Vary your workouts, somedays walk, somedays do the bike, some-days do the treadmill, elliptical, and so forth. On one of those days, do weights and body sculpturing. Each workouts, works different parts of the body and it also keep you from getting bored with the same routine.
7. Be patient and stay off the scale, your clothes will tell, if you lost or gained weight.
8. Read your bible, get disciplined in the Lord, once you do that, you'll see, like me, we have the power do all things in Christ, for He's the one who strengthen us; He'll have you back in shape in no time.
9. Pray away those pounds, allow the Holy Spirit to come in and do its thing!

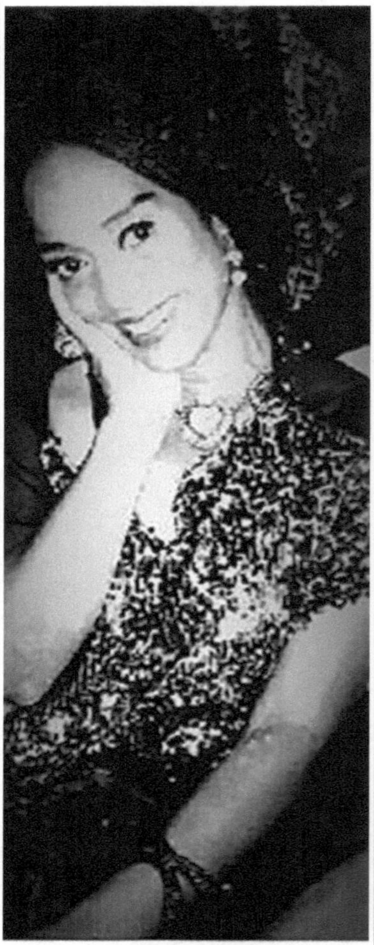

You can reach your weight loss goals, but it will require determination, account-ability and patience.

 Miss Asondra StarN'air

10. Love the body you're in, not everybody wants to be thin, however, you must realize your body is not your own it belongs to the Lord. Therefore you still must take excellent care of it weight loss or not.

Healthy Body, Healthy Mind, Work It All The Time!

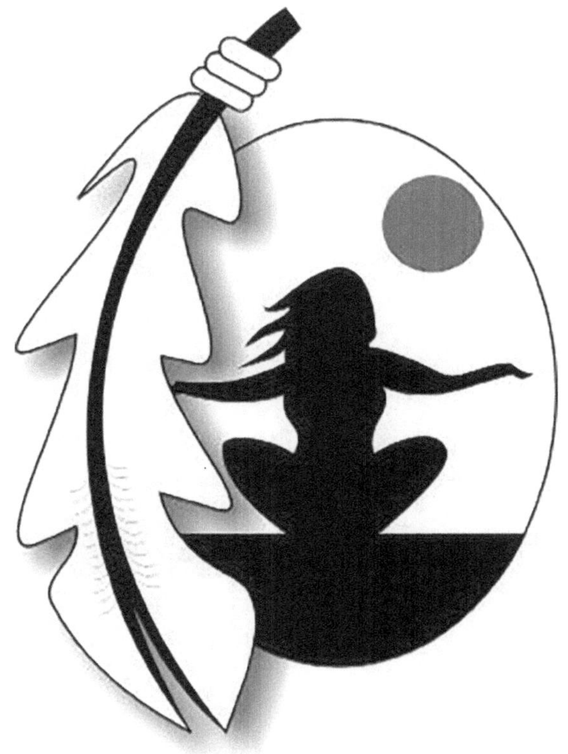

Normal Weight _______________________________________

Pregnancy Weight ____________________________________

Goal Weight ____

Goal Date ____

I can do all things in Christ, **"I Will Get Back In Shape!"**

SECTION XIII

Caregivers

Let's look at some other types of caregivers shall we!

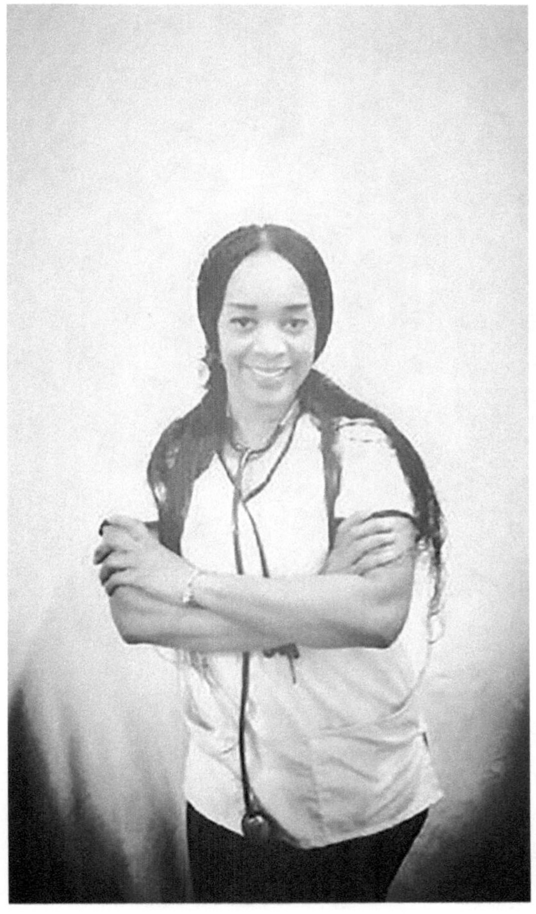

Family Care

Love You, Grandma, Say "Cheese!"

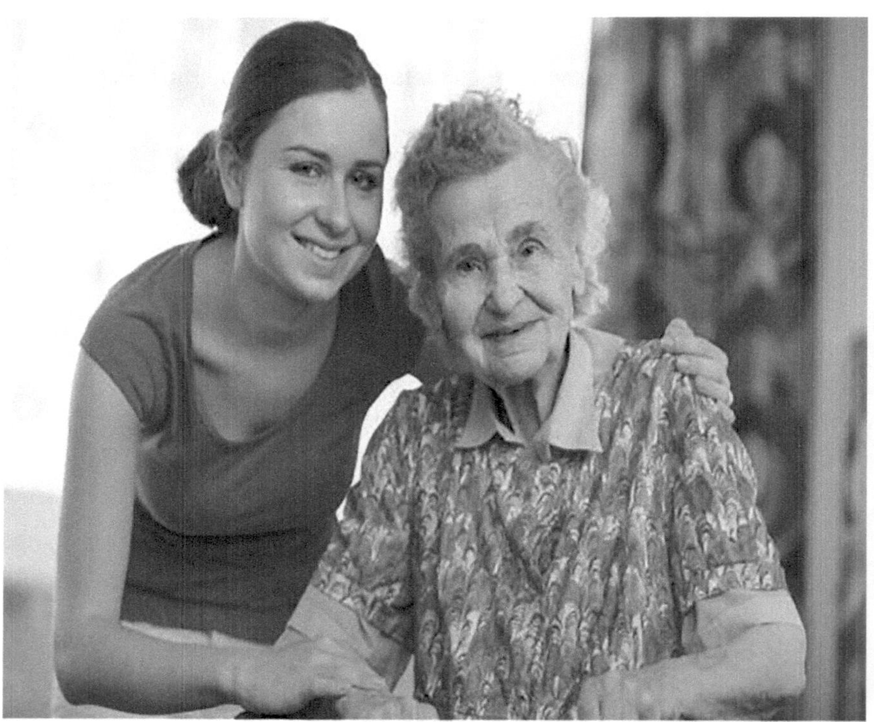

   Miss Asondra StarN'air

Family Care

Caring for a family member or close friend is due to happen at some point in our lives. For me, it was my dad. Without warning, a sudden illness emerged. Next thing I knew, I was a family care provider.

Never would have made it through without Jesus!

Some of you are now providing care for a loved one, and you are not alone. According to caregiver statistics, more than 65 million people (29 percent of the US population) are taking care of a chronically ill, disabled, or aged family member or friend on a regular basis.

Please remember to take care of yourself. Get plenty of rest and call on the name of the Lord. Allow him to strengthen and renew you.

Being a family caregiver can be overwhelming at times, but it's good to know Jesus is just a call away.

Welcome to the wonderful world of care-giving!

You Are one with us and In God we Trust.

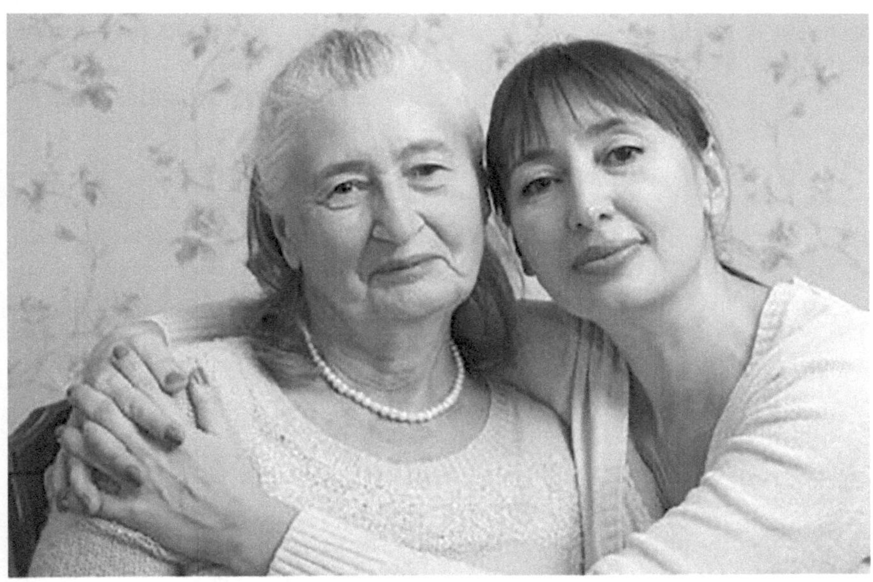

Presidential Proclamation National Family Caregivers Month 2015

NATIONAL FAMILY CAREGIVERS MONTH 2015

BY THE PRESIDENT OF THE UNITED STATES OF AMERICA

A PROCLAMATION

Day in and day out, selfless and loving Americans provide care and support to family members and friends in need. They are parents, spouses, children, siblings, relatives, and neighbors who uphold their unwavering commitment to ensure the lives of their loved ones shine bright with health, safety, and dignity. During National Family Caregivers Month, we rededicate ourselves to making sure our selfless caregivers have the support they need to maintain their own well-being and that of those they love.

One of the best measures of a country is how it treats its older citizens and people living with disabilities, and my Administration is dedicated to lifting up their lives and ensuring those who care for them get the support and recognition they deserve. Earlier this year, older Americans and caregivers, as well as their advocates, came together at the White House Conference on Aging, which provided an opportunity to discuss ways to identify and advance actions to improve quality of life for our Nation's elderly. Through the Affordable Care Act, we are providing more options to help older Americans remain in their homes as they age, and the law is giving caregivers the peace of mind of having access to quality, affordable health insurance. Additionally, I will keep pushing to make paid family leave available for every American, regardless of where they work—because no one should have to sacrifice a paycheck to care for a loved one.

When our men and women in uniform come home with wounds of war—seen or unseen—it is our solemn responsibility to ensure they get the benefits and attentive care they have earned and deserve. Caregivers in every corner of our country uphold this sacred promise with incredible devotion to their loved ones, and my Administration is committed to supporting them.

We have extended military caregiver leave to family members of eligible veterans dealing with serious illness or injury for up to 5 years after their service has ended, and we remain dedicated to providing greater flexibility

 MISS ASONDRA STARN'AIR

for our military families and for the members of our Armed Forces as they return home and handle the transition to civilian life.

For centuries, we have been driven by the belief that we all have certain obligations to one another. Every day, caregivers across our country answer this call and lift up the lives of loved ones who need additional support. During National Family Caregivers Month, let us honor their contributions and pledge to continue working toward a future where all caregivers know the same support and understanding they show for those they look after.

NOW, THEREFORE, I, BARACK OBAMA, President of the United States of America, by virtue of the authority vested in me by the Constitution and the laws of the United States, do hereby proclaim November 2015 as National Family Caregivers Month. I encourage all Americans to pay tribute to those who provide for the health and well-being of their family members, friends, and neighbors.

IN WITNESS WHEREOF, I have hereunto set my hand this thirtieth day of October, in the year of our Lord two thousand fifteen, and of the Independence of the United States of America the two hundred and fortieth.

BARACK OBAMA

Family Caregivers

And let us not grow weary of doing good, for in due season we will reap, if we do not give up. So then, as we have opportunity, let us do well to everyone, and especially to those who are of the household of faith. **Galatians 6: 9-10** There are millions and millions of Family Caregivers around the world "millions" You Are Not Alone "God" is here with you. He sees and knows all you are doing all the long hours you put in day after day, night after night. He wants you to call on him when things start to get hard, don't let anxiety and pressure overtake you, don't let that happen, Jesus reminds us in 1st Peter 'Cast all your worries and cares on the **LORD**, for he cares for you'.

Family caregiver just know this God is there to help every step of the way so please don't give up. Take a break if you need to but don't give up.

And this message is for the family members who can help out but won't, you are either too busy or too tired or whatever may be the excuse, hear what saith the Lord in 1 Timothy.

"But if anyone does not provide for his relative and especially for members of his household, he has denied the faith and is worse than an unbeliever."

So I encourage all members of the household to participate in the well beings of others "Do Good" and know that for those who love God all things work together for good, for those who are called according to his purpose. **Romans 8:28**

Amen!

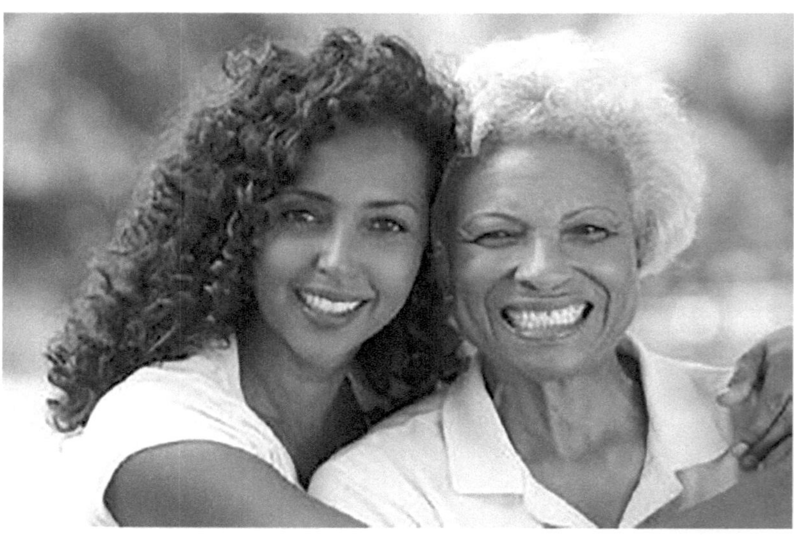

There are Many Rewards in Family Caregiving

Here are just a few and you can add to this list of rewards.

As mentioned earlier in my introduction, I was a family caregiver too and these are the rewards I received.

1. I learned I was stronger than I thought I was.
2. I learned new skills, had no idea I had natural nursing abilities. No idea!
3. Became an even more loving person, more companionate and caring.
4. My priorities changed, life was no longer about me, it became more about helping others.
5. I became even closer to my Dad/loved one.
6. I needed God more. Could not have held up during my father's terminal illness process without God guiding and holding me up.
7. I became a better person in every way.
8. I fully realized I could do all things in Christ who strengthens me. By the way that's **Philippian's 4:13.**
9. I wanted more of this kind and caring and loving so a few years later I changed careers became a fulltime Caregiver for those in need and have not looked back.
10. What Family Caregiving accomplished the most for me, it gave me a **"Jesus Heart"** and now I am taking everything I can think of with love putting in this book for you.

What about you, how have you been rewarded?

____
____
____
____
____
____

Family Care Journal

Being a family caregiver has __________________________

I take care of myself by __________________________

What I want God to know is _______________________________

____

____

____

____

____

____

____

My prayer for my loved one is _____________________________

____

____

____

____

____

____

____

____

____

The scriptures that help me the most during this time are: ______

____

____

____

____

____

____

____

____

My support also comes from _______________________

____

____

____

____

____

____

I also do fun things for myself like _______________

____

____

____

____

____

____

____

____

And I love _______________________________________

____

____

____

____

____

____

____

____

Being a child of God, I am thankful for ___________

____

____

____

____

____

____

 Miss Asondra StarN'air

What I have learned about myself from this caregiving experience is _______

____

____

____

____

____

____

____

What I love so much about the loved one I am taking care of is ___________

____

____

____

____

____

____

____

____

____

Our time together means so much _____________________________

____

____

____

____

____

____

____

____

____

My final thoughts are: ____
____
____
____
____
____
____
____
____

Resources and Contact Numbers

Name   Phone Number

________________________   ________________________
________________________   ________________________
________________________   ________________________
________________________   ________________________

So now faith, hope, and love abide, these three; but the greatest of these is
LOVE! 1 Corinthians 13:13

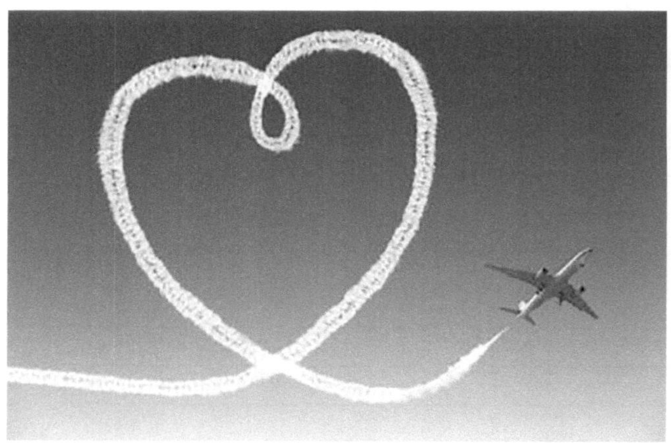

 Miss Asondra StarN'air

Foster Care

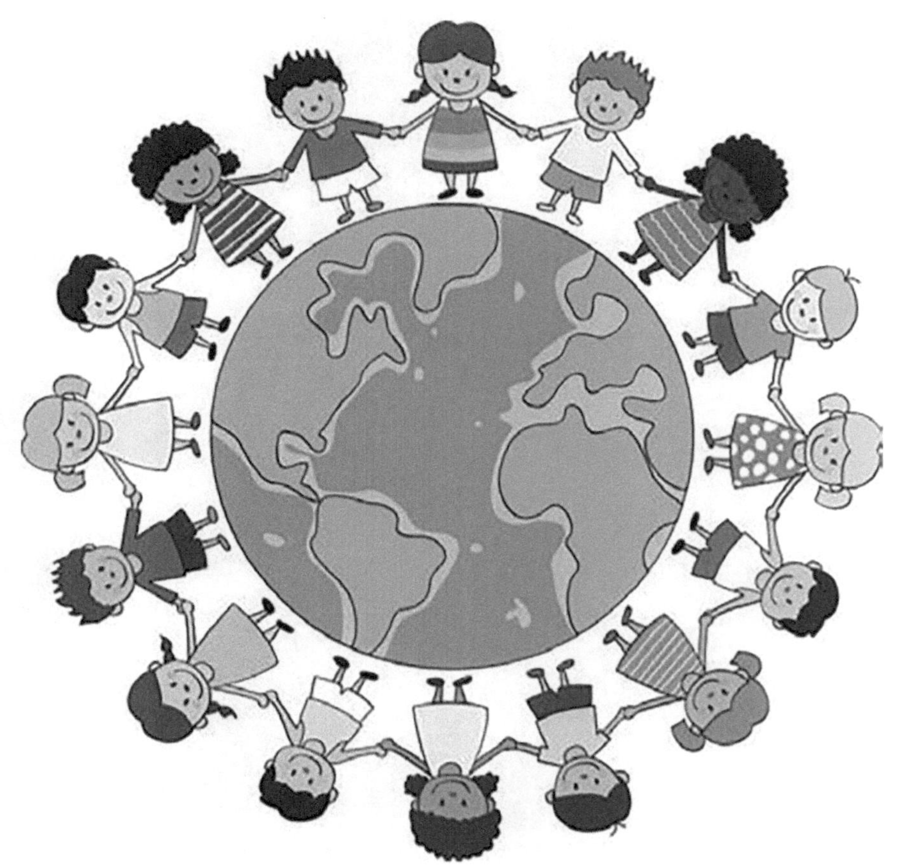

Be There!

Foster Care

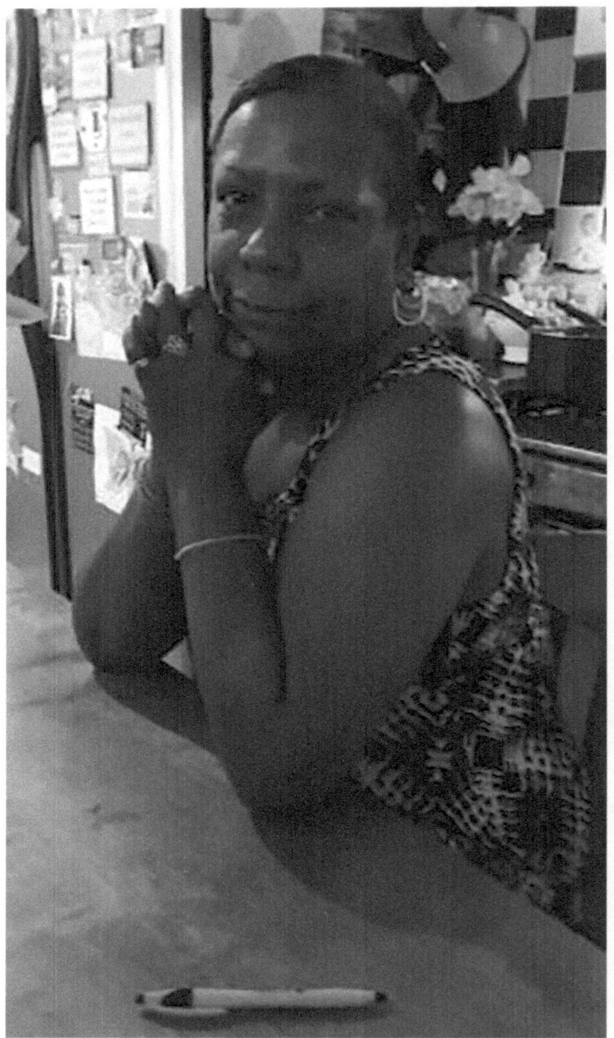

Amy Fortson

This page honors Ms Amy Fortson, you are an amazing foster care parent. We thank you for your contribution in making this world a better place for our children to live in. God bless you!

Please Help Us!

As we speak, we have a family crisis, today we have more than four hundred thousand children in the United States living in foster care and around one hundred thousand cannot return home to their biological parents according to Bethany Christian services.

That's why we need more caregivers who are willing to dedicate their time and heart to those in need. Contact your local child and family services for more instruction on how to become a foster care parent, you'll be glad you did.

I was a foster care parent too, I cared for two young boys they are now back home with their mom, doing well. Many of them do return home, that's always the goal, for families to get back together, reunite.

May is National Foster Care Month! it's a month set aside to acknowledge Foster care parents all over the world like **Amy Fortson** who have dedicated their lives to caring for those in need. **Thank You!**

May is a good month and **"May"** your **HEARTS** be open wide! Reach out to the less fortunate, Give them a loving home treat them as one of your own.

Caregivers We love you, we are so, so grateful that you are among us, may God bless you with all his might, may you always be taken care of every day and night.

In Jesus name **Amen!**

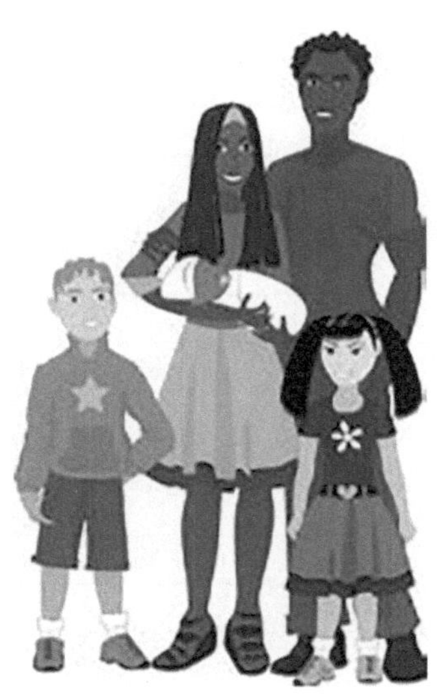

Foster Care Journal

Why I became a Foster Care parent _______________________________

____

____

____

____

____

____

____

____

____

What I hope to bring to this much needed area of caregiving is _______

____

____

____

____

____

____

____

____

____

____

____

My challenge of being a foster care parent are ___________________

____

____

____

____

____

____

____

____

My overall goal is to _______________________________________

____

____

____

____

This is the scripture that holds my life together: ________________

____

____

____

____

God has blessed me in so many ways since I became a foster parent ____

____

____

____

____

Foster Care, Be There!

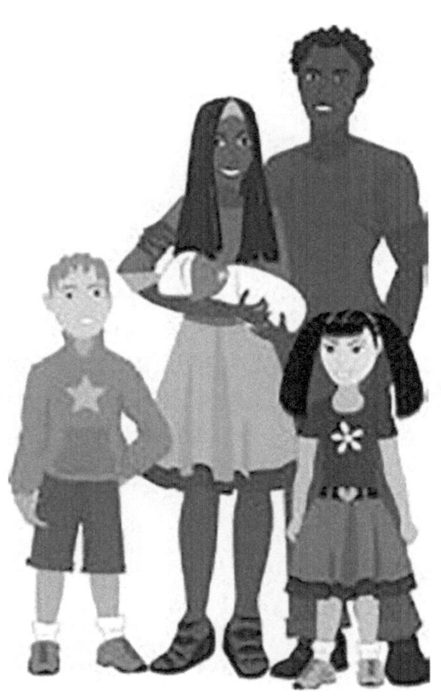

All My Children
List for Foster Care Parents

Name________________________________Age__________ Birthday____________

Name________________________________Age__________ Birthday____________

Name________________________________Age__________ Birthday____________

Name________________________________Age__________ Birthday____________

Name________________________________Age__________ Birthday____________

Name________________________________Age__________ Birthday____________

Name________________________________Age__________ Birthday____________

Name________________________________Age__________ Birthday____________

Name________________________________Age__________ Birthday____________

Name________________________________Age__________ Birthday____________

Name________________________________Age__________ Birthday____________

Name________________________________Age__________ Birthday____________

Name________________________________Age__________ Birthday____________

Name________________________________Age__________ Birthday____________

Name________________________________Age__________ Birthday____________

Name________________________________Age__________ Birthday____________

Name________________________________Age__________ Birthday____________

Name________________________________Age__________ Birthday____________

Name________________________________Age__________ Birthday____________

Name________________________________Age__________ Birthday____________

Name________________________________Age__________ Birthday____________

Name________________________________Age__________ Birthday____________

Name________________________________Age__________ Birthday____________

Name________________________________Age__________ Birthday____________

Name________________________________Age__________ Birthday____________

Name________________________________Age__________ Birthday____________

Name________________________________Age__________ Birthday____________

Daycare Providers

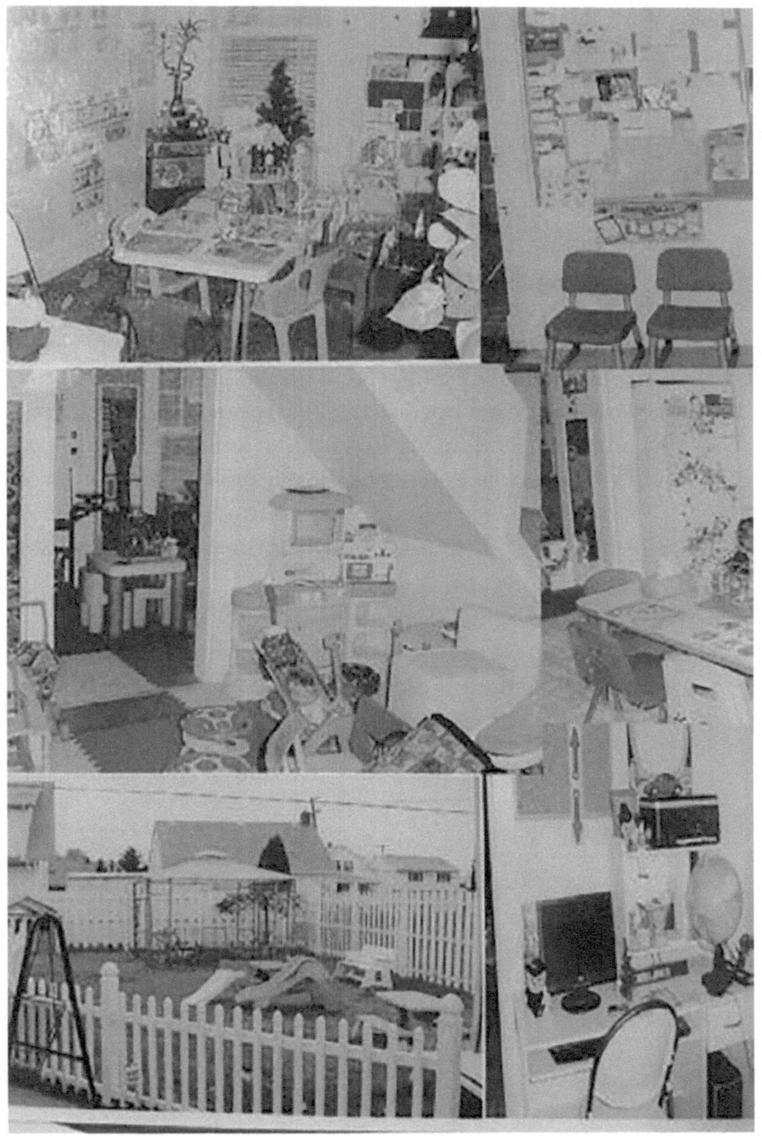

Former Jazzy Jazz Home Daycare Center

Daycare Providers

Hello, if you are a daycare provider, guess what? You are a caregiver too. Welcome to the world of care giving. There are many wonderful day-care centers and caregivers out there caring for children. Over the years home daycare providers and daycare center employees have become like family to many of our working moms and dads.

Today there are so many amazing caregivers out there that love what they do and can't imagine doing anything else. And the children love them too, I use to be one of you, I own and operated a daycare business for fourteen years and it was a joy nurturing and caring for children as I watched them develop and grow, it was an incredible experience for me and I'm sure for all of you.

What's also so wonderful too, families form tight bond with providers that can last for years and years.

Caregiving for small children is hard work, yet it's quite rewarding too. Here's what you do, Love and teach them well. **ABCDE "Step Up To Quality"!**

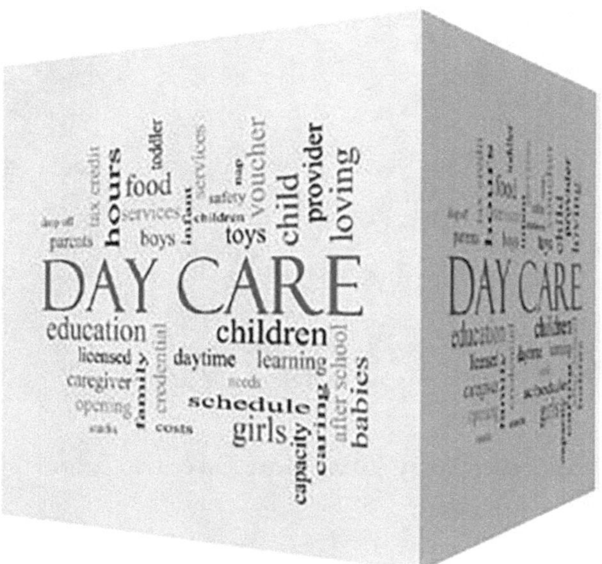

 Miss Asondra StarN'air

Child Care Providers

Step up to Quality! Step up to quality is a tiered quality-rating and improvement system for early learning and development programs. Birthed out of the state of Ohio and funded by the Ohio Department of Education (ODE) or the Ohio Department Of Job and Family Services. The Goal is simple, 'High Quality Care' for all children in daycare. For more information contact your state Job and family services department.

Now, in the tool box is a list of things needed to start your very own daycare home business if you are new in the field. All it takes is a little patience and rearranging of your home and soon you will be up and running. My advice to new providers is to "Step Up to Quality" be a winner, provide the best care possible. Again, welcome to the world of Care-giving!

My Jazzy Jazz Home Daycare Business back in 2006

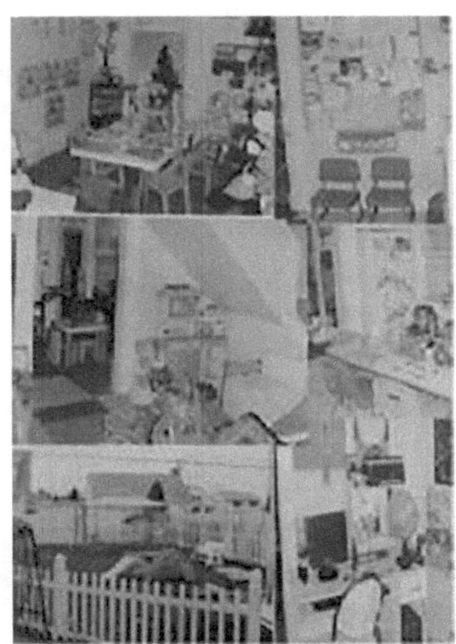

Care Giving at its Finest!

Tools You Can Use!

Open for Business!

Here's What You'll Need:

- City Inspection
- License
- CPR/First Aide
- Emergency Evacuation Plan
- Daycare Handbook
- Employee Hand Book for / Centers& Type A
- Accountant/Optional
- Food Program
- Continuing Education
- Daycare Name
- Adequate Space
- Case Worker
- Pre-School Material
- Dog or Cat shot Records
- Background Check
- Age Appropriate Toys and Materials.
- First Aide Kit
- Outside Play area
- Inside Play Area
- Child/Adult ratio
- Diaper Changing Area
- Posted Emergency Numbers
- Business Management Skills and Record Keeping System in place

CPR for Infants and Children

If you are alone with the unconscious infant give 2 minutes of **CPR** before calling 911.

Time is of the essence when dealing with **CPR** especially for infants, permanent brain damage or death can occur within minutes if a baby's blood flow stops. So no time to be scared to do **CPR**, you MUST do **CPR**! Many times the need for **CPR** happens after drowning, suffocation, Chocking, and in children it may be due to some other injuries.

CPR involves Rescue Breathing, which provides oxygen to the lungs and Chest compressions, that helps keep the blood flowing.

Anyone working with children should be certified, anyone who is a parent too, should be certified. And anyone who is neither should be certified!

CPR saves lives, we never know in life what we may be faced with, mightiest well be prepared to help The **Zero** and be a **Hero**!

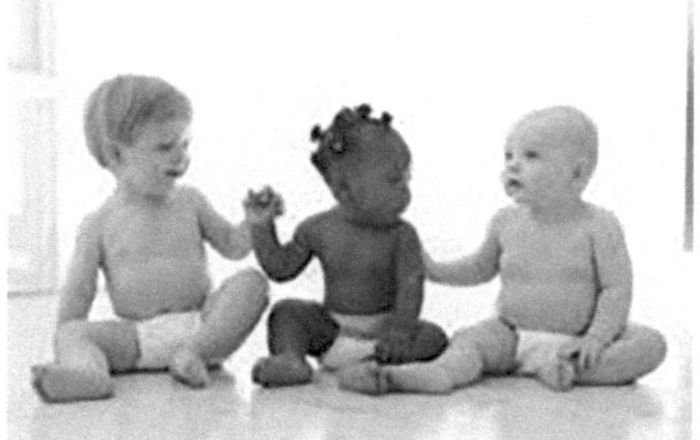

You can do it **CPR**

First   Check the scene
Check the victim
Call for help

Second If the child is not responding Put phone on speaker mode **LISTEN** to disputer, Start **CPR**

If you do not have a phone, here's what you do.

1. Shout and tap if the child does not respond, isn't breathing or is breathing but not normal. position the baby on its back and start **CPR**
2. Give 30 gentle chest compressions at a rate of 100 to -120 / minutes. Use two of three fingers, place those fingers directly in the center of the child's chest just below the nipples. Now press down about one – third the depth of the chest, which is about 1 and a half inches.
3. Open the air way by tilting the head back, lift the chin up. Gently do not tilt the child head back too far.
4. If the chest doesn't rise, open airway again and repeat all **CPR** steps until help arrives. We are caregivers we **MUST** help save lives.
5. Just remember to stay:

**Calm, Cool and Collected
"You Got This!"**

You Can Do It!

Child Care Journal for Caregivers

Why I became a child care provider ____

____

____

____

____

____

____

____

____

____

____I have been a child care provider for

____

What I love about taking care of children is _______________________________

____

____

____

____

____

____

____

____

____

____

The most challenging areas are ____

____

____

____

____

____

____

____

My overall goal is to ____

____

____

____

____

____

____

The scripture I use to keep me strong and focus is _______________

____

____

____

____

____

____

____

I love what do because ____

____

____

____

____

____

____

____

I Am Blessed!

 MISS ASONDRA STARN'AIR

All My Children's "Caregivers" List for Childcare Providers

Name_____________________________Age__________ Birthday____________
Name_____________________________Age__________ Birthday____________
Name_____________________________Age__________ Birthday____________
Name_____________________________Age__________ Birthday____________
Name_____________________________Age__________ Birthday____________
Name_____________________________Age__________ Birthday____________
Name_____________________________Age__________ Birthday____________
Name_____________________________Age__________ Birthday____________
Name_____________________________Age__________ Birthday____________
Name_____________________________Age__________ Birthday____________
Name_____________________________Age__________ Birthday____________
Name_____________________________Age__________ Birthday____________
Name_____________________________Age__________ Birthday____________
Name_____________________________Age__________ Birthday____________
Name_____________________________Age__________ Birthday____________
Name_____________________________Age__________ Birthday____________
Name_____________________________Age__________ Birthday____________
Name_____________________________Age__________ Birthday____________
Name_____________________________Age__________ Birthday____________
Name_____________________________Age__________ Birthday____________
Name_____________________________Age__________ Birthday____________
Name_____________________________Age__________ Birthday____________
Name_____________________________Age__________ Birthday____________
Name_____________________________Age__________ Birthday____________
Name_____________________________Age__________ Birthday____________
Name_____________________________Age__________ Birthday____________
Name_____________________________Age__________ Birthday____________
Name_____________________________Age__________ Birthday____________
Name_____________________________Age__________ Birthday____________
Name_____________________________Age__________ Birthday____________
Name_____________________________Age__________ Birthday____________
Name_____________________________Age__________ Birthday____________
Name_____________________________Age__________ Birthday____________
Name_____________________________Age__________ Birthday____________

Name_____________________________________Age___________ Birthday____________
Name_____________________________________Age___________ Birthday____________
Name_____________________________________Age___________ Birthday____________
Name_____________________________________Age___________ Birthday____________
Name_____________________________________Age___________ Birthday____________
Name_____________________________________Age___________ Birthday____________
Name_____________________________________Age___________ Birthday____________
Name_____________________________________Age___________ Birthday____________
Name_____________________________________Age___________ Birthday____________
Name_____________________________________Age___________ Birthday____________
Name_____________________________________Age___________ Birthday____________
Name_____________________________________Age___________ Birthday____________
Name_____________________________________Age___________ Birthday____________
Name_____________________________________Age___________ Birthday____________
Name_____________________________________Age___________ Birthday____________
Name_____________________________________Age___________ Birthday____________
Name_____________________________________Age___________ Birthday____________
Name_____________________________________Age___________ Birthday____________
Name_____________________________________Age___________ Birthday____________
Name_____________________________________Age___________ Birthday____________
Name_____________________________________Age___________ Birthday____________
Name_____________________________________Age___________ Birthday____________
Name_____________________________________Age___________ Birthday____________
Name_____________________________________Age___________ Birthday____________
Name_____________________________________Age___________ Birthday____________
Name_____________________________________Age___________ Birthday____________
Name_____________________________________Age___________ Birthday____________
Name_____________________________________Age___________ Birthday____________
Name_____________________________________Age___________ Birthday____________
Name_____________________________________Age___________ Birthday____________
Name_____________________________________Age___________ Birthday____________
Name_____________________________________Age___________ Birthday____________
Name_____________________________________Age___________ Birthday____________
Name_____________________________________Age___________ Birthday____________
Name_____________________________________Age___________ Birthday____________
Name_____________________________________Age___________ Birthday____________
Name_____________________________________Age___________ Birthday____________
Name_____________________________________Age___________ Birthday____________
Name_____________________________________Age___________ Birthday____________
Name_____________________________________Age___________ Birthday____________

 Miss Asondra StarN'air

Name_____________________________________Age___________ Birthday___________
Name_____________________________________Age___________ Birthday___________
Name_____________________________________Age___________ Birthday___________
Name_____________________________________Age___________ Birthday___________
Name_____________________________________Age___________ Birthday___________
Name_____________________________________Age___________ Birthday___________
Name_____________________________________Age___________ Birthday___________
Name_____________________________________Age___________ Birthday___________
Name_____________________________________Age___________ Birthday___________
Name_____________________________________Age___________ Birthday___________
Name_____________________________________Age___________ Birthday___________
Name_____________________________________Age___________ Birthday___________
Name_____________________________________Age___________ Birthday___________
Name_____________________________________Age___________ Birthday___________
Name_____________________________________Age___________ Birthday___________
Name_____________________________________Age___________ Birthday___________
Name_____________________________________Age___________ Birthday___________
Name_____________________________________Age___________ Birthday___________
Name_____________________________________Age___________ Birthday___________
Name_____________________________________Age___________ Birthday___________
Name_____________________________________Age___________ Birthday___________
Name_____________________________________Age___________ Birthday___________
Name_____________________________________Age___________ Birthday___________
Name_____________________________________Age___________ Birthday___________
Name_____________________________________Age___________ Birthday___________
Name_____________________________________Age___________ Birthday___________
Name_____________________________________Age___________ Birthday___________
Name_____________________________________Age___________ Birthday___________
Name_____________________________________Age___________ Birthday___________
Name_____________________________________Age___________ Birthday___________
Name_____________________________________Age___________ Birthday___________
Name_____________________________________Age___________ Birthday___________
Name_____________________________________Age___________ Birthday___________
Name_____________________________________Age___________ Birthday___________
Name_____________________________________Age___________ Birthday___________
Name_____________________________________Age___________ Birthday___________
Name_____________________________________Age___________ Birthday___________
Name_____________________________________Age___________ Birthday___________
Name_____________________________________Age___________ Birthday___________
Name_____________________________________Age___________ Birthday___________
Name_____________________________________Age___________ Birthday___________
Name_____________________________________Age___________ Birthday___________

Parents' Names and Numbers for Future References

Name	Telephone Number	E-mail Address

 Miss Asondra StarN'air

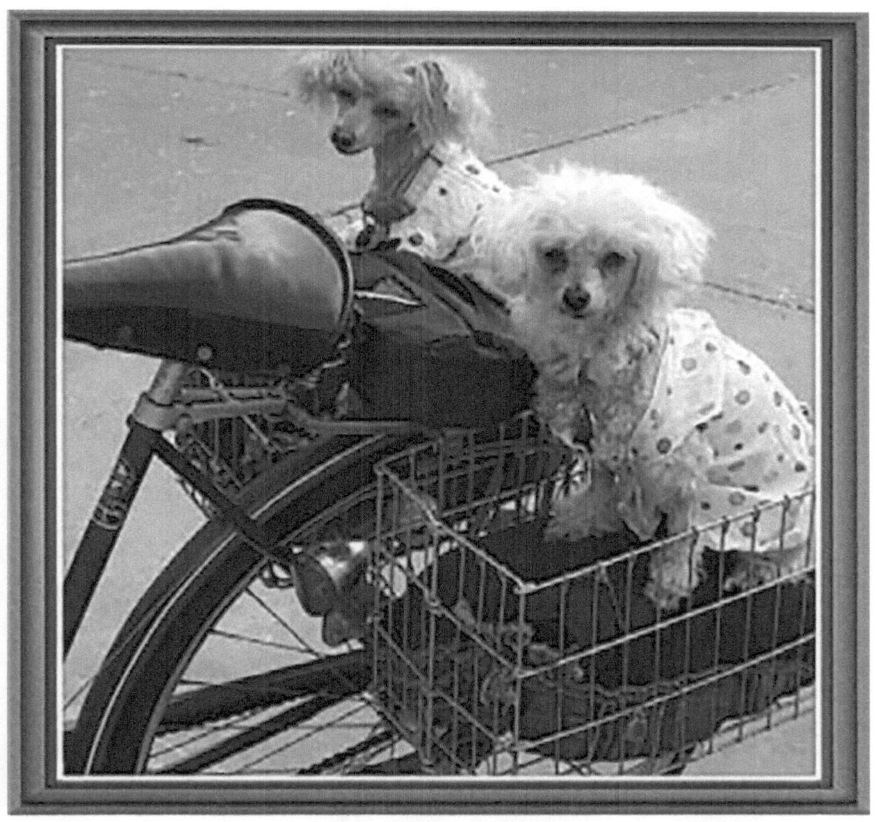

My Two Toy Poodles
Amanican Latt'e (R) and Mariah Autumn (L)

Miss Amanican Latt'e

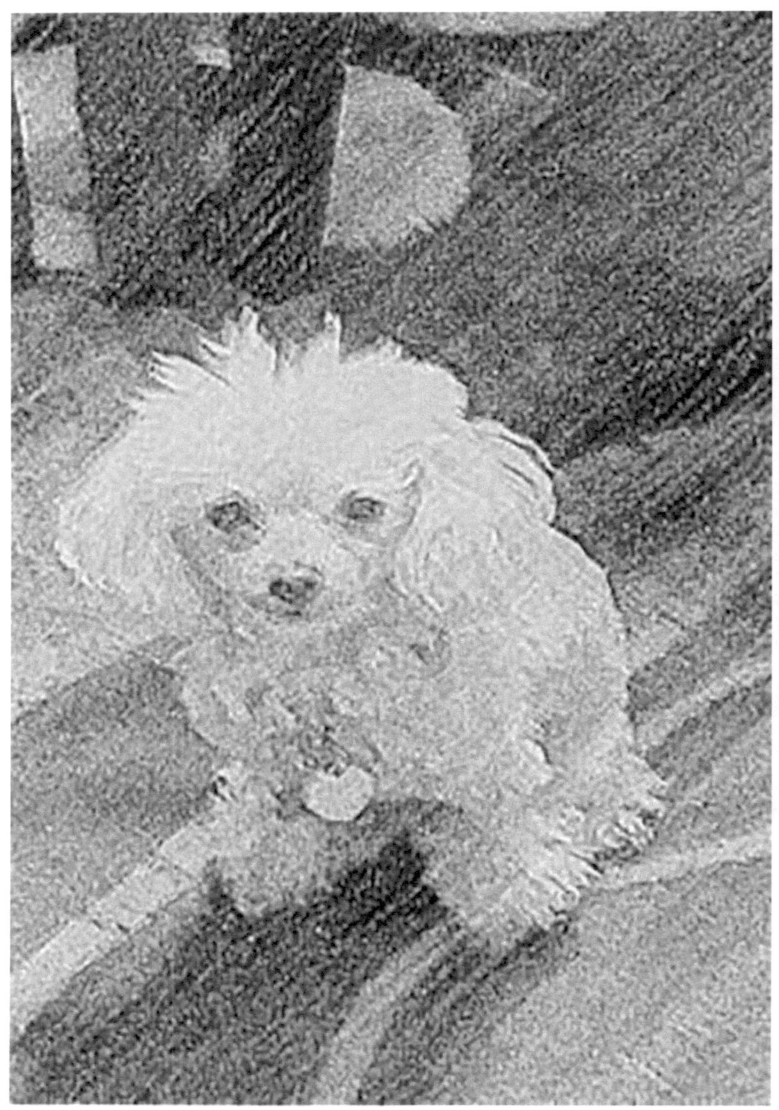

She's **Latt'e** in color, **"Miracle" doG** and **God** spelled backwards! She's wise, spiritual and all!

 MISS ASONDRA STARN'AIR

Miss Mariah Autumn

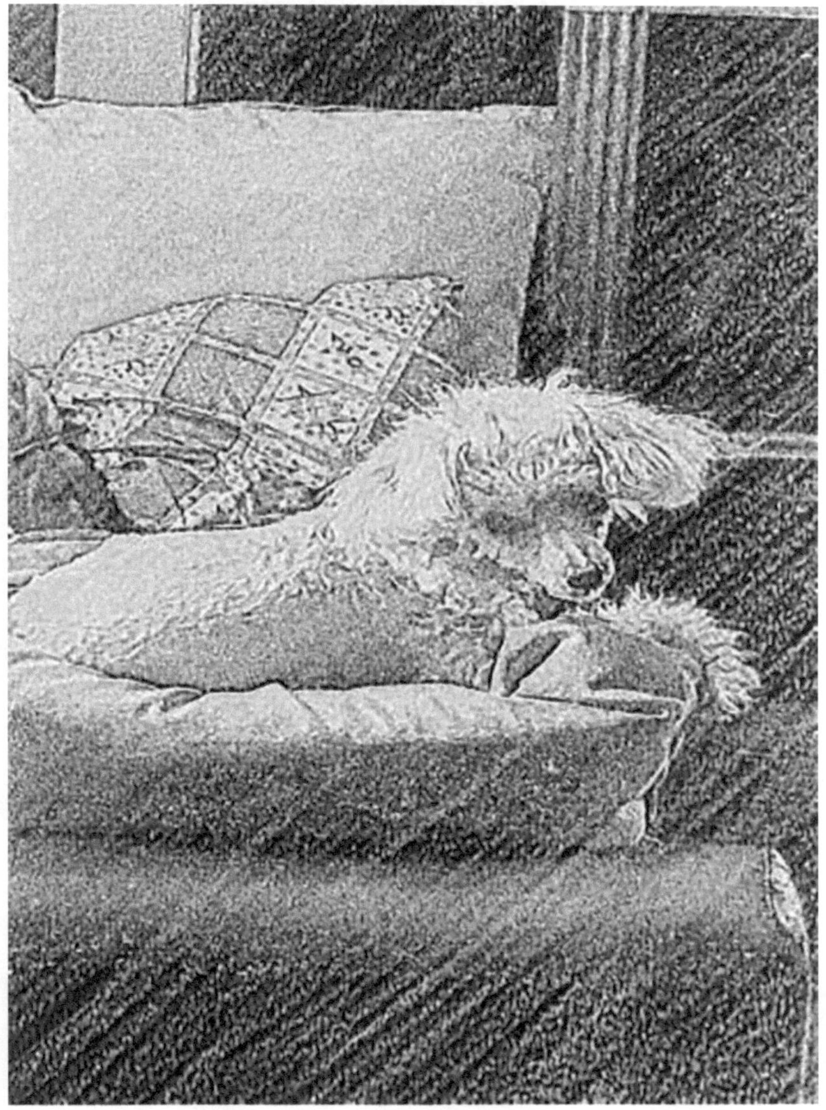

She is **Autumn** in color, and **'Fall'** is my favorite
season, God gave her this color for a reason!

Pet Parents/Caregivers

Did you know that **"DoG"** is **"God"** spelled backwards?

When this was pointed out to me, I was blown away! It confirmed my deep love for my dogs was not only natural but also a gift from **God** himself. Wow!

Dogs have what many of us don't have, and that's unconditional love—the kind Jesus speaks of. Our four legged friends can teach us a thing or two; mine have certainly taught me a lot.

If you are going to be a pet parent be an excellent one. Taking care of pets many time is just like taking care of children they are a full time responsibility as well.

That's why I entitled this page **"Pet Parents"**. You will be a parent /caregiver to that animal. And if you are a dog lover like me, you know in your heart they are part of the family. You mess with them, you mess with me. Remember **"doG" is "God"** spelled backward. I wouldn't go there if I were you; mistreating a dog or any animal today is totally inexcusable. There are new laws against it, and for good reason too. Domestic animals have hearts and souls, all animals do for that matter, but domestic animals like cats and dogs need us to love and take care of them the most, the way I see it from a pet parents prospective is **'Dogs Are Human Too!'**

They can hurt and feel you, they have a heart, eyes and ears, they bring us laughter, and calm our fears. Your pets love you, that's why I say **'Dogs Are Human Too!'**

Amanican Latte' and Mariah Autumn

My Two Toy Poodles!

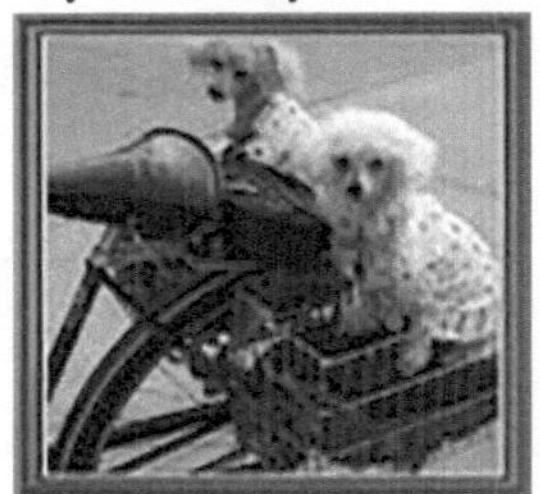

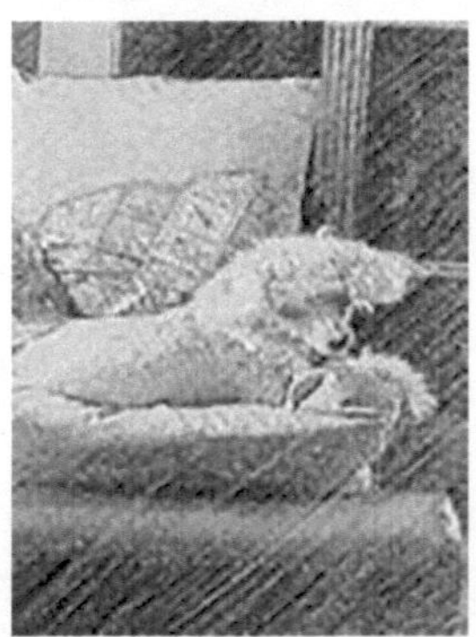

Mariah Autumn

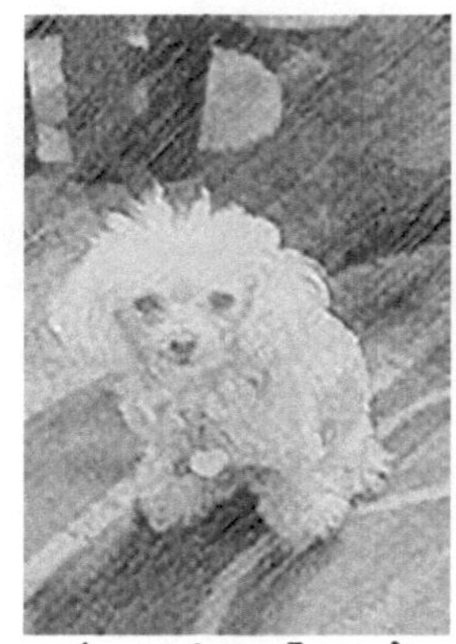

Amanican Latte'

Dogs Are Human Too!

Home, pets need one

Understand that they have needs too.

Maintenance they need to be bath and groomed.

Activities, all pets need something to do.

Neuter or spayed to reduce overpopulation.
If you really want to become humane, someone who will speak out against animal abuse, Add the E!

Education and respect for all animals.

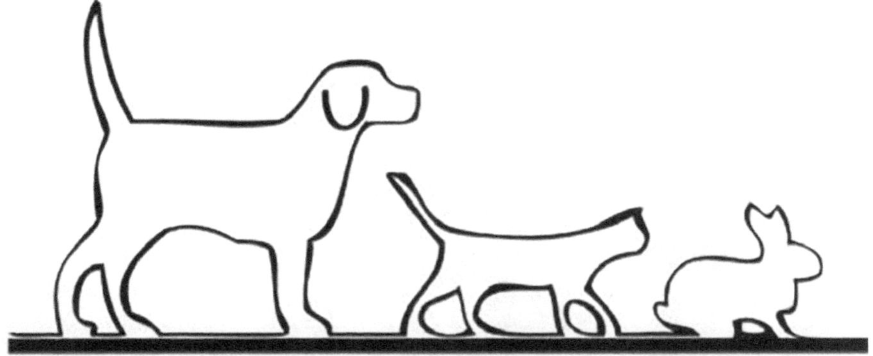

Pet Parent /Caregivers Memoir

First pet name ______________ Birthdate __________ Personality _______

____

____

____

____

____

____

____

____

____

What breed _________________ mixed with _________________ not mixed.

Color ____

Vet's name and location ____

Groomer's name and location _____________________________________

Brand name pet food ____

How has this pet inspired you? _____________________________________

____

In your wonderful words, tell why you loved being a pet parent/caregiver

____

____

____

____

____

____

____

____

____

Thank You For Being A Pet Parent!

 Miss Asondra StarN'air

Pet Canvas

Pet Parent /Caregivers Memoir

First pet name _______________ Birthdate __________ Personality _______

____

____

____

____

____

____

____

____

____

____

What breed _______________ mixed with _________________ Not mixed.

Color ____

Vet's name and location _______________________________________

Groomer's name and location ___________________________________

Brand name pet food ____

How has this pet inspired you? _________________________________

____

In your wonderful words, tell why you loved being a pet parent/caregiver

____

____

____

____

____

____

____

____

____

Thank you for being a pet parent!

Pet Canvas